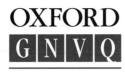

OXFORD
G N V Q

D1325103

Advanced
HEALTH &
SOCIAL CARE

CAMBRIDGE
TRAINING AND
CTAD
DEVELOPMENT
LTD

OXFORD
UNIVERSITY PRESS

OXFORD
UNIVERSITY PRESS

Great Clarendon Street, Oxford OX2 6DP

Oxford University Press is a department of the University of Oxford.
It furthers the University's objective of excellence in research, scholarship,
and education by publishing worldwide in

Oxford New York

Athens Auckland Bangkok Bogotá Buenos Aires Calcutta
Cape Town Chennai Dar es Salaam Delhi Florence Hong Kong Istanbul
Karachi Kuala Lumpur Madrid Melbourne Mexico City Mumbai
Nairobi Paris São Paulo Singapore Taipei Tokyo Toronto Warsaw
with associated companies in Berlin Ibadan

Oxford is a registered trade mark of Oxford University Press
in the UK and in certain other countries

British Library Cataloguing in Publication Data
Data available

ISBN 0-19-832826-5

Typeset and designed by Design Study, Bury St Edmunds
and Chris Lord Information Design, Brighton, East Sussex

Printed and bound by G. Canale & C., Italy

Thanks go to the following (first edition):
Addenbrooke's NHS Trust, Cambridge; Cambridge and Huntingdon Health Authority; Gill Betts; Boots the Chemist Ltd,
Cambridge; Centre 33 Young People's Counselling and Information Service, Cambridge; Emmaus Cambridge Community;
The Evelyn Hospital, Cambridge; Howard Fried-Booth; Lilian Gates; Granta Housing Society Ltd, Cambridge; Dr J. David Greaves;
Susan K. Greaves; Health Education Authority (physical activity team), London; Debra Howard; Joint Colleges Nursery,
Cambridge; Lifespan Healthcare Trust; Alison Monk; Papworth Hospital NHS Trust; Mr Rankine's Dental Surgery, Cambridge ;
Liz Redfern, education consultant (formerly assistant director of educational policy, English National Board); Sheila Stace, NVQ
consultant; Sid Stace, senior social worker. Thanks also go to the many other organisations and individuals who contributed
examples, case studies and other material.

Contributors to the second edition include:
Meg Holland, Jan Newman, Jane Hodges, Sid Stace, Sheila Stace, Abigail Masterson, Sally Lane,
Deavon Baker Oxley, Nicola von Schreiber

Thanks for permission to reproduce photos/extracts go to:

Age Concern (photos pp50, 52, 75, 168, 317); Anthony Bevins
(extract p.247); Ashbourne Ltd (photo p47); British Medical
Association (extract p.279); CNRI, Science Photo Library (photo
p.139); Commission for Racial Equality (homepage pp60, 63,
extract from 'Race through the 90's' p.54, 55); Contact a Family
(leaflet p.276); Dept. of Health (homepage p.47, leaflet p.78,
extract p.300); Equal Opportunities Commission (homepage pp
20, 25, equal pay poster p.26); Equal Opportunities Review
(extracts pp26, 28); Family Policy Studies Centre (statistics
pp198, 200); Forte plc (photo pp102, 322, 330); Josh Good
(photos pp73, 114, 237, 242, 273, 275); GPMU (logo p.45);

The Guardian (extracts pp9, 12, 18, 30); HMSO (Children Act
logo p.298); Manfred Kage, Science Photo Library (photo p.139);
MIND (logo p.296, extract p.297); NCVO (logo p294); National
Extension College (NEC) (photo pp42, 54); National Schizophrenia
Fellowship (extract p.297); National Union of Teachers (logo
p.45); NSPCC (extract p.294); NUM (logo p.45); Observer
(extract p.288); Office of National Statistics (statistics p.200);
Baroness Jill Pitkeathley, Past Chief Executive, National Carers'
Association (extract p.273); Pre-School Learning Alliance (logo
p.267), Public Health Laboratory Service (graph p325); Social
Services Inspectorate (extract p.245).

Contents

ABOUT THE BOOK

This book contains the information you need to complete the six mandatory units of your Advanced Health and Social Care GNVQ.

How it's organised

This book is organised in units and sections, like the GNVQ, so it's easy to find the information you need at any point in your course. Each section is divided into chapters. They cover all the topics in the section, using the same headings as the GNVQ specifications. At the end of each section there are some key questions, so you can check your knowledge and prepare for the unit tests. There are also suggestions for an assignment, which will help you produce the evidence you need for your portfolio. There are also key skills signposted at the end of each unit to help you identify the vocational requirements that your portfolio evidence can fulfil.

What's in it

The book presents information in several different ways so it's interesting to read and easy to understand. Some information is given in the words of people who actually work in health and social care jobs – for example, a social worker in child protection, a ward nurse in a hospital, or a care assistant in a residential home. There are definitions of important words like 'discrimination' or 'advocate'. There are illustrations and diagrams, and extracts from news reports and relevant pieces of legislation. Case studies go into detail by examining different individual's experiences with health and social care services. And there are photographs showing different care settings and the people who work in them.

How to use the book

Decide which part you want to read. For example, you can go straight to any section and read through the relevant chapters. You can find the information about any topic by looking at the list of contents at the front of the book and deciding which chapter looks most useful. Or you can use the index at the back to find the page reference for a specific topic or organisation.

As well as information, the book has suggestions for things you can do to help you learn about health and social care in a practical way. Discussion points suggest topics that you can think about and discuss with other people – other students on your course, your tutor or teacher, friends, family, people who work in health and social care. Activity boxes ask you to do things like prepare a leaflet about equal opportunity, identify tissues from a micrograph, design questions for a primary research interview, and so on. They will help you to get a real life picture of what it's like to work in the health and social care industry.

When you've finished a section, try answering the key questions at the end. You may want to make notes of your answers and use them when you're preparing for the unit tests. The assignment at the end of each section suggests what you can do to produce evidence for your portfolio. You might want to make an action plan for each assignment to help you plan and carry out the work.

Other resources

By itself this book is an important and valuable source of information for your GNVQ studies. It should also help you use other resources effectively. For example, it suggests that you should find out more information about some topics, such as different aspects of legislation or current issues in medical practice. You might be able to get this extra information in a local library or health centre, from the Internet, or from other books about health and social care. It also asks you to investigate the industry yourself, by visiting facilities, reading about it in magazines or watching relevant programmes on television.

Over to you

It's your GNVQ and your job to make the best of the opportunity to learn about health and social care. Use this book in whatever way helps you most. For example, you could:

- look at the contents page to give you the whole picture
- use the index to find out specific bits of information
- read a chapter at a time to help you understand a topic
- look at the assignment before starting a section so you know what you have to do
- turn things on their head and start with the key questions to see how much previous knowledge you have about a section.

It's over to you now. Good luck.

UNIT **1**

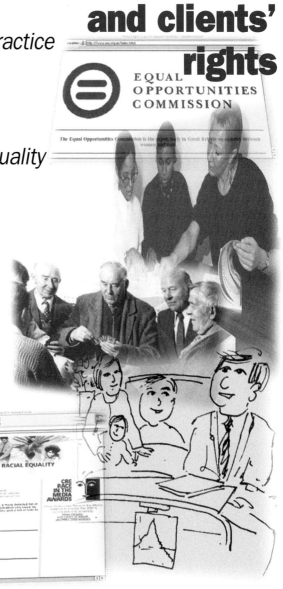

**Equal
opportunities
and clients'
rights**

3

About this unit

In this unit you will learn how to recognise discriminatory practices and how to judge when to intervene to safeguard clients' rights. You will learn that people who work in the health and social care sector need to know how equal opportunities have an impact on individuals, groups and society and the legal framework for this work.

You need to appreciate the ethical issues in equal opportunities and how these core values lie at the heart of all health and social care practice.

66 *There is no room for the social exclusion of anyone in our society. We must all work together to ensure that the poorest and most vulnerable people in our society get the services, help and opportunities to make the most of their lives.* 99

Dr Mo Mowlam, 1999, as coordinator of social exclusion unit policies across government

66 *When I was young, early last century, things were very different to today. I was one of seven children, although one of my younger sisters was deaf and put into an institution. The rest of us went to school, but left as soon as possible so we could earn some money. I worked in our local Woolworth's, which I loved, and I was made a supervisor by the time I was 20. My younger brother worked there too as a storeman, and was paid more than me – but then I suppose he was doing a man's job. When I was 21 and got married I had to give up my job, as married women weren't allowed to work when men were unemployed. I'm amazed when I see the things women take for granted today.* 99

a 90-year-old patient

66 *At my first school I was the only disabled kid and I had to leave at the end of Year 2 because I was leaving the infants and the junior school had lots of steps. When I first came here there were no ramps up to the huts, just steps. I could go up the steps on my sticks, but not in a wheelchair. Sometimes Mr Collins had to lift me up. There are ramps now, though . . . The toilets can be a problem too, you might have to go to one some way away if you need to use a catheter.* 99

Kamaldeep Singh, a primary school pupil with spina bifida (Times Educational Supplement)

66 *There was a case last year with the very difficult death of someone's partner. During the bereavement follow-up it became clear that the surviving partner wanted to make a formal complaint about the patient's treatment. It also became clear that it was hoped by some staff that counselling would persuade him not to do so. But counselling isn't about calming situations down, or putting things right. It is about the patient exploring what is going on. During counselling he looked at what he had to gain and what he would lose emotionally if he went ahead. He came to the conclusion that it would help him to vent his feelings and he went ahead. It was his decision.* 99

head of medical counselling and family support

Promoting equality

Promoting equality needs to be set into the context in which health and social care practitioners work: including information about discrimination and how this works for vulnerable and disadvantaged individuals and groups. In this section you will look at ethical issues concerned with supporting the rights of clients, boundaries that apply to clients' rights and how they are interpreted, and how resources may influence the effectiveness of policies that aim to promote client rights.

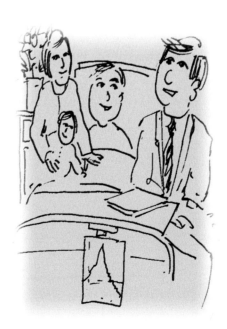

1.1.1 **Rights within health and social care**

We all have certain basic rights, such as:

- life
- health and support
- safety and security
- employment and an income
- education and personal development.

These rights are enshrined in national legislation and international conventions, such as the Human Rights Act 1999 and the European Convention on Human Rights.

Rights are a positive concept because they imply that every person is entitled to be treated as an individual, having their principles, values and cultures respected and able to have as good a quality of life as possible without restricting other people's rights. Where rights are ignored, individuals can be described as:

- discriminated against
- exploited
- oppressed or repressed.

66 *The older people I support are often frail, sick and vulnerable – not in a good position to assert their rights. Many feel that they are shuffled backwards and forwards from hospital bed to home, and their children see them as a burden rather than as individuals. I try to talk to them as equals and individuals, to find out what they really want and need. However old and weak they are, they have fundamental rights to make choices, maintain their privacy and dignity, and, as far as possible, to think and act as independent human beings.* 99

social worker

The concept of rights is particularly important for individuals or groups of people who may not be able to speak for or defend themselves. For us all, and for our government and international organisations, to give active support to enabling those who are vulnerable or disadvantaged to exercise their rights is important. Many people who come in contact with or rely on health and social care services will be those whose rights have been neglected or abused. Health and social care practitioners are expected to respect and promote their rights.

1.1.2 Discrimination

Being treated equally can mean a number of things, such as:

- being treated the same as everyone else
- being given the same chances as everyone else
- having the same rights as everyone else.

Discrimination is the practice of treating one person or group of people less fairly or less well than others.

Equalities legislation, and the policies of health and care organisations, is directed at ensuring that people are treated equally and reducing the amount of discrimination against individuals or groups. Discrimination can mean both negative and positive ways in which people are treated differently. It more usually has the negative meaning.

From an early age we make judgements about different individuals. Some of these judgements are based on rational choices but others are based on:

- our previous experience which may be negative
- the influence of our family and friends
- local myths or distortions in the media.

Prejudice is an unreasonable dislike of a person or group of people based on a prejudgement rather than knowledge. It is usually linked with the attitudes and behaviour that results from this prejudgement.

These judgements can be based on characteristics that the individual cannot change, such as their race, gender, age or disability, or they would find it offensive to be expected to change, such as their religion. This unreasonable dislike is called prejudice.

Prejudices can be positive. For example, contestants on a TV programme like *Blind Date* who say they're a nurse may get a spontaneous round of applause from the audience, based on the prejudice that nurses are caring, self-sacrificing people. But more often, prejudices, founded on ignorance rather than real knowledge of what people are like, are negative.

Prejudice often leads to stereotyping where a person is seen as a category and not an individual.

A **stereotype** is a fixed general image or set of characteristics that a lot of people believe represent a particular type of person or thing – for example, all Frenchmen wear berets and smoke smelly cigarettes.

Children learn their stereotypes of people from the world around them – from parents, friends, television programmes, books, films, songs and comics. They learn to group people together and form opinions about them based on their colour, national origin, age, sex or job. These opinions are prejudices – preconceived ideas of what a person, or a group of people, will be like.

DISCUSSION POINT

Almost everyone will have experienced discrimination at some time in their life – whether it was being told you couldn't do something because you were a girl or a child, or being teased or even physically abused because of your hair colour, ethnic origin or culture. Discuss occasions when you have felt discriminated against. Who discriminated against you? What do you think caused the discrimination?

Then think of an occasion when you have discriminated against someone else. What prejudice caused you to discriminate? What stereotype do you think created your prejudice?

ACTIVITY

1 Take a quick look at these pictures. Jot down the first two or three words that spring to mind about each one.

2 Which one would you think:

- runs their own business and drives a brand new top-of-its-range car?
- is studying electronics?
- is anxiously waiting for a cheque to arrive on Friday?
- uses a wheelchair?
- adores two daughters?
- has to attend Magistrates Court in the morning?
- was born on the other side of the world where English is not the first language?

The answers are at the end of this unit (page 68)

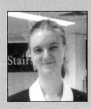 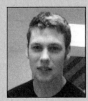 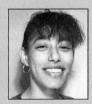 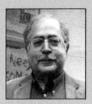 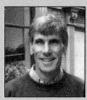 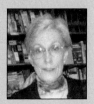

Discrimination can be applied in a positive way, such as:

- reserving seats on public transport for older people, disabled people and those with small children
- actively seeking to recruit new staff who are over 50
- celebrating Muslim and Jewish festivals in a crèche.

More usually it means that an individual or their group is treated less well. Discrimination can operate on a personal level, so a landlord will refuse to let to someone who is living as a single parent. It can be at an organisational level – for example, a company may be unlikely to promote women to be managers. It can also operate at a national level, such as apartheid in South Africa.

DISCUSSION POINT

Discrimination is often linked with power and status so that a more powerful person can abuse their power by denying another their rights. People working in health and social care frequently have power over the lives of clients. For example, many hold the key to access to a service because they can refer to a specialist or agree to services being provided. How do you think a practitioner could discriminate against a client? In what actions can a practitioner share their power with the client?

8

1.1.3 **The contexts for discrimination**

Discrimination takes place on three different levels:

- Individual discrimination is when people treat individuals differently because of stereotyping and prejudice – for example, name-calling, or avoiding someone with a disability.
- Societal discrimination is when stereotyping and prejudice are so accepted that they become part of the framework for society.
- Institutional discrimination occurs when discrimination, consciously or unconsciously, is built into practices and laws – for example, lack of access to buildings for people with disabilities, or the higher age of consent for homosexuals.

The Macpherson Inquiry Report into the murder of Stephen Lawrence found that institutional racism existed in the Metropolitan Police. It was defined as:

66 . . . the collective failure of an organisation to provide an appropriate and professional service to people because of their colour, culture or ethnic origin . . . It can be seen in processes, attitudes and behaviours through unwitting prejudice, ignorance, thoughtlessness and racial stereotyping which disadvantages minority ethnic people. **99**

The Crown Prosecution Service is to appoint a leading black member of 'the great and the good' to look into allegations of institutional racism, in an attempt to forestall a formal investigation by the Commission for Racial Equality.

The allegations of racism come from black lawyers in the Crown Prosecution Service who claim their promotion is blocked. Tribunals have found the service guilty of race discrimination and victimisation, and more cases are pending.

The Guardian, *Saturday 11 December 1999*

Another definition of institutional discrimination is 'inappropriate behaviour allowed by inappropriate systems'. This was the finding of the Crawford Report on institutional discrimination in Hackney Council. The Report referred to inappropriate behaviours as well as an absence of basic management practices.

Individual, institutional and societal discrimination can be either direct or indirect:

- Direct discrimination is behaviour that shows open prejudice against an individual or group – for example, making it clear that only women should apply for a job, or bullying.
- Indirect discrimination is less open and easy to spot than direct discrimination. It involves showing prejudice against an individual or group by avoidance, body language, or exclusion – for example, avoiding someone who is black, or not providing a crèche for workers with childcare needs.

Throughout this unit you will be considering examples of how discrimination is challenged at an individual, organisational and society level.

Equality in health and social care

Underpinning principles

Principles are fundamental beliefs that guide the way people behave. Individuals' principles form the basis of their personal code of conduct for life:

❝*I believe in animal welfare, non-violence and the sanctity of life so I don't eat meat.*❞

❝*I think there are too many people on the planet – I'm not going to have any children.*❞

In the same way, all societies have principles which control the way people behave towards each other. For example, two of the principles underpinning British society are that people shouldn't kill one another or be married to more than one person at the same time. Often laws enforce these principles – in this case, against murder and bigamy.

The principles of equality of opportunity have become increasingly important in Britain as it has become a more diverse, multicultural society: more women are working; disabled people's rights are more widely recognised. In line with this, a range of important legislation exists to promote equality and rights. This legislation is outlined in section 2.2.

All of this legislation is underpinned by three principles, which are essential in health and social care:

- equality of care
- individual rights
- individual choice.

Health and social care practitioners need to ensure that they implement these principles of equality of opportunity – following legislation when necessary – in every aspect of their work.

> ### DISCUSSION POINT
>
> How many principles can you think of which underpin the things you do – and don't do – from day to day? Which of these do you think are your own principles? Which have been passed on to you by the society you live in? Which of your principles do laws enforce?

Practitioners look to codes of ethics and their organisation's policies to guide them in putting the principles into practice. The Principles of Good Practice incorporated into the national occupational standards sets out the principles. This value base is described in section 1.3.2.

Principles of good practice

The national occupational standards for the health and social care sector are built on the following agreed principles of good practice:

- balancing people's rights with their responsibilities to others and to wider society and challenging those who affect the rights of others

- promoting the values of equality and diversity, acknowledging the personal beliefs and preferences of others and promoting anti-discriminatory practice

- maintaining the confidentiality of information provided that this does not place others at risk

- recognising the effect of the wider social, political and economic context on health and social wellbeing and on people's development

- enabling people to develop to their full potential, to be as autonomous and self-managing as possible and to have a voice and be heard

- recognising and promoting health and social wellbeing as a positive concept

- balancing the needs of people who use services with the resources available and exercising financial probity

- developing and maintaining effective relationships with people and maintaining the integrity of these relationships through setting appropriate role boundaries

- developing oneself and one's own practice to improve the quality of services offered

- working within statutory and organisational frameworks.

ACTIVITY

Think of a practical example of each principle in the caring services.

Individual choice

Bound up with the concept of individual rights is individual choice – people's freedom to have their own beliefs and preferences, to make their own decisions, and to take responsibility for themselves and those around them. Both equality of opportunity legislation and health and social care services aim to support this by promoting individuals' rights to lead their lives in the way they want.

Ethical issues and dilemmas

ACTIVITY

In the case of Thomas Creedon, who do you think was in the best position to decide the child's best interests? What action do you think should have been taken in the child's best interests?

Choose one of the following dilemmas.

■ A 70-year-old man is becoming increasingly frail and confused, but wants to stay at home. His family, who live 30 miles away, are concerned for his safety and think it would be in his best interests to go into residential care.

■ A 16-year-old girl was involved in a diving accident and is in a coma, which appears to be irreversible. The doctors want to switch off the life-support system, but her family is strongly opposed. The girl's organs could be used for transplants, saving other people's lives.

Make lists of the different moral arguments for and against taking action. Remember to consider the dilemma from the point of view of legal issues, health and social care practitioners, the person using healthcare/social services, their family and friends, and society as a whole. Talk to other people (including a health and social care practitioner if possible), to get their opinions. Then write a summary of the ethical dilemma facing the health and social care practitioners involved in each case.

An ethical dilemma involves making a decision when there is no clear-cut moral right or wrong. It may be that there is a conflict between different people's morals or beliefs, or that an issue is so complex or difficult to understand that it raises moral questions that are almost impossible to answer.

With people's lives and wellbeing in their hands, many health and social care practitioners face ethical issues and dilemmas as part of their day-to-day jobs.

DISCUSSION POINT

Have you experienced any ethical dilemmas in your life? Were your morals in conflict with someone else's? Was the issue so confusing that you couldn't make up your own mind? How did you resolve the ethical dilemma?

Agreeing the best interests of clients

The fundamental aim of practitioners is to act in the best interests of people using health and social services. However, is it always clear what those best interests are? All those involved will have their own views of a client's best interests, including:

■ different health and social care practitioners
■ the people using health and social services
■ their family and friends
■ the community in which the patients or clients live.

When making decisions about the best interests of people using health and social services, health and social care practitioners need to reach an agreement with all of these groups of people. This can mean carefully balancing a range of highly emotive issues and views, as in the following case:

66 *Thomas Creedon, a severely brain-damaged two-year-old who died recently, had been kept alive by medical interventions, including artificial feeding and hydration. His parents had argued that life-prolonging interventions were against their child's best interests. The doctors disagreed, saying that food and water were every human being's basic rights.*

Had the child survived, the issues would have gone to court. Apparently, the doctors had also stated that were the infant to develop an infection, they would not prolong his life with antibiotics. Nor, presumably, was the child put on a respirator when his breathing stopped, nor efforts made to institute CPR – cardiopulmonary resuscitation – when his heart stopped beating, even though these might have prolonged his life. **99**

The Guardian, *7 March 1996*

Confidentiality

66 *Confidentiality is the cornerstone of the centre. We have excellent links with Social Services and the Health Authority Services. Social Services tell young*

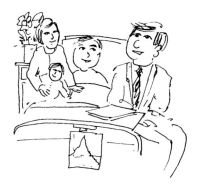

people about us – for example if they receive disclosures of sexual abuse they know we are here to talk to. It's their choice. **99**

senior worker (counselling), young people's counselling and information centre

A common dilemma faced by practitioners is deciding what information people need to know and who needs to know it.

Everyone has the right to enough information to make decisions about their treatment. For example, before signing a consent form for surgery, a patient needs to know the pros and cons of going ahead with the operation. Their surgeon should explain the operation using simple language, and make notes and draw diagrams for the patient. But should they go into the full details of potential problems if this may be upsetting or confusing?

Practitioners' responsibilities to give clients access to information is laid down in two main pieces of legislation:

- Access to Personal Files Act 1987 – this gives individuals the right to look at information local authorities (for example, social services departments) hold on them
- Access to Health Records Act 1990 – this gives individuals the right to look at their National Health Service (NHS) medical records.

To do their job well, practitioners will need to know information about their clients. Giving this information can be embarrassing and worrying, and people need to feel they can talk openly to their health and social care practitioners. This means trusting them to maintain the confidentiality of any information exchanged. Confidentiality is addressed in greater detail in unit 2.

DISCUSSION POINT

In which of the following situations do you think it is ethical for the health and social care practitioner to give information to people? What are the pros and cons in each case? What should the practitioner do next?

- A 14-year-old girl confides in the school nurse that she is pregnant, and the nurse has to decide whether to tell the girl's parents.

- An 85-year-old man is suffering from a terminal illness, and has been given a month to live. His doctor tells the man's children, and they beg the doctor not to tell their father.

- A depressed and disruptive teenage girl confesses to her social worker that she was raped a year ago. She asks for the information to be kept confidential, but the social worker feels the girl needs specialist support that she can't provide.

DISCUSSION POINT

A hospital doctor has just told a young father suffering from cancer that he has only three months to live. The man wants his last few months to be as happy and normal as possible, and asks the doctor not to tell his wife and children the truth. However, the man's wife is desperate to know what is really happening, and pleads with the doctor for information so she can come to terms with the situation and make plans for the future.

Talk about the different issues involved and the feelings and rights of all the people involved. What do you think the doctor should do?

As well as deciding what information to give, health and social care practitioners often face ethical dilemmas when it comes to passing on knowledge to other people. They have a responsibility to keep information confidential, but may feel the client's family has a right to know something. Or they may feel they can't cope with a case on their own, and decide to ask a colleague for advice.

13

Handling ethical issues

Every ethical issue and dilemma involves a unique set of circumstances, and has to be handled on its own terms. For example, it would be wrong to pass a blanket judgement that life-support systems should always be switched off after six months, or that all patients with mental health problems should be cared for in the community.

To help them approach the full range of ethical issues, health and social care practitioners have established different ways of handling dilemmas. These include:

- practitioners making individual decisions
- practitioners discussing issues with colleagues, clients and carers
- supervision by line managers
- setting up organisational policies and practices
- taking advice from representative bodies
- following government legislation
- improving training for health and social care practitioners
- establishing codes of practice on how to behave in particular situations.

Unit 2 puts theory into action and explores practical skills used in everyday communications with all the people involved.

DISCUSSION POINT

Think back to any ethical dilemmas you have faced in your life. How did you resolve them? Did you make a decision on your own? Or did you talk to other people or read information before making your decision?

ACTIVITY

Talk to a health or social care practitioner about some of the individual ethical decisions they make as part of their job. How do they reach these decisions? Are they comfortable with having to make decisions on their own?

Analysing different approaches to handling ethical issues

To evaluate the success of different approaches to handling ethical issues, it's useful to stand back and analyse particular cases. This can help health and social care organisations to:

- assess how well policies and practices are working, and decide whether they need updating
- confront any complaints or allegations of mistakes
- identify where improvements could be made.

1.1.6 **Boundaries to clients' rights**

❝*An important part of my job is making sure that children in need – who might suffer if they don't get help – are properly looked after. Whenever possible, I help families to bring up children in their own homes. I provide support in the form of home helps, nursery places for younger children, and sessions at a family centre. However, sometimes I believe children are in such danger that I have to go to court and ask for a Care or Supervision Order. This is always a terrible, heart-rending decision to make. Even if they are at risk, leaving home is a dreadful experience for a young child. Parents may be very distressed and angry that their family is being broken up. Other brothers and sisters may be badly affected. But ultimately, I have to put the risk to the child first. My main responsibility is to keep them safe.***❞**

social worker in child protection

In an ideal world we would all be free to act as we please. In practice, however, we surrender a range of freedoms for a wider social good, for example, driving on the left-hand side of the road (imagine the mayhem if we made our own decisions).

These agreements to surrender some of our liberties for a wider social good take two broad forms:

- those we do voluntarily because we feel it is right – i.e. not saying something which you know will offend someone
- those which are the subject of law and whose breach may lead to punishment, the extreme example being murder (which would deprive the victim of the right to life).

Workers in health and social care are dealing on a daily basis with people whose own choices might conflict with the rights of other clients or the workers. The choices may be contrary to the agreed plan of care for that client or challenging the organisation's decisions. You need to be able to identify the boundaries that apply to client rights and explain how policies to promote client rights are interpreted and used in practice. In particular you need to know when clients' wishes can be overruled, for example in cases concerning mental health or children.

Balancing the needs of individuals against those of others

In many cases, it's not enough to consider only the best interests of the person using health or social services. Decisions can also have repercussions for their family and friends, or for society as a whole. Before making decisions about the best course of action, practitioners need to assess whether:

- the person is at risk from their own behaviour
- the person is at risk from other people's actions
- their family, friends or carers are at risk from their behaviour
- society as a whole is at risk from their behaviour.

Handling conflicting values and beliefs

Everyone has their own set of values and beliefs. These may be affected by personal preference, religion or culture. Health and social care practitioners have a responsibility to recognise and respect these values and beliefs at all times – even when they are in conflict with their own or the organisation's practices.

A nurse working in an area with a large Muslim population explains the importance of understanding the values of people using health and social services:

66 *When I first came to work in this area, I found Muslim beliefs and practices very strange. Now I understand the significance of different customs and rituals, and I do all I can to support the families and friends involved. We recently had a Muslim patient who was dying. We moved him into a side room, where his many visitors could have more privacy, holy water could be given, and verses from the Qur'an could be read. When he died, I turned his face to the right, to symbolise turning to Mecca. I straightened his arms and legs, and closed his mouth and eyes. These simple things helped to comfort the bereaved family. I'm a Roman Catholic myself, but don't have any problem following Muslim practice. It's a mark of respect for the patients and their families.* 99

DISCUSSION POINT

Jehovah's Witnesses do not believe in blood transfusions. Even if a doctor says that a child will die during an operation if not given a blood transfusion, parents will not give consent, and doctors cannot intervene unless they have obtained a court order. How do you think this would affect the medical staff involved? Are there ever any circumstances in which you feel health and social care practitioners should be able to override the religious beliefs or cultural values of their clients?

1.1.7 **Restricting the liberty of individuals**

Restrictive legislation

The law regulates our daily lives in many ways. There are laws governing:

- the quality of food that we eat
- how we drive our cars and their road-worthiness
- the payment of taxes
- the health and safety of our workplaces.

In these circumstances the law acts as the oil of society, ensuring its smooth functioning and enabling the parts to work in harmony with each other. Imagine what would happen if there were no traffic laws telling us which side of the road to drive on. We all must surrender a degree of freedom to help us negotiate safely through our daily lives.

ACTIVITY

Think of three areas of the law, other than those given above, where we surrender a degree of freedom of choice. Write a brief report describing:

- what is given up
- who gains from it
- who decides what is to be given up
- the benefits which balance the losses.

For health and social care practitioners, a number of important laws relate to protecting people by restricting freedom. They cover three broad categories:

- people who put others at risk
- people who put themselves at risk
- people who are put at risk by others.

DISCUSSION POINT

Think about this case in the light of the three categories of risk given above. Into which category, or categories, would you place each of the four people mentioned?

Joan and Arthur Green are the parents of two children, Wayne and Samantha, aged eight and three. Arthur is a heavy drinker. When he is drunk he often beats his wife, occasionally to the point of unconsciousness. The children are frequent witnesses of the violence. Wayne has begun to bully his sister. Joan has become increasingly depressed and has stopped regularly feeding herself and the children. Alerted by neighbours, social workers and police enter the house. They find that Joan and the children are severely malnourished. Samantha has extensive bruising caused by Wayne hitting her.

17

1.1.8 **How resources may influence the implementation of equality**

❝ *The Government has a comprehensive programme to improve health and tackle health inequalities. Partnerships between the NHS, Local Authorities and other organisations are key to making our nation healthier, tackling social exclusion and reducing inequalities. Local action, including setting local inequalities targets, should be agreed as part of the Health Improvement Programme development process.* ❞

Modernising Health and Social Services,
National Priorities Guidance 2000/1–2002/3

Allocating resources

Another way in which individuals' rights can be restricted is through the allocation and level of resources. For example, a hospital may have a policy on waiting times at outpatient clinics, but because of lack of funding there are not enough staff to reduce waiting times to comply with the policy. Resources include staff. Decisions will be made about which client or patient will receive the service. There is, for instance, a shortage of educational psychologists; so children can wait a long time to receive their Statement for special education.

Since the introduction of the welfare state, people in Britain have come to expect the right to free health and social care on demand. However, resources have always been limited, and 'health rationing' is becoming an increasingly high-profile issue.

In section 5.4 you will find details of how funding is allocated in each health, social care and early years organisation. Health and social care organisations are given a finite amount of money, and have to work out how to balance the budget while providing a high-quality service. This means making decisions about how to allocate resources.

Schizophrenia drugs 'rationed'

David Brindle, Social Services Correspondent

Many psychiatrists are being prevented or deterred on cost grounds from prescribing drugs which can control schizophrenia, a survey suggests today.

The drugs cost up to £5.34 a day, or 66 times more than conventional medication — but that is dwarfed by the cost of in-patient treatment for a sufferer who breaks down and needs hospital admission.

Estimates put the lifetime costs of a schizophrenic needing long-term hospital care at £316,000, compared to £23,000 for a patient maintained in the community.

The results of the survey by the National Schizophrenia Fellowship and the Royal College of Psychiatrists are based on a questionnaire completed by 761 psychiatrists — some 59 per cent of those registered as working with patients in the community.

The aim of the survey was to establish attitudes to clozapine and risperidone — "new generation" generic drugs which are attracting growing, but not universal, endorsement for effectiveness in treating schizophrenia.

Clozapine, which is typically given to patients who respond poorly to other drugs, can have serious side-effects and requires regular blood monitoring. In contrast, risperidone is generally given as a first recourse and has fewer side-effects.

Although in Germany almost one in three people with schizophrenia is on clozapine, the survey found its use very limited in Britain.

Thirty-five per cent of the psychiatrists said they had no patients on Clozapine, and 25 per cent said they had none on risperidone. Most who prescribed it did so for fewer than five of their patients.

Forty-six per cent had been challenged about the cost of clozapine, £5.34 a day compared to 8p for a standard alternative, and 52 per cent had been challenged about risperidone, which costs £4.04.

Nine per cent said formal rationing was imposed on prescribing clozapine, and a further 14 per cent said informal limits existed. Similarly 3 per cent said there were formal limits on risperidone prescription and 11 per cent cited informal curbs. One psychiatrist said: "I have 150 patients who would benefit from clozapine, but I am only allowed to prescribe it to 20."

Chris Mihill
Medical Correspondent

The first birth to a surrogate mother funded by the NHS could follow discussions between a health authority and a test tube baby clinic over the help to be given to the infertile couple.

Previous surrogacy arrangements — where a woman bears a child for an infertile couple — have been private. It is not yet known whether the health authority would restrict funding to in vitro fertilisation treatment, or if it would pay the expenses of the surrogate mother.

John Parsons head of the Assisted Conception Unit at King's College Hospital, south London, yesterday revealed that his clinic had been told by a health authority that it would meet the cost of a surrogate pregnancy, although detailed discussions were continuing.

Mr Parsons said he believed that surrogate pregnancies should be available on the NHS as a last resort for infertile couples. His unit received four or five requests a year for IVF treatment for surrogate pregnancies. Each case was decided by the couple who wanted the baby or the prospective surrogate mother. He also refused to identify the health authority, although it is believed to be in the south of the country.

The treatment involves taking eggs and sperm from the would be parents, mixing them in a laboratory and implanting them in the surrogate mother. IVF costs about £2,000 per course of treatment.

Expenses for a surrogate mother would normally include loss of earnings, travel costs and clothing. Most surrogate mothers receive between £7,000 and £10,000.

The announcement came as the British Medical Association issued revised guidance to doctors, saying they should help patients involved in surrogate pregnancies, as counselling about the possible pitfalls would lessen the chances of arrangements going wrong.

Each case was decided by the hospitals ethics committee, after the couple and the surrogate mother had undergone psychological assessment and counselling.

Tim Hedgley, chairman of Issue, the fertility pressure group, said last night: "I think it is very good news. It is very forward thinking of the health authority. The authority is paying to alleviate stress and suffering in an infertile couple."

Extract from the *Guardian*

Senior managers balance the needs of one group of clients against another, and decide who should receive priority. This may mean tackling ethical dilemmas such as:

■ Is a heart operation on a child more important than a hip operation on an older person?

Because of limited resources, most people can no longer choose when, where and how they receive treatment and help. However, those who can afford to do so will still be able to make choices by buying private health care.

- Do you think this is fair?
- What ethical issues does this raise?

- Should resources be directed into buying vital new equipment, which might save hundreds, rather than continuing the treatment of a young person with leukaemia who has a slim chance of survival?
- Is it more important to take a child in danger of physical abuse into foster care, or to pay for home alterations for a physically disabled man of 30?

At an individual level it may mean that a patient or a client in one area may not receive a service or treatment which is available to someone living elsewhere. For example, a woman who had contracted hepatitis from a blood transfusion a decade ago has been refused a drug treatment that costs £4,000. If she lived in the neighbouring health authority, she would have the treatment.

ACTIVITY

What are people's views on health rationing? Compile a questionnaire to find out how your colleagues at school or college think resources should be allocated. For example, you might put together a list of different health problems, and ask people to rank them in order of importance. Or find out people's opinions on providing health care to older people and children, or to smokers with lung disease.

Write a short report on the results of your survey, presenting your statistical findings in bar charts and pie charts.

Key questions

1 Why is the concept of rights important in health and social care?

2 What are ethical issues?

3 What is the effect of the links between power and discrimination?

4 What is stereotyping?

5 What influences our judgements?

6 Whose views should be considered when agreeing the best interests of patients/clients?

7 What is health rationing?

8 What are the main advantages of discussing ethical dilemmas?

9 Name the three types of discrimination.

10 Name two pieces of legislation which social workers may use to restrict the liberty of clients.

SECTION **1.2**

Legislation, policies and codes of practice for promoting equality

It is illegal to discriminate against people because of their sex, cultural or ethnic origin, or disability. You need to know about the laws relating to equal opportunities and about the organisations responsible for establishing the legislation and ensuring it is up to date. Laws and related codes of practice, guidelines and charters are not necessarily the same throughout England, Scotland, Wales and Northern Ireland. Always find out what applies in your part of Britain.

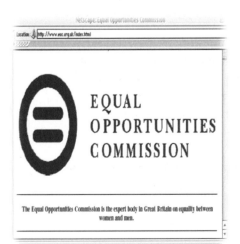

Netscape: Equal Opportunities Commission

Location: http://www.eoc.org.uk/index.html

EQUAL OPPORTUNITIES COMMISSION

The Equal Opportunities Commission is the expert body in Great Britain on equality between women and men.

Bullying and discrimination have no place in today's work environment. Government has a role in stamping out discrimination and harassment and must lead on promoting diversity and equality of opportunity. We are working to transform Britain. Transform it into a society which is inclusive and prosperous, where equality of opportunity is a reality for everybody.

Ian McCartney, Cabinet Office Minister, announcing a major package of cross-governmental initiatives on equal opportunities at a conference on combating workplace bullying, 30 November 1999

While women make up almost half of the workforce, the gulf remains between what is regarded as 'women's work' and 'men's work', which restricts opportunities for both sexes. Challenging these gender stereotypes will be a key priority for the EOC in the new century.

Julie Mellor, Chair of the Equal Opportunities Commission, December 1999, launching Women and Men at the Millennium

If we are to achieve equality and diversity, it is not sufficient to make the right noises and subscribe to the right principles. Equality is not achieved by treating people equally. This is one of the fundamental principles of disability discrimination legislation to which I have devoted much of my time recently through my role on the Disability Rights Task Force and the National Disability Council. Equality of opportunity entails treating people differently, keeping individuals' individual circumstances in mind.

David Grayson CBE, Chairman, The National Disability Council, October 1999

1.2.1 Making sense of the law

Government produces a Green Paper outlining issues under consideration or asks an organisation to produce a report

After discussion and consultation, the government publishes a White Paper outlining proposed legislation

A bill is produced, giving details of the legislation. This may be:
- a Government Bill
- a Private Member's Bill (sponsored by an individual MP).

This is then:
- debated in parliament
- passed by the House of Commons
- passed by the House of Lords
- given royal assent

ACT OF PARLIAMENT

Equal opportunities legislation makes it illegal to discriminate against a person because of their race, sex or disability. We are all protected from infringement of our rights by laws such as the:
- Sex Discrimination Acts 1975 and 1986
- Equal Pay Acts 1975 (to be incorporated for the Twenty-First century within a single Sex Equality Act)
- Race Relation Act 1976
- Disability Discrimination Act 1995 and 1999
- Fair Employment (NI) Act 1989.

You need to understand why those using health and social care services may be vulnerable to infringement of their rights and know about the current laws:
- which aim to protect people regardless of their race, sex, religion, sexual orientation or disability
- which apply to care and early years settings.

There are also charters that identify entitlement to services and define national standards, for example the Citizen's Charter and the Patient's Charter. You need to be familiar with these and know how to identify if the standards they promote are being achieved by knowing how to:
- apply the laws in different types of setting
- identify codes of practice and policies, for example equal opportunities · policies, bullying policies, sexual harassment policies
- identify quality assurance procedures and monitoring.

Acts of Parliament

Health, social care and early years services have legal status through Acts of Parliament which define what must be done, what may be done and what must not be done. Statutory services can only act (powers and duties) in ways laid down by the legislation. Some services must be provided ('mandatory' services) and individuals have a statutory entitlement to them. More often legislation gives powers to provide certain services if authorities so decide. These services are called 'discretionary' and may give rise to variations in what is available at the local level.

Acts of Parliament do not usually set out details of how the service or facility will be provided. This is given in the Statutory Instrument, Directions or Approvals where government ministers are able to specify matters such as:
- who and what actions or services are covered by the legislation
- how the rights or duties are to be carried out
- sanctions and penalties
- organisations responsible for implementing the rights, actions or services.

Precedence	Means	Does
First	*Act of Parliament* (primary legislation)	Places duties or powers
Second	*Statutory Instrument* (secondary or delegated legislation)	Regulations which can place duties or powers
	Directions under an Act of Parliament	Delegated legislation Places duties
	Approvals made under an Act of Parliament	Places duties
	Guidance, National Standards and *codes of practice*	Some guidance is explicit under legislation whereas other guidance is issued by government departments to guide authorities
Third	*Circular Guidance*	A statement of government policy to guide authorities

Guidance and codes of practice

Most of the detailed explanation of what is required locally is contained within Guidance and codes of practice, issued by the Department of Health or Department for Education and Employment (for early years services). Both departments issue circulars that cover:

■ information about departmental policies
■ details of how changes in legislation are to be implemented
■ details of national funding available
■ assistance on planning and developing services.

Although Guidance and circulars do not have the same legal force as Acts of Parliament, failure to implement them can be used by the courts or health service and local government commissioners to criticise the government, the NHS or local councils for not providing services 'as intended by Parliament'.

Circulars

Circulars are the means by which the Department of Health informs the NHS and local authorities about its policy for health and social care. They may set out the details of national funding available for services or how changes in legislation are to be implemented. Circulars are useful to authorities when planning, developing and defending their policies against any challenge.

Variations under the law

Refinements to the various laws are constantly being made through:

- case law decisions
- codes of practice and charters
- manifesto priorities of new governments
- Statutory Instruments and new Acts of Parliament.

Case law has been particularly important for equal opportunities legislation as individuals and groups have tested the scope and effectiveness of the legislation. You will find a few examples of such cases in this section. Newspapers and journals frequently report cases so that you could follow how equal opportunities legislation is being clarified and interpreted.

Key groups

The following groups of people all contribute to the formation of equality of opportunity.

- **Pressure groups** – campaign on issues such as rights for people with disabilities and rights for homosexual people. By raising awareness of issues and demanding action, they bring concerns into the public eye and onto MPs' agenda. Once a Green Paper or report has been drafted, pressure groups may be consulted for their opinions on the issues that concern them.
- **Publicly funded bodies** — the Equal Opportunities Commission and the Commission for Racial Equality are two examples. They both receive a grant from the Home Office. They review equality of opportunity legislation and make recommendations to the government for changing it.
- **Political parties** – are represented in Parliament (for example Conservatives, Labour, Liberal Democrats, Scottish National, Plaid Cymru, Ulster Unionist). Each has particular policies and concerns which they aim to promote by influencing legislation.
- **Members of Parliament (MPs)** – debate and vote on bills introducing new laws, and have the final say in whether legislation is passed. They are influenced by the wishes of their political party, and the needs and concerns of their electorate (the people they represent).
- **Devolved Authorities** – since 1999, in addition to the parliament in Westminster, Scotland and Wales have significant new devolved legislatures.
- **European Union (EU)** – British law is now increasingly coming into line with European Union directives. European law has had a major effect on British equality of opportunity legislation.

1.2.2 **Equal opportunity legislation**

Much of the focus of equal opportunities legislation is directed to treatment at work and the provision of goods and services. The major pieces of legislation concern:

- sex
- race
- disability
- religion (in Northern Ireland).

Other legislation has provided employees with greater protection in terms of:

- pay and work conditions
- health and safety
- harassment and bullying.

In 1998 the Human Rights Act was passed, bringing into British law the European Convention on Human Rights. This means that both practice and new and existing laws will be judged by British Courts under the Act that will have paramountcy. Parliament will be under an obligation to ensure that all new legislation meets the requirements of the Act.

Equality of the sexes

The Equal Pay Act 1970 in Northern Ireland was the first equality of opportunity legislation related to the sexes. This was extended to the rest of the UK in 1975 in the Sex Discrimination Act. This made it unlawful to discriminate against people because of their sex or marital status in:

- employment (recruitment and promotion of both full-time and part-time staff)
- training
- education
- providing housing, goods, facilities and services
- advertising.

At the same time, the Employment Protection Act 1975 gave women the right to take paid maternity leave and then return to work after having a baby.

The Sex Discrimination Act recognises three types of discrimination:

- direct discrimination – when one person is treated less favourably than another on the grounds of their sex
- indirect discrimination – when unnecessary conditions are applied which disadvantage one sex
- victimisation – when an employer treats an employee less favourably because they have made complaints of sex discrimination in the past.

Reinstatement recommended

Winn v Northwedge Ltd

A Bristol industrial tribunal (Chair: C F Sara) recommends the reinstatement of a female bouncer who was dismissed because of her sex.

Jacky Winn was the only female among five bouncers employed by Northwedge Ltd at a Trowbridge nightclub. In February 1995, the company took a policy decision not to employ female bouncers and Ms Winn was offered bar work. She refused the offer and was dismissed. The company admitted sex discrimination. The industrial tribunal awarded £2,416 compensation, including £1500 for injury to feelings. It also considered it appropriate to recommend reinstatement, to take effect from two weeks of the hearing date.

ACTIVITY

The Sex Discrimination Act 1975 set up the Equal Opportunities Commission (EOC) to promote and enforce equal opportunities for women and men. Write to the EOC for up-to-date information on progress with the proposals for *Equality in the Twenty-first Century*. (The EOC address is at the end of this unit.) If you have access to the Internet, visit the EOC web site (*http://www.eoc.org.uk/html/eoc_overview.html*).

Use this information to produce your own leaflet advising a hospital, nursing home or childcare centre on its responsibilities to treat women and men equally. The leaflet should:

■ summarise the original Equal Pay and Sex Discrimination Acts and their most recent changes

■ advise the organisation on its responsibilities towards staff and clients under both Acts

■ indicate the possible future changes.

Equality in the Twenty-first Century

At the turn of the century, Britain undertook a comprehensive review of equal opportunities legislation: *Equality in the Twenty-first Century* proposed that the Government amend and replace the Sex Discrimination and Equal Pay Acts within a single Sex Equality Act. Proposals included:

■ changing the emphasis from combating discrimination to promoting the positive 'right to equal treatment'

■ making employers responsible for reviewing their pay systems and taking action to close the pay gap between men and women (at the time this book was published, men averaged 20% higher pay than women for comparable work)

■ giving public bodies responsibility to promote equal opportunities

■ simplifying and improving legal rights and remedies (what does this mean for pregnant women?)

■ extending protection to include sexual orientation and gender reassignment

■ other issues that might arise in the future.

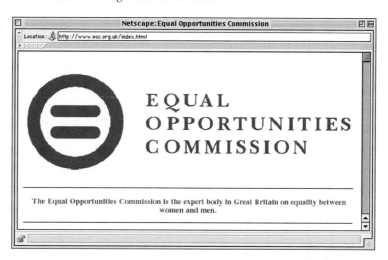

The Equal Opportunities Commission is the expert body in Great Britain on equality between women and men.

Equal pay

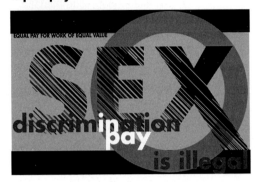

The Equal Pay Act 1975 was introduced to eliminate discrimination between the rates of pay and terms of contract offered to men and women. Since being amended in 1984, the main focus of the legislation has become 'equal pay for work of equal value'. In the past, women had to prove that a man was being paid more for the same job to claim discrimination. But now, women doing jobs in which few men are employed (for example, sewing machinists and cleaners) can claim equal pay if they believe that men doing jobs which are similar in demand are paid more.

To assess whether jobs are of equal value, a job evaluation study is carried out, as in the following case study.

ACTIVITY

Look at the information you collected from the Equal Opportunities Commission on the Equal Pay Act. Under the Act, what are the responsibilities of organisations such as North Yorkshire County Council in the case study shown here? What are the responsibilities of individuals, such as the catering assistants?

MARKET FORCES NO DEFENCE

Ratcliffe and others v North Yorkshire County Council

The work of catering assistants (or 'dinner ladies') in North Yorkshire had been rated as equivalent to that of road-sweepers and refuse collectors under the local government job evaluation scheme. However, following compulsory competitive tendering, the council took the view that in order to compete with private contractors, it needed to reduce the catering assistants' pay. The catering assistants complained that this contravened the Equal Pay Act.

Their claim was upheld by the House of Lords who found that the reduction in pay arose out of economic and social factors which led to the catering staff being almost exclusively women, who were prepared to accept lower rates of pay. Giving the decision for the Lords, Lord Slynn said: 'Though conscious of the difficult problem facing the employers in seeking to compete with a rival tenderer, I am satisfied that to reduce the women's wages below that of their male counterparts was the very kind of discrimination in relation to pay which the Act sought to remove.'

(from Equal Opportunities Review, *Discrimination Case Law Digest)*

Legislation relating to race

The first legislation protecting individuals against racial discrimination was the Race Relations Act 1965 (amended in 1968). However, this left many loopholes in the law, and was replaced by the Race Relations Act 1976.

The 1976 Act protects individuals against discrimination when:

- applying for jobs
- at work
- buying a home
- renting accommodation
- buying goods or services (from banks, restaurants, shops and so on)
- in education and training
- joining a club.

The Act states that it is unlawful to discriminate on the grounds of colour, race, nationality or ethnic origin. It makes it an offence to incite racial hatred. The Commission for Racial Equality (CRE) was set up to enforce the Act and give advice on improving equal opportunities for people from minority ethnic groups.

Discrimination, prejudice and racism

The Race Relations Act deals with racial discrimination, not prejudice. It is concerned with people's actions and the effects of their actions, not their intentions.

- Prejudice literally means 'prejudging' someone – knowing next to nothing about them but jumping to conclusions because of some characteristic, like their appearance.
- Discrimination occurs when someone is treated less favourably because of that characteristic – in the case of racial discrimination because of their racial, national or ethnic origins.
- Racism is the belief that some 'races' are superior to others – based on the false idea that different physical characteristics (like skin colour) or ethnic background make some people better or lesser than others.

Racial discrimination, like sex discrimination, is defined as direct, indirect and victimisation. Mr Singh, a Sikh, explains how he has been the victim of all three types of discrimination at different stages of his life:

66 *As a child, I was indirectly discriminated against by a school which refused to make an exception to the school rule of wearing a cap. As I had to wear a turban, this indirectly excluded me from the school. Since starting work I've suffered direct discrimination, being turned down for a transfer to a different (all-white) section because I 'wouldn't fit in'. I complained to the management, they apologised and the transfer went ahead. But since then I've been branded as a trouble-maker, and turned down for two promotions I know I should have got.* 99

The Race Relations Act covers colour, ethnic group and national origin, but not religion – although some religious groups, such as Sikhs and Jews, have been identified by tribunals or courts as ethnic groups.

Review of the Race Relations Act

At the time of writing there is a debate between the CRE and the Government about possible changes to the law on race relations. You will need to keep in touch with developments.

ACTIVITY

Prepare a resource file of information on the Race Relations Act and the Public Order Act. Find out more about the following organisations and how they can help:

- Commission for Racial Equality
- Institute of Race Relations
- your local Racial Equality Council
- Joint Council for the Welfare of Immigrants
- Liberty
- local Citizens Advice Bureaux
- local law centres
- libraries.

ACTIVITY

Read the following accounts of two discrimination cases. Select one and note the elements where organisational policy and/or practice fell short of required standards. How did this result in direct or indirect discrimination? Where is there evidence that an equal opportunities audit should have taken place? How might such an audit have prevented expensive litigation? Prepare an action checklist on what the organisation should be doing now to prevent a recurrence of discrimination.

Case law press report Tuesday 23 November 1999

MAJOR RETAILER GUILTY OF DISCRIMINATION

Manmohan Bawa, a highly successful, prize-winning store manager who secured substantial increases in the sales at various stores he was responsible for, was promoted to run the Currys Tottenham superstore in North London. After nearly one and half years in the position, he was suddenly removed by his then area manager and replaced with a white manager from a store with a poor record. The area manager, the tribunal said, 'had no compunction about antagonising' Mr Bawa, having decided to move him from the superstore because of his race.

After Mr Bawa put in a complaint of racial discrimination to the employment tribunal, his then area manager, in the words of the tribunal, sought to 'stamp his authority on [Mr Bawa] in an aggressive manner to forestall any similar difficulties arising between them'. The area manager, the tribunal said, has 'simply decided to find fault' with Mr Bawa and engaged in a 'campaign' against him.

The tribunal added that it was satisfied that the area manager 'felt able to do this as he works in a company which maintains a glass ceiling through which managers from ethnic minorities have only rarely in the past been able to break and above which there have not been any ethnic minority managers for some time'.

It rejected claims by senior managers from the company that they did not know that Mr Bawa had put in the discrimination complaint, saying: 'it appeared inconceivable to the tribunal that senior managers would not inform each other about and consider matters of importance in their areas; a complaint of discrimination must be just such a matter.'

JOHNSON V (1) ARMITAGE (2) MARSDEN (3) HM PRISON SERVICE

From mid-1991 to March 1993, Claude Johnson, a prison officer at Brixton prison, was ostracised by fellow prison officers following his complaint about the manhandling of a black prisoner by officers. He was also warned about his sickness absence, although a white officer with a poorer record was not warned; he was frequently detailed for particular work, but when he arrived at work was given non-detailed duties; and he was reported for leaving duty early, although it was customary to do so, and given a warning.

An industrial tribunal found that Mr Johnson had suffered a campaign of appalling treatment, ruling that he had been unlawfully discriminated against on racial grounds and awarded damages. The tribunal said that, where individuals are found to have committed unlawful acts of discrimination, they should be liable for their acts and not rely on their employers to bear complete responsibility.

(from *Equal Opportunities Review*, Discrimination Case Law Digest)

Legislation relating to disability

Although there has been legislation aimed at ensuring employment for disabled people since 1944 (The Disabled Persons Employment Act), equal opportunity legislation on a par with that for sex and race is recent. The Chronically Sick and Disabled Persons Act 1970 required local authorities to identify people with disabilities in order to provide them with information about services. A further Act in 1986 gave disabled people the right to have their needs assessed, to be represented by a friend and their needs monitored and reviewed. Both these Acts related to a disabled person's right to health and social care.

In 1995, after much consultation and debate, The Disability Discrimination Act gave disabled people new rights in the areas of:
- employment
- access to goods, facilities and services
- buying or renting land or property.

The Act also required schools, colleges and universities to provide information for disabled people and allowed the Government to set minimum access standards for new taxis, trains and buses. It set up the National Disability Council (NDC) in January 1996, and a corresponding Northern Ireland Disability Council (NIDC). NDC was an independent body to advise the Secretary of State on measures to reduce or eliminate discrimination against disabled people and on the operation of the Disability Discrimination Act. The NDC has been replaced by a Disability Rights Commission with powers similar to those of the Equal Opportunities Commission and the Commission for Racial Equality.

Although the Discrimination Act was passed in 1995, a number of its provisions have had delayed implementation. So, although health and social services providers have been required not to refuse services or offer a worse standard of service since 1996, they had:
- until October 1999 to take reasonable steps to change their practices which make it impossible for a disabled person to use a service
- until 2004 to take reasonable steps to remove, alter or avoid physical barriers to access to a service or facilities.

It is too early for sufficient cases to clarify the law. In the case study on the following page, the application of the Act to a person with a mental illness illustrates how the Act works.

ACTIVITY

Collect information about the Disability Discrimination Act. Contact the National Disability Council or the Royal Association for Disability and Rehabilitation.

Produce a checklist for health and social care organisations of key points of the legislation, summarising especially the most recent requirements of the Act. Highlight any changes you think they should consider. Consider the possible impact on resources for health and social care organisations in relation to the Act.

Leading construction group John Laing yesterday admitted unlawfully discriminating against a man it had intended to appoint its company secretary, after rejecting him when it emerged that he had a history of schizophrenia.

In the first case of its kind, the group agreed to pay undisclosed damages to Andrew Watkiss, who has had no mental illness for eight years and holds a senior post as assistant company secretary at Unigate, the leading dairy group. He applied for the post at John Laing and was offered the job in January 1999, subject to a medical.

During the examination, he acknowledged that he had been diagnosed with schizophrenia in 1980 and had suffered three breakdowns between then and 1991. Although he had since been perfectly able to manage the condition with medication, the company withdrew the job offer on 'medical' grounds that the post would be too stressful for him.

Mr Watkiss challenged the decision under the Disability Discrimination Act, which had not previously been used successfully against recruitment prejudice on mental health grounds.

John Laing has now settled the case, with its admission of culpability written into the employment tribunal record. The financial terms of the settlement are being kept confidential but compensation is likely to be substantial as it includes both injury to feelings and future loss of earnings for Mr Watkiss, aged 46.

He said yesterday that John Laing's attitude had been in marked contrast to that of Unigate, which had taken him on within a year of his last admission to hospital. Since then, he had experienced no mental illness.

"John Laing sent out a very negative message, so I hope this outcome will make employers more aware and open to people with this sort of mental health problem," said Mr Watkiss, who lives in London and is a fellow of the Institute of Chartered Secretaries and Administrators.

The mental health charity Mind said that about 70% of people with mental health problems were deterred from applying for jobs because they feared unfair treatment.

The Guardian, *Friday 24 December 1999*

1.2.3 **Some key phrases**

Formal investigation

The Commission for Racial Equality may on its own initiative conduct formal investigations of organisations or individuals where there is evidence that discrimination may have taken place – for example where a discriminatory advertisement has been published. Notice must be given that a formal investigation is to take place. This is usually done by taking space in a newspaper. If the investigation is concerned with named persons, those individuals would need to be given separate notice. If the commission is satisfied that a contravention of the Race Relations Act has taken place, it may issue a non-discrimination notice. In essence, the notice will require the person or organisation to which it is served to comply with specified provisions of the Act.

Genuine occupational qualifications

It is possible lawfully to discriminate in recruitment for employment in circumstances where being someone of a particular sex or racial origin is a 'genuine occupational qualification' (often abbreviated to GOQ). The specific circumstances are:

- for reasons of authenticity
- to provide personal and welfare services
- for reasons of decency and privacy
- because of the nature of the establishment.

Positive action

Where there is evidence of under-representation of a particular group in an organisation or work area, an employer may take positive action through advertising and training to enable members of the less represented group to take advantage of the recruitment and promotion processes. Positive action under these circumstances is lawful.

Positive discrimination

Positive discrimination occurs when an employer chooses a woman or a person from a minority ethnic group, for example, during recruitment, promotion or dismissal because of their sex or colour rather than their ability. Positive discrimination under the Sex Discrimination and Race Relations Acts is unlawful. Under the Disability Discrimination Act, positive discrimination is allowed where all other factors are equal.

Vicarious liability

All employers are held initially responsible for any discriminatory acts of their employees except where they have taken clear steps to ensure that discrimination does not take place. Under the Sex Discrimination and Race Relations Acts, individuals are also held responsible. If, therefore, an unlawful discriminatory action took place, both the employer and employee are likely to be held responsible.

31

Victimisation

Victimisation is treating a person less favourably because that person has asserted rights, or helped another to assert their rights, or because they are suspected of doing either of these things.

ACTIVITY

Decide whether each of the situations listed below is a case of direct discrimination, indirect discrimination or victimisation, or whether no discrimination has taken place. Explain your decision in each case.

- a job advertisement asking for an 'experienced male actor to play the part of King Lear'
- a job advertisement asking for an 'experienced waitress'
- an interviewer asking a woman candidate about her childcare arrangements
- a male teacher being repeatedly passed over for promotion after giving evidence in a sex discrimination case
- a single-sex boys' school refusing to accept a female pupil

1.2.4 **Other employment initiatives**

A great deal of European Union legislation and codes of practice – especially under the Social Chapter – is bringing about changes in pay and employment which apply to the UK.

Other government pay and employment initiatives helping towards family-friendly employment include:

- Employment Rights Act 1996 – strengthened protection where people have been forced to leave a job because of an employer's conduct
- Working Time Regulations – protects people from the hazards of working excessive hours (see *http://www.dti.gov.uk/IR/work_time_regs/index.htm*)
- Employment Relations Act – increases rights to maternity, paternity and other parental leave and a right to reasonable time off for domestic emergencies (see *http://www.dti.gov.uk/IR/erbill.htm*)
- Working Families Tax Credit and Childcare Tax Credit – provides improved financial support to working families and additional help with the costs of childcare (see *http://www.dfee.gov.uk/childcare/content5.htm*)
- National Childcare strategy – aims to ensure good quality affordable childcare for children aged 0–14 in every neighbourhood (see *http://www.dfee.gov.uk/childcare/content1.htm*).

Initiatives like the Minimum Pay legislation introduced at the beginning of 1999 had greatest impact on those receiving the lowest levels of pay. This includes many workers in health and social care, and some of the most vulnerable people in society, predominant users of health and social services. Issues such as reviewing the pay levels set and any possible adverse impact of the legislation, especially on small businesses and non-profit-making organisations, will continue to be important. Many bodies will be pressing their particular case with the Government as developments continue.

ACTIVITY

If you have access to the Internet, find out from the web site of central government the most current proposals and legislation concerning pay. If you are based in Northern Ireland, Wales or Scotland, conduct research for your own area. Considerable changes to the legislation concerning pay are taking place.

ACTIVITY

Draw out all the information relevant to employment from the research material on equality of opportunity legislation you have collected so far. Produce a poster, summarising the legislation relating to the employment of:

- men and women
- people of all races, colours, and ethnic and national origins
- disabled people.

ACTIVITY

Carry out a media search for two weeks, collecting news reports, features and advertisements related to equality of opportunity legislation. Organise the information according to whether it relates to sex, race, disability, pay or employment.

Legislation against harassment and bullying

An employee has the right to terminate their employment without notice under contract law if, because of the employer's conduct, they consider themselves to have been constructively dismissed. If an employer harasses an employee, or knows of their harassment and fails to take reasonable steps to stop it or prevent its recurrence, the employee may be entitled to treat this as a breach of the implied contractual terms of trust and confidence. In the event of a serious breach, the employee is entitled to resign and claim constructive dismissal.

Employees who believe themselves to have been harassed because of, for example, their age, marital status, religious conviction or because they are gay or lesbian, may also be entitled to claim unfair or constructive dismissal under the Employment Relations Act.

Reference to harassment and bullying is contained within all the main equality and anti-discrimination Acts. But the Protection from Harassment Act 1997 introduced a new offence of harassment which includes alarming someone or causing them distress. The conduct must occur at least twice and can either be harassment by action or by words. The criminal penalty for harassment under this legislation is imprisonment for a maximum of six months or a maximum fine of £5,000.

Sexual harassment could include:
- unwarranted, intrusive or persistent questioning about a person's marital status, sexual interests or orientation
- telling lewd jokes or making remarks that contain innuendo
- suggesting that sexual favours may enhance a person's career or that not offering sexual favours may adversely affect their career.

Racial harassment could include:
- racially derogatory or stereotyped remarks and statements
- displaying or circulating racially offensive material e.g. graffiti.

Bullying could include:
- shouting or similar aggressive behaviour towards a colleague
- ignoring successes but consistently highlighting small failures.

Health and Safety at Work Act (1974)

According to this Act, all employers have a duty so far as is 'reasonably practicable' to ensure the health, safety and welfare of their employees. Harassment and bullying at work are increasingly recognised as a serious health hazard because of the stress they can cause. An employee who is under stress is less effective and more likely to act erratically or carelessly, putting themselves and others at risk.

If an employer fails to respond to complaints about harassment and the complainant's health and ability to work suffer as a result, like any other health and safety issue, employees are entitled to pursue this through internal procedures, the relevant statutory enforcement bodies or the civil courts.

Employees who believe themselves to have been harassed because of, for example, their age, marital status, religious conviction, disability or because they are gay or lesbian, may also choose to pursue their complaint citing the Health and Safety at Work Act.

ACTIVITY

Contact a health or social care organisation in your area, for example a local health trust, clinic, social services department or care facility. Ask if you may have a copy of their equal opportunities policy. Based on the information you collect, make a chart summarising their policy for:

- equal treatment of men and women
- equal treatment of people of all colours, races, ethnic and national origins
- equal treatment of people with disabilities
- equal pay for their staff
- equal employment opportunities for all.

Do they also refer to other areas of possible discrimination such as religion, age or sexuality? (In England, for example, these are not always included in the law.) Colour-code your chart to show which policies relate to the way the organisation treats clients, which relate to the way it treats its staff and which relate to both.

DISCUSSION POINT

In a situation at work where employees may face abuse from their colleagues, what steps can employers take to prevent discrimination?

Other legislation bearing on individual rights

There are other laws relevant to the work of health and social care practitioners. Some of this legislation is covered in unit 5, while unit 2 explains the:

- Access to Personal Files Act 1987
- Access to Health Records Act 1990
- Data Protection Act 1998.

All the above Acts cover confidentiality of information and access to information.

Other Acts that affect individual rights include:

- The Public Interest Disclosure Act 1998 (known to some as the 'Whistleblower's Charter'). This provides protection for workers who disclose information about a colleague in the public interest. Such information includes when a criminal offence has been/is being/is likely to be committed; when a person has failed, is failing or is likely to fail to comply with a legal obligation.
- The Human Rights Act 1998. This incorporates most of the articles of the European Convention of Human Rights. It enables any individual in the UK who considers themselves to have been a victim of a human rights violation to challenge a public authority (e.g. local or central government, the courts, the police) in the courts or tribunals.
- The Rehabilitation of Offenders Act 1974. This Act allows for certain criminal convictions to become 'spent' after a period of time determined by the length of the sentence received. However, many posts working with children, young people and vulnerable adults are exempted.
- Care Standards Act 2000. This sets up a General Social Care Council and tightens the restrictions on people who work with children and vulnerable adults.

Inconsistencies under the law

Although equality of opportunity legislation is in place to safeguard equal rights, loopholes and inconsistencies in the laws themselves can perpetuate and even create inequalities. For example:

- The Race Relations Act covers colour, ethnic group and national origin, but not religion (although as mentioned earlier some religious groups are protected under the law because it's assumed that people professing the religion belong to a minority ethnic group).
- The Sex Discrimination Act does not apply to some aspects of employment in the armed forces. Special measures apply for ministers of religion, the police, prison officers and athletes playing competitive sports.
- Many disabled people feel that equality of opportunity legislation does not give them the same rights under the law as other groups in society and that even with recent changes, the legislation doesn't make adequate allowance for the particular needs of those with disabilities.

There are many inconsistencies to do with age limits – within the UK, and between the UK and other parts of the EU and the rest of the world.

DISCUSSION POINT

Why do you think inconsistency in the law exists concerning age constraints and matters of sex and sexuality? Whose principles is the legislation reflecting?

1.2.5 **Redress under the law**

ACTIVITY

Look into the procedure for taking action if an employee alleges discrimination and wishes to seek redress under the law. What are the time limits for taking action? What is the role of the Advisory, Conciliation and Arbitration Service (ACAS), which was set up to settle industrial disputes, in trying to help the employee and employer reach an agreement without going to a tribunal? What are the advantages for an employee of taking a discrimination case to an employment tribunal? Can you think of any possible disadvantages?

Employment Rights (Dispute Resolution) Act 1998

In April 1998, the Employment Rights (Dispute Resolution) Act 1998 was passed. It amends legislation relating to the resolution of individual employment disputes. Such disputes are usually linked to the requirements of one or more of the following Acts:

- the Sex Discrimination Act 1975
- the Race Relations Act 1976
- the Trade Union and Labour Relations (Consolidation) Act 1992
- the Disability Discrimination Act 1995
- the Employment Tribunals Act 1996
- the Employment Rights Act 1996.

If a complaint about discrimination cannot be resolved within the organisation, individuals have the right to seek redress through legal systems. This can mean taking a complaint to:

- a county court in England or Wales
- a sheriff court in Scotland
- an employment tribunal.

For useful sites on tribunals and the latest guidance on dispute resolution see *http://www.employmentcomplaints.com/*. Look at HelpNET, a site for those taking job-related complaints to the employment tribunals. The site is dedicated to those who have lost their jobs or are experiencing problems at their jobs and are presenting job complaints to the employment tribunals.

Complaints about discrimination outside employment are dealt with in the courts. If the court finds that discrimination did occur, it can award damages.

Employment tribunals

An employment tribunal hears most cases of sex, disability or race discrimination. The tribunal is made up of a legally qualified chairperson and two lay members who have knowledge or experience of industry or commerce. At the tribunal both complainants and respondents may put their case themselves or be represented by another person (for example, a solicitor, a trade union representative). If the tribunal finds in favour of the complainant it may invoke:

- an order declaring the rights of the parties
- an order requiring the respondent to pay the complainant compensation (there is currently no limit to the amount of compensation that can be awarded).

When a tribunal is deciding on a figure for damages, it may consider both tangible and intangible considerations, such as:

- loss of earnings
- injured feelings
- a recommendation that the respondent take a particular course of action to reduce the adverse effect of discrimination on the complainant.

Application of the law

There is a lot of equality of opportunity legislation in the UK. But how equal are people's rights under the law? And how consistently is legislation interpreted and enforced? Even when people's rights under the law are consistent, legislation is not always interpreted and applied consistently.

Some equality of opportunity laws are almost ignored. For example, legislation which was introduced in the 1940s making it a legal requirement for employers with a staff of over 20 people to employ 3 per cent disabled people was rarely enforced and there were only a handful of prosecutions over the years.

In other areas people choose to ignore, or misinterpret, the legislation. Laws provide a starting point but they need positive action if they are to be put into effect. Employers may develop an equal opportunity policy supporting equal rights for women, but still not offer facilities such as crèches and flexible working arrangements to meet a parent's needs.

1.2.6 National variations in equal opportunities law

As a result of differences in the legal systems in England, Wales, Scotland and Northern Ireland, there are also major inconsistencies between equality of opportunity legislation in different parts of Britain. Legislation often includes explanations of how the Act applies in Scotland, and sometimes a separate Act is passed. Northern Ireland has its own legislation, which is introduced by Order in Council. Acts that apply in the rest of the UK don't always have a related Order in Northern Ireland; for example, the Education (Handicapped Children) Act 1981 focuses on the integration of children with special needs into mainstream schools in England and Wales, while the Education (Scotland) Act 1981 has the same function in Scotland, but there is no comparable Act in Northern Ireland. In the same way, the Fair Employment Act (NI) only applies in Northern Ireland, and there is no comparable legislation in the rest of the UK.

Legal reform and devolution

In all these areas, the law is undergoing reform and development. This is inevitable a few years after a change of government in the UK and as European influences become stronger. The turn of a century and the start of a new millennium gave extra impetus.

Although this book aims to give you up-to-date information and highlight known areas of imminent change, it cannot be regarded as a definitive legal statement. You should follow up the sources of information given – especially the Internet contacts – to find out the current situation.

An additional complexity is that in 1999 devolution of significant powers was granted to:

- the Scottish Parliament
- the National Assembly of Wales
- the Northern Ireland Executive.

Devolution allows divergence in policy-making to address local needs and priorities. Gradually these three devolved authorities will review and reform existing legislation and bring in their own laws and codes of practice.

In all matters of the law, it is important for you to be aware of any variations that might apply in your part of the UK and at the time of your study. Even where no reference is made in this book to special provision in Scotland, Wales or Northern Ireland, you should always assume that there may be specific laws. So make sure if you live in one of these countries.

Northern Ireland

From 1 October 1999, the Equality Commission for Northern Ireland took over the functions and responsibilities of the Equal Opportunities Commission for Northern Ireland, the Commission for Racial Equality for Northern Ireland, the Fair Employment Commission and the Northern Ireland Disability Council. The Commission has important responsibilities for the statutory duty on all public bodies to promote equality of opportunity no matter what an individual's:

- religion
- political opinion
- sex
- race
- age
- marital status
- sexual orientation
- disability
- position in respect of dependants.

The Public Order Act 1986 in Northern Ireland and the Public Order (NI) Order 1987 strengthened the law on race by making it an offence to incite racial hatred by threatening, abusive or insulting words or behaviour intended to stir up racial hatred. This includes producing or possessing material in writing, on video or on audio tape.

Scotland and Wales

The devolved parliaments in Wales, Scotland and Northern Ireland include race relations in their priority. At the time of writing they were reviewing their equal opportunities legislation and codes of practice as one of their priorities. Watch out for further information! A good way of keeping up to date with changing legislation is via the Internet if you are able to get access. A good web site to start with is *http://www.cre.gov.uk/law.*

ACTIVITY

Find other examples of inconsistencies in equality of opportunity rights between the four parts of the UK. Check whether any such regional variations are likely to apply to your geographical location.

1.2.7 Application of equal opportunities legislation to use of health and social care

In addition to being discriminated against because of their sex, race or disability, health and social care clients will be further affected because they have low status as a result of:

- age
- the nature of their disability
- their health status
- their family status, such as being a single parent
- religion
- employment status
- low income
- where they live.

All this means that health and social care practitioners must be aware of the effect that double or multiple discrimination has on their clients. Their employers will have developed equal opportunity policies which spell out how client rights will be implemented. In the next section, you can see how organisations take this further.

Health and social care organisations are required to offer their services in a way that puts service users first. The Mental Health Act, the Children Act and NHS and Community Care Act set out their duty to do so. Unit 5 covers these Acts. The expectations of health and social care organisations and those who work in them is strengthened further by the Human Rights Act.

1.2.8 Charters and codes of practice

Over the last decade, the government has encouraged and expected health and social services to have written statements of what those who use them can expect. At national level the government published:

- the Citizen's Charter, which aims to improve the quality and choice of public services
- the Patient's Charter, which sets out what patients should expect from their health service
- the Parent's Charter, focusing on education and the rights of parents to choose a school for their children.

At local level, most organisations will have developed statements on how their services will be offered and to whom, and targets for their performance.

These charters cover:

■ information about services available

■ how practitioners will treat patients and clients

■ what goods or services a client is entitled to

■ how clients will be involved in decisions made about them

■ how clients can complain and seek redress

■ commitments to monitoring and reviewing, with targets for performance and a process for publishing information from monitoring.

The following extract is taken from the 1993–94 community care plan for Northumberland. It lays down guidelines on care priorities and how practitioners should allocate resources.

Category **A**:

help will always be offered to resolve problems in these areas if a solution is feasible and within the powers of the Authorities.

Getting into and out of bed; getting dressed and undressed; moving between your bed and a chair.

Washing your hands and face daily; looking after your body (e.g. getting your hair and nails cut, shaving); getting washed all over at least once a fortnight (more often if you need to for your health). Getting clean clothes and bedclothes, and keeping your home clean and well-maintained enough to avoid harm to your health.

Looking after your health by eating and drinking adequately, keeping warm, and taking medication appropriately. Carrying out bodily functions in a dignified and hygienic way; changing position often enough to avoid bedsores or other problems.

Avoiding preventable risks, such as risk of falls and burns; getting help in emergencies and letting people into your home safely.

Getting at least two hours a day free from care or self-care tasks. If you are a carer, getting at least two hours a week away from the person you care for.

Making your needs and views known; understanding your health condition; being properly prepared for the care or self-care tasks you carry out; knowing about your benefit entitlements.

Avoiding:

● Degrading treatment, extreme isolation or avoidable pain

● Harming yourself or other people

● The collapse of your relationships with the people you live with

● Significant harm to children, or children taking inappropriate responsibilities for care.

Category **B**:

social services or health resources should usually be available, if required, to resolve problems in these areas.

Living in your own home.

Keeping your home free from smells and grime. Basic money management.

Feeling confident about future support if current arrangements break down. If you are a carer, getting a few days each year away from caring.

Maintaining key friendships and contacts. Free from other people's rules about how you should live.

Sharing a bedroom with your partner if you wish to.

Reading, writing, watching TV, and listening to the radio (or equivalents if these are not possible). Finding satisfying and productive occupation if you are not able to work or study.

Avoiding:

● severe difficulty with basic tasks

● avoidable discomfort

● constant exhaustion

● difficulty coping with major crises such as bereavement.

Key questions

1 Name one piece of equality of opportunity legislation relating to each of the following: sex, race, disability, pay, employment.

2 Give three responsibilities of organisations under the Sex Discrimination Act.

3 List five situations in which the Race Relations Act protects against discrimination on the grounds of race.

4 Give three responsibilities of organisations under the Disability Discrimination Act.

5 What is the main focus of the Equal Pay Act?

6 Explain why there are inconsistencies in equality of opportunity legislation in different parts of the UK, and give two examples.

7 Give three examples of behaviour that would count as sexual or racial harassment under the Protection from Harassment Act 1997.

8 Why are clients likely to experience double or multiple discrimination?

9 What are the effects of the Devolution Act 1999?

SECTION **1.3**

How care organisations promote equality

Health and social care practitioners need to identify how individuals' rights are promoted and maintained through day-to-day practice. Charters and policies are produced by many care organisations, and procedures and systems support good practice and protect individuals. You will need to consider equal opportunities issues for all employees working in health and social care and how care practitioners can apply the care value base.

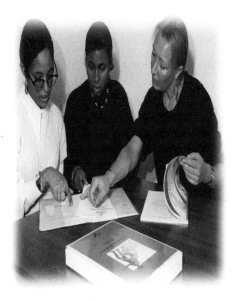

We are not forgetting that staff in the NHS who are disabled must also be treated with equal value and respect. It is important that we have a workforce that represents the diverse community that uses the services we provide. In trying to achieve this, the skills, experience and potential of disabled people must not be ignored. To help and encourage NHS employers in recruiting and retaining disabled people, a good practice guide 'Looking Beyond Labels' has been published. We want to see the NHS use the advice it gives on designing jobs around what people can do and offer – and so help remove any barriers to employment within the NHS which disabled people may face.

John Hutton, Minister for Health, on the launch of Welcoming Patients With Disabilities, speaking on the International Day for Disabled People, December 1999

Article 13 of the Amsterdam Treaty could lead to race equality legislation across the EU. Article 13 should eventually provide citizens with a legal instrument to use against discrimination based on race, sex, religion or belief, disability, age or sexual orientation – but it will need a major campaign both within and outside the European Parliament.

Claude Moraes, The Guardian, December 1999

Our equal opportunities policy aims to ensure that all the children are treated equally. It's something we're acutely aware of and all staff know that if they feel the policy is not being complied with completely in any area they can bring the matter directly to me or my deputy. We bring in multicultural activities as a matter of course so that the children understand that other people may be different in some way but they are still equal.

head of private day nursery and childcare centre

1.3.1 **Organisational responsibilities**

Equality of opportunity legislation places responsibilities on both organisations and individuals to ensure the fair treatment of everyone who comes in contact with them. In health and social care organisations, equality of opportunity practices exist to ensure fair treatment:

- of employees (e.g. in terms of recruitment, working conditions, training, promotion)
- of everyone using health or social care services (e.g. the quality of care they receive must be free from discrimination).

To put equality of opportunity legislation into practice, all health and social care organisations – from regional offices and health authorities to dental practices and residential homes – should have a clear policy for putting equalities into place. The policy will deal with:

- being an employer
- giving staff training and support to promote good practice
- promoting clients' equality and protecting them from abuse and exploitation.

Managers must make sure that staff know about the policy, and provide guidelines and support to help them implement it. In turn, employees must make an effort to understand and promote equal opportunities in everything they do.

Organisations often have rules, procedures and policies that restrict equal opportunities. They try to eliminate:

- stereotyping – where the general organisational culture reinforces beliefs about a group or practice which goes beyond the available evidence
- prejudice – either organisational prejudice for, or against, something
- subjectivity – favouring people we identify because they have the qualities we have or would like to have. Subjectivity can be a big barrier to equal opportunities during job interviews and selection, promotion and assessment for career and professional development.

Without these policies and procedures being in place, existing organisational cultures may lead to:

- arbitrary employee selection criteria – for example, asking for higher qualifications than the job demands for the organisation's convenience (perhaps to cut down on number of applicants) or assuming that jobs and working conditions must conform to a pattern which may disadvantage, deter or bar those with commitments outside work
- unsatisfactory procedures – rules and policies which do not take account of equal opportunities, the procedures may create or fail to stop indirect discrimination, unlawful direct discrimination or victimisation.

Employment practice

You will find details of legislation relating to employment in section 1.2. In addition, employers are encouraged by government departments to put in place policies and procedures which encourage equality and diversity. For example, the Department for Education and Employment (DfEE) has produced an equal opportunities 'toolkit' of recommendations for small organisations and departments of large organisations to help them check their equal opportunities performance with respect to their employees and improve it if necessary.

Equal Opportunities ToolKit: a ten-point plan

1 Develop an equal opportunities policy, embracing recruitment, promotion and training.

2 Set an action plan including targets, so that you and your staff have a clear idea of what can be achieved and by when.

3 Provide equal opportunities training for all staff to help people, including management, throughout your organisation to understand the importance of equal opportunities, and provide additional training for staff who recruit, select and train your employees.

4 Monitor the present position to establish your starting point, and monitor progress in achieving objectives to identify successes and shortfalls.

5 Review recruitment, selection, promotion and training procedures regularly to ensure that good intentions are being put into practice.

6 Draw up clear and justifiable job criteria and ensure these are objective and job-related.

7 Offer pre-employment training, where appropriate, to prepare potential job applicants for selection tests and interviews and positive action training to help under-represented groups.

8 Consider your organisation's image; do you encourage applications from under-represented groups and feature women, ethnic minority staff and people with disabilities in recruitment literature, or could you be seen as an employer who marginalises these groups?

9 Consider flexible working, career breaks, provision of childcare facilities etc., to help women in particular meet domestic responsibilities and pursue their occupations; and the provision of practical help and advice for people with disabilities.

10 Develop links with local community groups, organisations and schools, and so reach out to a wider pool of potential recruits.

The *Equal Opportunities ToolKit* is available free from DfEE publications in Sudbury, Suffolk.

Professional associations and trade unions also offer advice on good employment practice. The Royal College of Nursing (RCN), for example, has launched a campaign for 'employee-friendly policies' to promote a balance between work and life for all nurses regardless of sex and whether or not they are carers. The extract illustrates the coverage. You can find out more by contacting the Royal College of Nursing or visiting their web site (*http://www.rcn.org.uk*).

Having a life: the Royal College of Nursing campaign for employee-friendly policies

Flexible working – employment practices initially instigated by employers to meet changes in demand for services – such as: • flexi-time • part-time working • job-share • self-rostering • special shifts • voluntary reduced working time • annual hours contracts • term-time or school holiday contracts • non-standard full-time working week (which can coincidentally be employee-friendly practices as well).

Employee-friendly policies help employees achieve a balance between the responsibilities of work and life outside work. Research suggests that the most successful employee-friendly workplaces are those that take a strategic rather than ad hoc approach offering a number of examples of initiatives to support: • child care • carers of friends and relatives • a healthy work/life balance and the development of wider interests.

Changes in attitudes towards work and family life and demographic shifts in the general population and the workforce mean that employment practices must change. Employment practices must enable organisations to secure the workforce they need and allow people with increasingly complex lives to participate in paid work.

There is also a shortage of nurses – estimated at around 15,000 in England alone – the worst for 25 years, while demand for health care increases. Employee-friendly working arrangements can help to recruit and retain skilled and experienced staff, ensuring the delivery of high-quality nursing services.

Professional bodies, such as the British Medical Association and British Association of Social Workers, and trade unions offer advice to their members. They also provide information, support and legal advice if individuals making a complaint need help to present their case to their employer, and to attend hearings and meetings as a witness. Employees who have experienced discrimination in the workplace and are following internal complaints or grievance procedures can enlist the help of their trade union representative.

Supporting employee good practice

Equal opportunities legislation and policies are integral to good day-to-day practice in health and social care. However, discrimination, especially indirect discrimination, can be subtle, deep-seated and insidious. Much discrimination occurs as a result of a lack of awareness but there does not have to be an 'intention' for acts to be discriminatory.

Because of its possible impact on clients, managers should always take appropriate action where any member of staff is suspected of discrimination. All employers are held initially responsible for any discriminatory acts of their employees except where they have taken clear steps to ensure that discrimination does not take place. Managers can be answerable personally to an employment tribunal for complaints of discrimination by their staff. Under the Sex Discrimination and Race Relations Acts individuals are also held responsible. If an unlawful discriminatory act took place, the employee may also be held personally responsible.

Methods of developing good practice include training programmes, awareness-raising and setting goals and targets for good practice, thereby demonstrating not just the penalties of poor practice but also the benefits to be gained from good practice.

Remember to distinguish between:

- practice – what is done/day-to-day working methods; models of appropriate attitudes and behaviour for health and social care workers are often referred to as 'models of good practice' and may be published in codes of practice
- procedures – how things should be done; procedures may be identified in organisational procedural statements or handbooks
- legislation – the law e.g. Acts of Parliament, regulations and statutory instruments.

Training

Confidence in handling the issues arising from the need for equality of opportunity usually comes through experience. However, professional, vocational and skills training can help practitioners to:

- learn new skills in analysing and handling equal opportunities issues
- reinforce their knowledge and understanding
- gain a wider perspective
- find out about professional codes of practice.

Induction training and professional and vocational qualifications give new health and social care practitioners an opportunity to explore equal opportunities issues and learn the ground rules of handling dilemmas. Continuing professional training should then support the practitioners' development of skills and understanding as they handle equal opportunities ethical issues in practice. Training may also be needed to explain and share equal opportunities policies and procedures within an organisation.

Promoting equality for clients

Many health and social care organisations, from hospitals and doctors' surgeries to health authorities and social services departments, have their own policies and practices for handling ethical and equal opportunities issues. These may include:

- charters which establish guidelines for acting in the best interests of clients, assessing risks, giving information, maintaining confidentiality, respecting personal values and beliefs
- training programmes for staff, to help them handle ethical issues
- guidelines on how to allocate resources between different areas.

Section 1.2 explores charters and codes of practice more fully.

NHS organisations were guided by the original Patient's Charter and its successor the new NHS Charter, which aims to improve the quality of health

---

ACTIVITY

Talk to a health or social care practitioner to find out whether they have received any professional training on equal opportunities. If they have, what did it cover? How useful was it in practice? If they haven't, what training would be useful?

ACTIVITY

Over a two-week period, collect as many reports as you can on health and social care cases involving equal opportunities dilemmas. Look in newspapers, magazines and specialist journals, and listen for news items on television and radio. Compile a scrapbook on the different cases you have found, and choose one to focus on in more detail.

Write a short report on the case you have chosen, analysing the way the dilemma was handled.

and social care services offered to the general public. The Charter sets out patients' rights and the standards of service they can expect to receive, including equality of care and individual choice:

66 *You can expect the NHS to respect your privacy, dignity and religious and cultural beliefs at all times and in all places. For example, meals should suit your dietary and religious needs.* 99

Many health and social care services are developing their own equal opportunity policies based on the standards laid down in the Patient's Charter. As an important part of this, they usually include guidelines on how people using health and social services can complain when they feel they have been discriminated against.

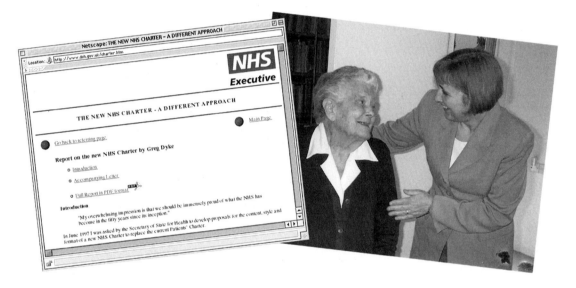

Health authorities and the Community Health Council deal with complaints about the National Health Service.

1.3.2 **Values in care practice**

When National Vocational Qualifications (NVQs) were established, the then Care Sector Consortium established a Value Base of Care Practice, which laid down a set of values and principles to follow, and gave health and social care practitioners clear guidelines on ethical issues for the first time. These principles are still valid quality indicators.

The Value Base has five elements:

The elements	Practitioners should
1 Promotion of anti-discriminatory practice	■ identify and fight their own prejudices ■ never stereotype individuals ■ use language that clients can understand.
2 Maintaining confidentiality of information	■ respect clients' requests for confidentiality as far as possible ■ explain who will have access to information.
3 Promoting and supporting individual rights to dignity, independence, choice and health and safety	■ encourage clients to be independent ■ recognise clients' rights and choice ■ encourage individuals to express their needs and wishes.
4 Acknowledging individuals' personal beliefs and identity	■ recognise and support clients' rights to beliefs ■ encourage individuals to express personal beliefs and preferences, as long as they do not affect the rights of others.
5 Supporting individuals through effective communication	■ communicate in a way which is appropriate for individual clients (level of understanding, language and so on) ■ check that people using healthcare/social services understand information ■ develop their listening skills ■ recognise the importance of non-verbal communication.

ACTIVITY

Investigate the Value Base of Care Practice. Produce your own summary of the Value Base in the form of a simple leaflet for care practitioners, summarising the main equal opportunities issues and how they should be handled.

Applying the care value base

❝ *We always called our doctor 'Sir' and wouldn't have dreamt of questioning anything he said. He was much cleverer than the rest of us, and we trusted him completely.* ❞

89-year-old man

Although the general public's respect for the medical profession may not be as heartfelt as in the past, people still place enormous trust in health and social care workers. People usually need health or social care support when they are vulnerable in some way – perhaps as a result of illness, frailty, financial problems or homelessness. They may be worried about the future, not understand what is happening to them and feel powerless to solve their problems.

In contrast, health and social care practitioners are in a powerful position. They have specialist knowledge, understand how the care system works, and often know personal details about the client's health and lifestyle. The decisions practitioners make can transform – sometimes even save or destroy – people's lives.

Because of this, people need to know that they can trust health and social care practitioners to:

- act in their best interests
- make decisions only after assessing risks to individuals and groups
- give them all the information they need
- respect the confidentiality of information they provide
- empower them – give them the freedom and knowledge they need to make decisions and maintain their independence.

These are health and social care practitioners' basic professional responsibilities to act 'ethically' – to behave in a morally correct way in their dealings with people using healthcare/social services.

DISCUSSION POINT

What health or social care services have you used during your life (for example, doctors, dentists or social workers)? Who do you feel has had the power in these relationships? What responsibilities do you feel health and social care workers have as a result of the trust you place in them?

Key questions

1 What is the difference between practice and procedures?

2 What is the Value Base of Care Practice? What are the five main areas it covers?

3 What should health and social care organisations have in place to ensure the clients' equality is promoted?

4 What does training do to support clients' equality?

5 Which organisations support employees when they believe that their employer has discriminated against them?

6 List four different actions an employer can take in order to become 'employee-friendly'.

SECTION **1.4**

The effects of discriminatory practices on individuals

People working in health and social care must treat all clients equally and must not discriminate unfairly. It is important that you know what the effect will be for a client if a practitioner discriminates against them. You should be able to identify non-oppressive practice and how it can add to a client's self-esteem and self-worth.

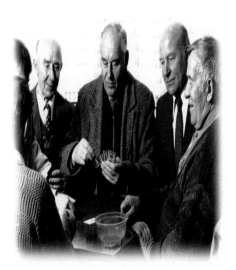

> **❝** *I was forced to retire from my job at 65, when I was perfectly healthy and happy. Since then, my life has gone downhill. I've got less money, and find it hard to fill my days. I don't like having to draw a pension – I see people looking at me when I go to collect my money, and am sure they feel I'm a drain on society. Even my family seem to think I've had a personality transplant since I hit 70 – they're always telling me to slow down and to 'grow old gracefully'! My daughter actually told me off for standing on a chair to change a light bulb the other day. I just wish they could see that I'm exactly the same person as I was 20 years ago, not some stereotype of a frail, semi-senile old man.* **❞**

75-year-old man

> **❝** *When my boss first ridiculed me for being an 'incompetent girl' I knew he was wrong and was angry. But as time went on, and he carried on putting me down, I began to lose confidence in myself. A nagging voice at the back of my mind started saying that perhaps he was right. Because I was nervous, I made more mistakes. Over the course of a couple of months I went from being a self-confident person to feeling helpless and worthless.* **❞**

woman who suffered sex discrimination in the workplace

1.4.1 Discriminatory practice and its effect

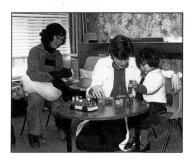

Section 1.1 describes how we make judgements about people. Often this does not matter until our attitudes are shown in our behaviour and we begin to act on our stereotyping and prejudices. The behaviour may be overt or directly discriminating, when we show our prejudices against an individual by ignoring, bullying or restricting choices. At least as potent but much less easy to spot is indirect discrimination, where we show prejudice by avoidance, exclusion or body language:

❝*It's not what you say, but the way you say it – or whether you even talk at all.*❞

Practitioners must be aware of how this translation of their attitudes into behaviour takes place.

As individuals, health and social care practitioners must take steps to avoid both direct and indirect discrimination, by:
- thinking about the language they use
- making an effort to understand clients' religious practices, customs, diet and language needs
- not showing anger, frustration or dislike through their body language or tone of voice
- treating all clients equally, regardless of age, sex or specific health problems.

Health and social care practitioners are not clones, and all have their own opinions and feelings. However, they have a responsibility not to allow their personal prejudices to affect the quality of care they provide.

Who is discriminated against?

Most discrimination is against groups who have low status in society, or who are in a minority. As well as sex, race and disability, discrimination can also be based on:
- age
- the nature of the disability
- family status
- health status
- religion
- sexuality
- educational disadvantage
- people whose first language is not English.

Other individuals are also vulnerable to discrimination because of their personal attitudes and circumstances. By heightening awareness of the risks of discrimination and understanding the effects it is likely to have on individuals, health and social care practitioners can consciously counter the negative affects of the prejudices and judgements humans cannot help making. Heightened sensitivity forms a foundation for developing the practical skills in communicating with patients and clients. This is covered in unit 2.

Social values

Often the individuals and groups affected reflect the social values at the time. For example, 100 years ago women could not vote, many white people had never seen a black person and people with disabilities were considered freaks. At the beginning of the Twenty-first Century, women play a fuller part in decision-making, black people are visible in most communities and many children with disabilities are educated in the same schools as their able-bodied peers. Equal opportunity legislation has been put in place and behaving in a discriminatory way is no longer socially acceptable.

Age

Discrimination based on age is widespread. This usually affects the two ends of the age range – children and older people.

The traditional view of children is that they should be seen and not heard. This means that their views are not sought and their choices, worries and complaints unheard – they are not told or consulted about decisions being made on their behalf. More seriously, their neglect, abuse and harm by adults goes unchallenged. The Children Act 1989 addresses this issue and, together with other developments in child protection, sets the framework for health and social care practitioners (see page 298).

Older people are often pigeonholed as being frail, silly or dependent on their children. Alternatively they are seen as grumpy and ill-mannered, like Victor Meldrew in *One Foot in the Grave*.

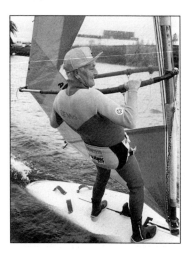

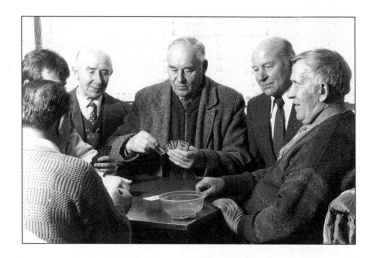

The nature of the disability

Although attitudes have changed towards disabled people, some disabilities are still seen as socially unacceptable. For example, people with learning difficulties are still not accepted in some public places. There is growing evidence that they can be abused and harmed by others who take advantage of their vulnerability.

Family status

The government and employers like to see themselves as family-friendly. Some families are less acceptable than others. Single parents, especially younger single mothers, can be stigmatised as being feckless and living off the state.

Health status

Certain illnesses are not always acceptable. People with mental ill-health are particularly affected by prejudice and discrimination. Despite one person in four experiencing some kind of mental health problem during the course of a year, attitudes are such that many people hide this problem.

Sexuality

In the UK, many people are prejudiced against sexual relationships that don't conform to the conventional heterosexual pattern. Until the 1960s, gay men and lesbians were treated as mentally ill, and homosexuality was illegal. People today are more tolerant, but discrimination still exists:

- the age of consent is higher for homosexuals than for heterosexuals
- gay men and lesbians miss out on job opportunities – for example, they were barred from military careers
- they may face verbal or physical abuse in everyday life.

The spread of HIV and AIDS – originally seen by many as a 'gay disease' – increased the suspicion and prejudice encountered by gay men. Heterosexuals can also face discrimination if their sexual behaviour is seen as promiscuous or outside the 'norm'. But who decides what the 'norm' is?

Some cases of discrimination on the grounds of sexual orientation have been successfully brought before the European Court of Human Rights. In 1999 the Court issued a clarification on the law on gay men and lesbians in the armed forces, recognising the value of every citizen – regardless of their sex or sexual orientation – and the contribution they can make to the armed services. This spurred calls for the government to legislate against discrimination on the grounds of sexual orientation and challenged homophobia.

Multiple disadvantage and discrimination

Although the law focuses on specific groups who are most in need of equal opportunities legislation, and this book similarly catalogues groups who are most vulnerable, the situation is worse for people who fall into several categories. An example might be a woman from a minority ethnic group, with a low level of education, who lacks literacy skills and who is becoming older. Patients, clients and staff are not one-dimensional individuals and may therefore be vulnerable to more than one kind of discrimination and harassment. Health and social care practitioners should aim to reflect this in their equal opportunities policies and ensure that their monitoring categories, publicity and resources reflect the complexity and diversity of individuals who make up the local community.

ACTIVITY

Other groups which can be discriminated against are:

- people who need help with literacy and numeracy
- people whose language is not English
- people who are homeless.

Choose one of these groups and find out:

- the number of people in this group
- what type of discrimination they may face
- what measures health and social care organisations take to meliorate this discrimination.

1.4.2 **The effects of discrimination**

Being discriminated against can create a range of reactions:

❝*I feel furious at the injustice of being ignored because I'm a woman.*❞

❝*I feel frustrated that people don't see I'm just the same inside as I was when I was 30.*❞

❝*It really gets me down, being constantly told I'm not as good as my white colleagues. After a while it makes me start to wonder whether it's true.*❞

❝*At first I was angry at being passed over for promotion because of my disability. Now I'm just bored with my job, and can't be bothered to fight any more.*❞

All of these emotional responses are a natural reaction to prejudice and discrimination.

In practical terms, individual and societal discrimination can also:
■ affect individuals' rights
■ restrict individuals' opportunities.

Discrimination affects individuals' wellbeing in terms of:
■ social and economic status
■ health
■ self-esteem and sense of empowerment
■ personal development and relationships
■ employability.

Social and economic status

People who are discriminated against usually have a low status in society. This affects their social and economic status, as follows:
■ they may not be able to find a job, get promotion and follow their career path
■ they may live in poor housing
■ they may have restricted educational opportunities and access to recreation and leisure activities.

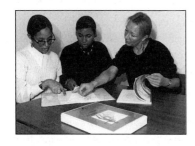

Almost half the ethnic minority population of the UK were born in Britain, and nearly three-quarters are British citizens. Yet many are still treated as outsiders, facing discrimination in employment, housing and education, as well as day-to-day verbal and physical abuse.

Meena, a young Asian woman with eight GCSEs and three A levels, went for an interview at an insurance firm where her friend, Sally, worked:

❝*I didn't get the job. But Sally told me they said that when firms are downsizing, it was important to give jobs to your own. Now, tell me, what does that mean? I was born here, I speak with a Brummie accent. My grandfather, like so many others, died fighting for this country – he was in Italy – we even have a letter from his commander about how brave he was. My mother works in the health service, my father in insurance. They've never collected a penny in benefits, and have paid taxes for 25 years. Dad won't even let me go on the dole. So what does 'your own' mean?"*

(from *Race Through the 90s*, published by the Commission for Racial Equality and BBC Radio 1)

Health

People with illness and disability may be discriminated against just because of their condition but there may be additional discrimination because they receive worse standards of health care than the general population. This can be because:

- there are other priorities for resources and staff
- practitioners feel that they have brought about their own illness, by smoking or drinking or drug misuse
- the individual does not know any difference.

People who are discriminated against can find their health affected. Bullying at work is a major contributor to the level of absence from work because of stress. This very clearly links with self-esteem.

Self-esteem and empowerment

If people are constantly told they're not capable of doing something, they can start to believe it. They lose their sense of control over a situation, feel powerless and eventually give up trying.

A care assistant explains how she tries to sustain people's motivation to live an independent life:

" Quite often I visit elderly people who are letting their independence slip away from them. Once they're forced to give up work, they slowly fall into the stereotype of an 'old person'. Their family and friends start seeing them as frail and feeble, advise them to slow down, and tell them what they should and shouldn't be doing. The problem is often compounded by physical problems, which make them lose confidence in their abilities. They are treated like an old person, and they start believing that is what they are. They feel helpless and weak, and lose their motivation to fight for their independence – in some cases, even their will to live. Part of my job is to help them rediscover their motivation by giving them small tasks to achieve from day to day – perhaps visiting a friend, or playing a game of cards. With achievable goals to strive towards, they regain some confidence and enthusiasm."

Self-esteem is a person's good opinion of themselves – their sense of self-worth. Loss of self-esteem is a common reaction to repeated discrimination.

People who have lost self-esteem as a result of discrimination are less likely to claim their rights in society. Those who have a low sense of self-worth as a result of discrimination tend to believe that they get what they deserve.

In March 2000, the Audit Commission published a report on provision of prosthesis, aids and adaptation by the NHS and Social Services Department. They found that the service was inadequate because there were delays in delivery, insensitivity in meeting the needs of patients and a failure to understand the importance of their service for promoting a quality of life.

ACTIVITY

Talk to someone you know who has been discriminated against, for example because they are black, gay, disabled or female. Ask them what emotional effect the discrimination had on them. Did it influence their motivation? Did they lose self-esteem?

With the permission of your interviewee, write a short case report focusing on the emotional effects of discrimination.

A consequence of this lack of self-worth is that people now lack confidence in their ability to make choices and take control over their own lives. The term for this is 'disempowerment' and is the opposite to what practitioners should be promoting with their clients.

Personal development and relationships

Everyone needs opportunities to develop their identity, beliefs and values, their understanding of the world and their talents. They need to acquire life skills and the ability to make relationships with others. If you are discriminated against, you will be:

- unrecognised as an individual
- have your beliefs and values belittled, ignored or denied
- restricted in your access to education, employment and recreation
- limited in your opportunities to develop and improve your skills so that you can have as independent a life as possible.

> It is estimated that 2% of the UK population have a learning disability. Some jobs and training programmes have traditionally been considered 'suitable' for people with learning difficulties. This can result in people's skills and capabilities being underestimated, or their aspirations being ignored. Staff responsible for finding someone with a learning difficulty a work placement may be tempted to opt for less challenging opportunities in order to 'protect' those with learning difficulties. But evidence suggests that many people with mild or moderate learning difficulties do better in open employment than in a sheltered environment. They are more likely to realise their potential, even though some will require additional support, particularly at the start of the job. They may also take longer to achieve certain outcomes.

Being able to begin and keep friendships and to get on with others around us is essential for our wellbeing. If you lack self-confidence and feel you are worthless, you will find making relationships difficult.

Attitudes towards older people or people with disabilities have often restricted their opportunities for relationships, particularly sexual ones. Until recently, residential homes made few arrangements for married couples. Practitioners working with people with learning difficulties discouraged young people to become couples – often with the support of the parents.

ACTIVITY

Think about your hopes for the future. How do you think other people's attitudes could affect whether you achieve your hopes?

Employability

This is very closely related to social and economic status and to personal development.

1.4.3 How non-oppressive practice can encourage self-esteem and self-worth

66 *Illness and disease are great levellers and no particular respecters of background or race. As the NHS treats the illness or disease, the personal circumstances of the patient comes second.* 99

Felim, a ward nurse

Most health and social care practitioners come into contact with a wide range of people in the course of their work. All of these people have a right to receive care and treatment of an equal quality. Health and social care practitioners can then put equality of care into practice by:

- encouraging everybody – regardless of sex, race, religion, age, disability or sexual orientation – to make the most of the services on offer
- responding to every individual as a human being of equal value
- not discriminating against an individual on any grounds.

Empowering people using health or social services

It is easy for practitioners to assume a position of power in their relationships with people using health or social services, especially where an individual is particularly vulnerable or ill. Even where they may be dependent on the practitioner, it is important that clients are empowered to make decisions about their care and take control of their lives. This is called 'empowerment'. Simple decisions, such as what to wear, who to sit next to at dinner and what to watch on TV, help a person to maintain independence and dignity.

> **DISCUSSION POINT**
>
> If you were a GP, what practical steps could you take to ensure equality of care for the following people?
>
> - an 85-year-old man with Alzheimer's disease
> - a child with Down's syndrome
> - a young woman with HIV
> - a man who does not speak English.

> **DISCUSSION POINT**
>
> Read the following conversation between Joanna (a care assistant), and Mrs Clark (an older woman living in sheltered accommodation).
>
> Joanna: Now come on, Mrs C. You know you like a nice cup of tea at 5 o'clock. Drink it up.
>
> Mrs Clark: Do you think I could have another spoon of sugar? I like two sugars in my tea.
>
> Joanna: (Sighs) We're getting confused again. Your son told me you had one sugar.
>
> Mrs Clark: Oh. (Takes a mouthful of tea and screws her face up.)
>
> Joanna: Then when you've finished that, we'll get you into your nightie in time for *Neighbours*.
>
> Mrs Clark: But it's only 5! I wanted to pop next door to see how Jenny's feeling today. And I don't like that silly *Neighbours* anyway.
>
> Joanna: Look, the council's not made of money you know. I'm only here until 6, so we've got to get you ready for bed before I go. And I thought it would be nice for us to sit down cosily and watch telly together for half an hour.
>
> Mrs Clark: Oh well, if you say so.
>
> Talk about the conversation. How many different ways does Joanna deny Mrs Clark her individual rights and choices? Could the organisation she works for do anything to help empower Mrs Clark?

ADVOCACY

Advocacy schemes protect the interests of disabled or disadvantaged people by making their views known. It may be suitable for people with learning difficulties, those with language disabilities or mental health problems, or those from minority groups who may lack the opportunity to participate in the management and delivery of services on which they may be dependent.

Effective advocacy:

- allows the voice of clients to be heard
- helps clients obtain the support they are entitled to and understand their rights
- gives clients the information they need to make informed choices
- helps eradicate conflict of interest within a service
- enables feedback from clients to policy-planners, commissioners and others involved in service development.

A number of different, often complementary, modes of advocacy exist: formal, professional, voluntary and self-advocacy. An advocate is usually a volunteer who becomes involved with a person with a disadvantage, becomes their friend, speaks up on their behalf and represents their interests. Advocacy projects may receive some funding from health or social services to enable them to identify those in need of support, recruit and train advocates, and match them to partners. However, as advocacy schemes need to operate independently from service-providing agencies, conflict of interest should be kept to a minimum.

ACTIVITY

Investigate modern codes of practice, such as those issued to nurses, social workers and residential homes. Choose one, and compare it to the Declaration of Geneva for doctors, shown on the next page. Summarise the ethical issues covered by each code, and decide which you think would be more useful to health and social care practitioners.

To promote empowerment, practitioners should:

- identify the personal beliefs and values of their clients
- respect the individual needs and choices of each client
- treat each client as an individual and avoid stereotyping
- take into account the individual's feelings, opinions and beliefs.

Information and knowledge are the keys to empowerment. Without understanding their situation and different options open to them, people cannot make choices. People's rights to be given information in order to play an active role in their own health and social care are laid down in professional codes of practice.

The following version of the Hippocratic Oath, the traditional ethical code for doctors – known as the Declaration of Geneva – was drawn up by the World Medical Association in 1948, and updated in 1968.

PLEDGE

At the time of being admitted a member of the medical profession:

- I solemnly pledge myself to consecrate my life to the service of humanity;

- I will give my teachers the respect and gratitude which is their due;

- I will practise my profession with conscience and dignity;

- The health of my patient will be my first consideration;

- I will respect the secrets which are confided in me, even after the patient has died;

- I will maintain by all the means in my power, the honour and the noble traditions of the medical profession;

- My colleagues will be my brothers;

- I will not permit considerations of religion, nationality, race, party politics or social standing to intervene between my duty and my patient;

- I will maintain the utmost respect for human life from the time of conception; even under threat I will not use my medical knowledge contrary to the laws of humanity.

People can only make sensible decisions and choices if they have full, accurate information on their situation. For example, a parent asked to give permission for their child to have an operation needs to know the exact risks and benefits of surgery in order to make the right decision. This aspect of health and social care is taken up in unit 2.

Key questions

1 What part does language play in discrimination?

2 Give four steps which practitioners can take to avoid discrimination.

3 Name four bases for discrimination, other than gender, race and disability.

4 What effect can discrimination have on someone's health?

5 How can people with learning difficulties be affected by discrimination?

6 What is empowerment?

7 List the areas of a person's wellbeing that can be affected by discrimination.

SECTION **1.5**

Sources of support and guidance

You need to know about the role and key functions of organisations that challenge discrimination and act on the behalf of, and support, individuals. In this section you will find out about the various commissions, agencies, councils and other organisations involved in challenging discrimination.

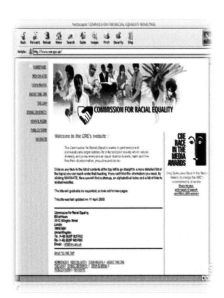

Many employers won't touch people with a barge pole if there is any mention of mental health problems. Sometimes that's fair enough, where people are still ill, but the essential thing is that people have to be treated on their merits and not on the basis of stereotypical views.

solicitor in a case of unlawful recruitment discrimination against a senior executive with controlled schizophrenia, The Guardian, December 1999

As family structures change dramatically, women and men now expect to be in paid work and manage their caring responsibilities. British dads work the longest hours in Europe, which is a serious issue for parents who are struggling to maintain a healthy balance between work and family life.

Julie Mellor, Chair of the Equal Opportunities Commission, December 1999, launching Women and Men at the Millennium

When dispensing prescriptions it doesn't matter who is seen – we would not divulge any detail of their prescription outside the company.

pharmacist

Staff and patients do not always understand that counselling is about a free exploration of the issues rather than directive advice giving; so it is possible to be asked to persuade people to behave in a particular kind of way. Ethically, that is not my role – my role is to enable my patients to make their own choices.

head of medical counselling and family support

One of the organisation's stated aims is that everyone should be accorded equal respect, regardless of race, colour, creed or sex. By the same token, we don't believe in positive discrimination. Everyone is judged on his or her own merits. We maintain the Declaration of Human Rights.

community coordinator for homeless people

1.5.1 **Regulatory and other bodies**

A wide range of organisations is available to give detailed advice and up-to-date information, nationally and locally. Libraries and librarians are an invaluable help, but this is an area where the Internet comes into its own. In this section web site addresses are provided where possible. However, while every effort has been made to ensure these are accurate, numbers and addresses do change and you may have to do some research to get the required details.

The main regulatory bodies associated with equal opportunities legislation are an important source of information and support. These are independent 'watchdogs'. They can offer an objective opinion on cases where grievances can't be settled through complaints procedures within an organisation or through professional bodies such as trade unions.

Regulatory body	How can it help?
Equal Opportunities Commission (EOC)	Ensures effective enforcement of the Sex Discrimination Act and the Equal Pay Act, and promotes equal opportunities between the sexes. It carries out formal investigations into complaints of sex discrimination, and in some cases helps individuals to prepare and conduct complaints in tribunals and courts.
Commission for Racial Equality (CRE)	Ensures effective enforcement of the Race Relations Act, and promotes equal opportunities for all, regardless of colour, race and ethnic or national origin. It has the power to advise and assist individuals taking cases to court.
Ombudsmen and women	Consider complaints from individuals who feel they have been treated unfairly in receiving a service. There is a Health Service Ombudsman who deals specifically with complaints about the NHS. The Ombudsman investigates complaints and seeks redress in cases of discrimination and wrongful treatment.
Citizens Advice Bureaux (CAB) and law centres	Provide information and advice for individuals on ways to seek redress for discrimination.
Advertising Standards Authority	Deals with complaints about discrimination in advertising on radio or television and in printed material.
Broadcasting Complaints Commission	Deals with complaints about discrimination in television and radio programmes.
Press Complaints Commission	Handles complaints about material printed in newspapers and magazines.
Police Complaints Commission	If individuals have complaints about discriminatory treatment by the police, they can contact the Police Complaints Commission who will investigate the case and seek redress.

Equal Opportunities Commission (EOC)

The EOC was set up under the Sex Discrimination Act 1975 to:

- work towards the elimination of discrimination
- promote equality of opportunity between men and women
- keep the Sex Discrimination Act under review.

61

The commission may conduct formal investigations of organisations or individuals where there is evidence that discrimination may have taken place – for example where a discriminatory advertisement has been published. It may provide assistance to individuals who are making a complaint under the Act where:

- the case raises a question of principle
- it is unreasonable for the individual to act unaided (if the case is complex)
- some other special consideration applies.

In these circumstances the commission may:

- give advice
- seek a settlement
- arrange for legal advice, assistance or representation.

The commission publishes a code of practice that offers guidance on the elimination of discrimination in employment and the promotion of equality of opportunity between men and women. Note: At the time of publication the EOC's document *Equality in the Twenty-first Century* was under consultation and was due to be published in 2000.

Contact details

The Equal Opportunities Commission (EOC), Overseas House, Quay Street, Manchester M3 3HN, tel. (0161) 833 9244 e-mail *info@eoc.org.uk* web site *http://www.eoc.org.uk/*.

Commission for Racial Equality (CRE)

The Commission for Racial Equality (CRE) was set up under the Race Relations Act 1976. It has similar powers and functions to the Equal Opportunities Commission. It was set up to:

- work towards the elimination of discrimination
- promote equality of opportunity and good relations between persons of different racial groups
- review the Race Relations Act 1976.

The commission publishes a code of practice offering guidance on the responsibilities of:

- employers
- individual employees
- trade unions
- employment agencies.

Ethnic diversity

The CRE devotes part of its web site to:

- facts and figures showing how different ethnic groups are affected in employment and unemployment, housing and homelessness, education, criminal justice

Assignment

Investigate how clients' rights are promoted and how vulnerable clients are provided for in one health care, social care or early years setting. Your investigation should cover:

- at least one code of practice or charter of rights used in the chosen setting
- at least one piece of legislation or policy that affects clients' or workers' rights
- how an organisation supports clients and workers in promoting equal rights.

Key skills

You can use the work you are doing for this part of your GNVQ to collect and develop evidence for the following key skills at level 3.

when you	you can collect evidence for
	communication
examine your own attitudes and prejudices, engage in discussion on how care workers can implement best practice, and take part in simulations	key skill C3.1a contribute to a group discussion about a complex subject
research one code of practice or charter of rights and one piece of legislation which affects clients' rights or workers' rights; find out how an organisation supports clients and workers	key skill C3.2 read and synthesise information from two extended documents about a complex subject; one of these documents should include a least one image
describe one code of practice or charter of rights and one piece of legislation which affects clients' rights or workers' rights; describe the effects of discriminatory practices on individuals	key skill C3.3 write two different types of document about complex subjects; one piece of writing should be an extended document and include at least one image
	information technology
research into organisations that challenge discrimination and act on the behalf of, and support, individuals	key skill IT3.1 plan, and use different sources to search for, and select, information required for two different purposes

when you	you can collect evidence for
	improving own learning and performance
set targets for learning and revision when preparing for external assessment	key skill LP3.1 agree targets and plan how these will be met, using support from appropriate others
prepare and revise for external assessment	key skill LP3.2 use the plan, seeking and using feedback and support from relevant sources to help meet the targets, and use different ways of learning to meet new demands
review performance and agree methods for improvements	key skill LP3.3 review progress in meeting targets, establishing evidence of achievements, and agree action for improving performance
	working with others
plan an investigation of practice in a range of different types of care and early years setting	key skill WO3.1 plan the activity with others, agreeing objectives, responsibilities and working arrangements
investigate practice in a range of different types of care and early years setting	key skill WO3.2 work towards achieving the agreed objectives seeking to establish and maintain cooperative working relationships in meeting responsibilities
review the success of the investigation	key skill WO3.3 review the activity with others against the agreed objective and agree ways of enhancing collaborative work

UNIT 2

Communicating in health and social care

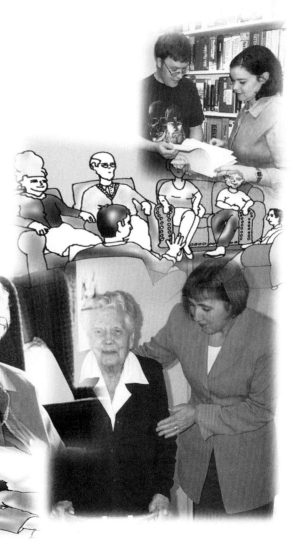

About this unit

Good communication is central to the helping relationship, in which an imbalance of power is inherent. Through being aware of their role and of how communication skills can tackle this imbalance, practitioners seek to empower clients and produce a more equal relationship.

In this unit you are given the opportunity to learn and practise communication skills. Health and social care professionals need good communication skills to help them develop relationships with people and show individuals that they are valued. Effective communication also has implications for an individual's wellbeing.

You will learn about:
- the types of interaction used in health and social care settings
- the effective skills that improve communication
- how communication with individuals and with groups can help you to value people as individuals
- factors that enhance and inhibit interaction and their potential effects on an individual's health and wellbeing
- the methods used to evaluate interactions
- other information and communications issues – privacy, confidentiality and written communications
- the importance of maintaining client confidentiality.

This unit links with unit 1 Equal opportunities and clients' rights.

66 *No professional speciality can work in isolation if integrated holistic care is to be delivered.* 99

nurse manager

66 *I like to listen. I have learnt a great deal from listening carefully. Most people never listen.* 99

Ernest Hemingway

66 *You have to let patients know what is going to be happening to them and reassure them. We both have a role – the dentist and I both try to do our bit to put people at ease. The approach can be a bit different with children – you can often distract them and take their minds off it by talking to them about things they like. Today I had a child who was having his tooth out. I knew he liked football because I asked his Mum. So I asked him what team he supported and he was off. His mind switched away from his worry to his main passion and he kept calm. The treatment was a much better experience for him than it could have been. By the time it was done he was surprised it wasn't so bad.* 99

dental assistant

Types of interaction

Working in health and social care, you will need to communicate with managers, colleagues, other professionals and relatives as well as with clients. You will take part in one-to-one interactions with clients and other professionals, and group interactions such as case conferences, group work and staff meetings.

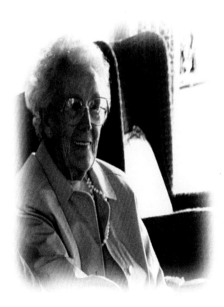

2.1.1 **Why is communication important?**

Interpersonal interaction – communication between at least two people – is crucial to effective health and social care. Without good communication, health and social care workers will not understand clients' beliefs and preferences and clients will not understand their rights and choices. Communication breakdowns can result in people not getting the support they need and being put at risk.

Communication is central to promoting equality and helping workers to learn about and understand other people. To communicate effectively you will need to:

■ recognise and overcome barriers to effective communication
■ adapt the way they communicate to meet the needs of individuals
■ develop good listening skills
■ recognise the importance of body language (non-verbal communication).

Every time a worker meets a client, they have an opportunity to:
■ establish mutual trust and respect
■ give and receive information
■ give advice
■ provide practical support.

Health and social care workers need to make the most of these opportunities.

A counsellor explains how he tries to optimise interaction with the people he meets:

66 *When people visit me, they are often nervous, embarrassed, angry or upset. I need to make sure I create a good atmosphere for them to talk in, putting them at ease and encouraging them to communicate. One of the first steps is to get the environment right – a warm room, comfy chairs, good lighting, no disruptive noise or disturbances, cups of coffee. I don't want to be seen as a figure of authority, so I try to sit alongside someone, rather than looking down on them from the other side of a desk. If I'm in my own office, I put the phone on divert. It's important to establish a good rapport with people. If it's the first time I've met someone, we have a general chat so I can get to know them and their interests. Then the next time I meet them, I pick up on some of these points to show that I'm interested in them as a person and put them at ease. It can be helpful if we share a common interest – I've got one client who loves opera, which I do too. During our conversation I listen carefully and try to increase their confidence in me as a listener, and in themselves as individuals with something valid to say. They will only speak openly if they feel I'm paying attention and not sitting in judgement.* 99

Sometimes a health or social care worker needs to take positive action with a client. One physiotherapist explains:

66 *I work in the community, visiting people to give physiotherapy in their own homes. I try to make every encounter as worthwhile as possible, and to maintain a good relationship with all my patients. Often I need to take positive steps to make the most of our interactions, such as suggesting we move to a quieter room if there's a TV on in the background, or moving some comfortable chairs in from another room. Sometimes I have to make a conscious effort to avoid stereotyping and imposing my set of values and beliefs on people. If I walk into a home which seems dirty and uncared for, I remind myself to approach the person as an individual whose choices and way of living are as valid as my own.* 99

ACTIVITY

List the different factors that the counsellor finds enhance interaction with clients. From your own experience as a speaker and listener, can you add to this list?

2.1.2 Where does communication take place?

Many interactions between health and social care workers and clients take place in a 'care setting' such as:

- the client's own home
- a day-care centre
- a clinic
- a residential home
- a hospital.

The atmosphere, facilities and practices in this environment can have a big impact on the client's reaction to the care given. The aim is for all interactions to be positive.

Care settings should:

- ensure the physical safety and security of clients
- provide emotional support, creating an environment which shows that clients are important and valued
- encourage social interaction
- give information about where to go and the roles of different members of staff
- include access, information and facilities for people with disabilities
- be functional, with appropriate toilet and washing facilities, catering provision, seating, lighting, heating.

Health and social care workers need to be aware of the impact of the care setting, and do all they can to make the environment friendly and comfortable. However, the steps they can take are obviously limited by the financial resources and time at their disposal.

The client's home

In many cases, the client's own home is an ideal setting – they are in control of their own environment, and can decide about the activities of daily living such as where to sit, the temperature of the room, what to watch on TV, when to eat, wash and sleep. The worker must fit in with this routine and environment, rather than impose their own schedule and values. This way they become aware of the client's needs and preferences as an individual, and are likely to respect their privacy.

However, some people feel that workers coming in and out of their home are an intrusion – an invasion of their personal space. People who are used to looking after themselves may find it difficult to accept the help offered by home carers, and resent their presence. As a result, relationships with carers can become strained and this will affect the quality of care given and accepted.

DISCUSSION POINT

❝**I feel ashamed of the way I live today. I'm so embarrassed when my home help arrives because the place is always topsy-turvy. I can't get around to keep it tidy, or bend over to clean the bathroom, or move the vacuum cleaner about. My furniture has become shabby and stained, but I can't afford to replace it. I feel like she's looking down on me because I can't look after myself any more. I sometimes think I'd be better off in a home.**❞

Miss Crownley, 75 years old

Why do you think Miss Crownley is finding it hard to accept home care? If you were her care assistant, how could you make her more at ease about the situation? Where would effective communication come into your approach?

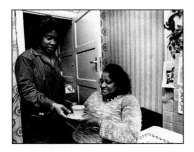

Day-care centres

For many clients, particularly older people, day centres offer a welcome opportunity to spend time away from home in the company of others. In most cases, transport is provided to and from the centre, and people are able to spend the day talking, taking part in activities, and sharing a meal. However, as with other care settings, day centres can have both positive and negative effects.

Clinics

Clinics, which provide medical services for the whole community, need to create an environment that is instantly friendly and welcoming.

People visiting a clinic often feel vulnerable or afraid because they are unwell. A comfortable waiting area can go a long way towards putting people at ease by providing:

- a bright, clean and welcoming environment
- comfortable, good-quality seating
- magazines for people to read (care should be taken to provide materials in appropriate languages)
- toys for children to play with
- leaflets and posters providing medical information
- clearly signposted toilet facilities, with disabled access.

Residential care and nursing homes

Moving into a residential home can mean a distressing loss of independence, privacy and hope. Older people may feel they are being sent to a residential home to die. As a result, they may become withdrawn, depressed and lose their self-esteem.

The routines and rules of life in some residential homes can be dehumanising and depressing. Turning a poor residential setting into a good one is often a question of respecting people as individuals. Providing a comfortable environment automatically enhances people's self-esteem and sense of self-worth. Allowing people to make choices, rather than forcing them into rigid routines, helps them to maintain their independence.

Workers in residential homes can show respect for individuals by:

- giving them a choice of having a room of their own (not making them share a room)
- respecting their privacy (staff should never enter someone's room without knocking first)
- letting them bring their own pictures, pieces of furniture, plants, crockery and so on

DISCUSSION POINT

Which aspects from this list include some form of communication? Explain how effective communication between residential care workers and clients can have a big impact on the residents' experience of wellbeing. Give specific examples of interactions that would benefit their wellbeing.

ACTIVITY

Visit a hospital in your area, and investigate the possible effects that the environment has on patients. Think about how it might influence different groups, such as children, older people and adolescents. Observe the interactions taking place between patients and staff. How well do you think the hospital staff help to overcome the negative effects of the hospital care setting?

- letting them eat, wash, get up and go to bed when they want
- letting them sit where they want, in the type of chair they like
- providing them with any equipment they need to help them perform tasks independently
- letting them choose what they wear, and what they watch on television
- giving them a choice of menu, with options to suit particular diets
- letting them have access to the whole building.

Hospitals

People find going into hospital frightening. Often they are admitted to hospital suddenly, as the result of an accident or emergency. As well as having to cope with the pain of injuries and illness, they have to deal with the shock of being in an unfamiliar, intimidating environment. Even if people know in advance that they are going into hospital, they have to cope with the fear of pain and sense of helplessness. They are separated from their family and friends, and have to form new relationships with other patients and staff. Hospitals have cultures and languages of their own. It is essential that people:

- know why they are in hospital
- know what is going to happen and when
- are given information in a language they can understand
- feel that they are involved in the process.

2.1.3 **The purposes of communication**

Interactions take place between health and social care workers and:

- clients
- carers, relatives and friends
- other workers, employees and professionals in health and social care
- professionals in associated external services
- providers of various services and aspects of care
- members of community and voluntary groups.

What information do they exchange?

Clients and carers may need information from workers about:

- the purpose of the service being provided
- the standard and nature of service they can expect
- their rights to a service and what they are expected to do when they receive the service

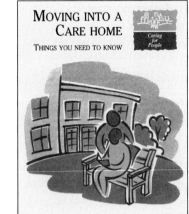

MOVING INTO A
CARE HOME

THINGS YOU NEED TO KNOW

Caring for People

- how decisions are reached and who takes the decisions
- how they can complain
- what is expected of them
- alternatives that may be available.

In the past, care settings did little to dispel the anxiety of people arriving for the first time. Today, workers try to counter clients' fear of the unknown by giving them information about the organisation. Many produce documents that include:

- maps or plans of the building and grounds
- organisational charts explaining the structures and roles of staff
- details of daily routines (mealtimes, menus, leisure facilities)
- information for visitors.

Workers need information from clients about:

- personal details (age, name, address, next of kin)
- history and current circumstances
- the service they are seeking
- relationships and support networks
- likes and dislikes.

Workers exchange information between each other such as:

- details of clients
- concerns about a client
- specialist knowledge from one professional to another
- changes in practice
- details of treatment or intervention.

To be useful, information should be:

- given at right time
- presented in simple language (and in other languages if appropriate)
- offered with help if people need clarification.

A starting point for exchange of information includes:

- which services and workers are already being provided
- whether there is a carer involved and the level of care they are providing
- what social or peer groups are supporting the client.

When is information exchanged?

Workers may need to provide or exchange informative advice and support:

- during needs assessment
- when discussing service options
- when they advise clients about decisions concerning their care
- when exchanging views on the services provided
- when care plans are evaluated and modified.

A relaxed atmosphere is necessary to allow the client or carer to express their views clearly.

Why communicate information?

Workers exchange information with clients, their carers or with each other so that they can:

- understand the client's needs
- relate the needs to the organisation's policies
- agree what can be done to help.

Communication of information during assessment should be simple, quick and informal if possible, and should focus on the client. The worker listens, observes and clarifies what they are being told or shown and then records any agreements made about the assessment of needs.

Communicating to explain procedures

Prospective clients and carers need information about the services available and whether they are eligible for them.

Healthcare organisations have procedures for responding to requests for advice, assistance and services. Not everyone asking for information will be eligible for a formal assessment. Questions at this stage are usually limited to what is thought essential:

- finding out what the enquirer wants to know
- the name, address and telephone number of the potential client
- whether there's been any previous contact with the organisation
- the urgency of the assistance being sought
- a convenient time for follow-up
- any other information which would help further contact, such as whether there are any language or other communication difficulties.

People may be distressed, hostile or anxious when asking for assistance. Reception staff and those answering the telephone can help by making allowances for this.

Communicating to promote relationships and offer support

People in need of health and social care may feel anxious, embarrassed, inadequate or depressed. On the surface, their needs may be for physical care, medical treatment or help with daily tasks. But all clients have emotional needs and these can only be met through professional yet warm, supportive, caring relationships. However effectively or efficiently a service is provided, if emotional needs are neglected, the services cannot be seen as of the highest standard of health or social care.

Matt, who receives physiotherapy at home twice a week, describes his experiences:

66 My physiotherapist comes to my house every Monday and Thursday to treat me, and he's very good. I'm slowly becoming more mobile, and the pain is less intense. I certainly can't complain about the service I'm getting. But he just doesn't seem interested in me, or want to offer anything apart from physical help. I'm stuck in the house all day and I often feel lonely and bored until my girlfriend gets home from work. It would be great if we could have a chat – I don't expect us to be best mates or anything, but it would be nice if I could look forward to him coming. Instead, I just feel like I'm a nuisance – he makes me feel useless. 99

People gain from professional caring relationships by increased health and social wellbeing. Since workers aim to act in the best interest of clients, this may mean simply making people's everyday lives as pleasant and comfortable as possible.

Even if the ultimate goal is to improve health and social wellbeing, caring relationships can be negative for clients. A common negative effect is the creation of dependence. Clients who feel forced to accept help – whether it's 'meals on wheels' or hospital care – do lose some control over their lives. Some clients find this difficult to accept, and become angry or lose self-confidence because of their loss of independence; others may slip into a pattern of dependence easily and start to become institutionalised or overreliant on their carers.

Workers can sometimes create anxiety in a client. Many workers are under stress and may not have the time or resources to give clients the individual attention they need. In extreme cases, clients may be neglected or even physically harmed (for example, by hitting or pushing). More often, harassed workers may lose their temper, show dislike or disapproval, or humiliate a client in front of others. All of these acts are abusive. They abuse the power that exists in the caring relationship. As a result, clients may become:

■ severely fearful
■ lacking in confidence
■ increasingly dependent
■ withdrawn and depressed.

Getting to know clients and assess their needs

Whatever the level of the work involved, a relationship of some kind needs to be established between the worker and client. If the worker is to assess the needs of their client, this will involve developing knowledge of the client not only as a case, but as a person. A relationship must also be based on trust and confidence that the information will not be misused. The role of assessment in the delivery of service is discussed in unit 5.

Communicating to negotiate and liaise

Liaison with clients

Within care planning, workers should encourage the client's participation by:

- providing information about the services available and offering choices and options
- giving an opportunity for clients to communicate their feelings, views and preferences
- encouraging them to comment on the services proposed
- enabling them to take an active part in their care
- asking them about the service provided and enabling them to take an active part in monitoring
- involving them in reviewing their care plan.

Liaison with carers

Carers (discussed fully in unit 5) now have a right to be assessed separately from clients. The communication listed above is relevant to carers as well. Workers must take consultations with carers seriously, check their understanding and keep their promises.

Liaison with colleagues and other professionals

Health and social care workers do not operate in isolation, but as members of teams and networks. The teams might be:

- the staff in a residential home
- field social work team
- members of a health practice
- the wards staff in a hospital
- a group of volunteers in a befriending scheme.

Networks will involve others, linked professionals and, while sharing some of the purposes of liaison with the team, will also involve:

- the sharing of information from different sources
- the bringing together of different services in a common plan
- negotiation to obtain resources
- joined training and learning.

This has become even more important with the emphasis now put on joint working between different practitioners in multidisciplinary teams and different agencies.

Promoting interaction between group members

Taking part in activities can be a good way of promoting interaction between people. Activities can be enjoyable and relaxing, providing a natural context for social interaction, whether:

- one-to-one
- with a small group of people
- with a larger group of people.

DISCUSSION POINT

Think of occasions when you have taken part in activities with other people, such as sport, drama or music. Did you find this a good way of forming relationships and communicating with people? Why?

For example, watching a TV programme and chatting about it can be a good way to get talking. Reading a story to a small group of children can encourage them to react and give their ideas. Taking part in group activity such as drama or sport can help a larger group of people get to know one another.

Client and carer networks and forums

Clients and carers can be helped to play a greater part in their care through client and carer networks. These are communication networks which:

- provide mutual support to members who share an illness, disability or situation
- provide information, advice and representation for individual members
- contribute to the planning and monitoring of services
- exchange views on the quality of services and campaign for better and different services.

ACTIVITY

Find out more about these communication networks for clients and carers. Make contact with the Carers' National Association and ask for details of a forum. Identify the purposes, types and methods of communication used by the participants. Write a brief report explaining the role of the forum and the importance of communication to the participants.

Key questions

1 How does interaction influence health and social wellbeing? Give an example of a positive and a negative interaction.

2 How can workers in residential homes communicate respect for their residents?

3 State five purposes of interactions in health and social care.

4 List five different groups of worker within or linked to health or social care you may need to exchange information with.

5 What communication needs do carers have? How can they be met?

6 What is the purpose of client and carer networks?

ACTIVITY

Choose a common social situation (a party, common room, café) and make notes on people's use of:

- language (words when speaking)
- tone, pitch, volume of speech
- listening skills
- touch
- physical closeness to one another
- eye contact
- posture
- mirroring.

What do these show you about the people involved, and their relationships with each other?

If people are comfortable with each other and communicating well, they often copy each other's body language. This is called mirroring, and helps to create rapport.

Health and social care workers also need to be aware of differences between cultures and age groups. A nod or shake of the head or a thumbs-up sign may mean different things to people from different cultures.

Body language is particularly important when interacting with young children, who can't rely on spoken language. Often children use gestures and facial expressions with less inhibition than adults, and are able to express their feelings more freely through body language. Health and social care workers need to be aware of this when watching a child's body language, and when using non-verbal communication themselves.

The way in which you dress can also impact on the way in which others perceive you. You would be unlikely, if you are male, to wear a suit and tie to work with young children. On the other hand a social worker who attended a Family Proceedings Court in jeans and T-shirt would probably be listened to less sympathetically than if he or she were dressed formally.

UNIT

2

SECTION **2.2**

Think about:

- what your face is showing

  Use your eyes, nose, mouth and brow to express emotion – smile if it's good news, look serious and sad if it's bad news, frown if it's unclear.

- your gestures

  Nodding, shaking the head and shrugging can be useful ways to reinforce what you're saying in language – but remember, gestures can mean different things in different cultures.

- your body position

  Try to look relaxed – if you look as if you're nervous, the patient definitely will be! Relax your muscles, sit with your hands loose in your lap, or stand with your arms by your sides; never clench your fists!

- your posture

  Maintaining an open posture, with arms and legs unfolded, leaning forward slightly, gives the impression that you're friendly and welcoming; a closed posture, with legs crossed and arms folded, gives the impression that you're unwelcoming and defensive.

- mirroring

  If people are communicating well, they mirror each other's body language, so try leaning the same way as the person you're talking to, moving your head the same way, copying their gestures – it can create instant rapport! But don't make it too obvious what you're doing – they may think you're mimicking them.

- your position in relation to others

  Don't intrude on their personal space – but remember, people from some cultures (Latin America, Africa, Arab countries) stand much closer than Westerners.

Emotional factors

66 *Listening is not merely not talking, though even that is beyond most of our powers; it means taking a vigorous human interest in what is being told us.* 99

Alice Duer Miller, poet and author

66 *You can't fake listening. It shows.* 99

Raquel Welch, actress

Workers need to be 'active listeners' to hear and understand what patients and colleagues are telling them. An active listener:

- gives full attention to the speaker
- makes appropriate eye contact with the speaker – not staring too hard, but with 'soft eyes'
- lets the other person speak without interrupting
- hears the words the speaker says
- responds to the non-verbal messages, the body language
- concentrates on understanding the messages
- responds in an appropriate way
- encourages the speaker to continue, by nodding and giving encouraging words and signs at appropriate places.

An active listener is interested in listening to what someone else is telling them and can interpret what they are hearing into something which will enable them to improve patient care. Workers need to have highly developed active listening skills. However well they can talk, if they can't listen actively and concentrate on understanding their clients' messages, they're unlikely to be effective communicators.

To summarise, a good listener is:

- relaxed
- understanding
- warm
- sincere
- respectful
- responsive.

A poor listener:

- imposes their own agenda
- does not see feeling as important
- interrupts or changes the subject
- gives inappropriate advice
- is patronising
- offloads their own experience.

Social factors

The very first meeting you have with someone will be an important one for both of you. If it gets off to a bad start, you will both carry the memory of that start and it will take a lot of undoing. On the other hand, get off to a good start and you may set the scene for a long and productive relationship. What will you do to get off to this good start?

- Give appropriate and welcoming body language.
- Show interest in the other person as an individual.

- Adjust your responses to fit with the other person (for example, you would use very different language with an elderly person from that you would use with a child).
- Ask the other person appropriate open-ended questions about themselves – recognising that, at a first meeting, it can be inappropriate or intrusive to be too probing or inquisitive.
- Make appropriate disclosures about yourself and your likes and dislikes designed to identify points of common interest or experience between yourselves.

This process of seeking points of common contact with someone is a basic skill used by people in the caring professions and is known as 'empathy'. Empathy doesn't mean that you have to agree with another person, but does mean that you're able to understand their point of view.

Of course, this process works well if you like the person. In this case there will be a basic sympathy between you. However, it's not unusual in care situations to find some clients who are less popular than others. Unpopular clients are often those who make the worker feel incompetent, unappreciated and uncomfortable because of their way of communicating. Workers may react by keeping contacts with these clients to a minimum – perhaps being distant, skimping on care or being actively unpleasant. This becomes a vicious cycle where relationships become worse and worse between the worker and the client. By being pleasant and supportive the worker can break this cycle. Often a manager or supervisor could help to suggest other strategies such as asking the client why they are unhappy with their care.

There are also considerable dangers where a client is treated unfairly by members of staff, or other clients, by being stereotyped or having a label put on them. There may be real (such as incontinence) or imaginary reasons (they may have had a dispute with someone which has caused others to take sides).

Almost everyone has positive points or a 'button' that can be 'pushed' to get them to talk in a positive and sympathetic way. Workers should try to seek these buttons and work on the positive. This does not mean that clients don't have negative aspects. Often, the need to change these factors may be a focus for work, but being able to challenge and change them will be more possible from the basis of a relationship.

It is also essential in one-to-one communication to be very carefully aware of the values of care and the need to apply equal opportunities approaches at all time. This means:

- showing respect for the client
- valuing the client as a person
- respecting the client's culture and not saying or doing anything that might undermine or insult that culture.

You can achieve this by, for example:

- asking them to teach you about their culture
- sharing with them aspects of yours.

In this way they can feel that a relationship is two-way and that they're contributing something to your knowledge and understanding.

Perhaps the most difficult situation can be when you have to deal with a prejudiced or bigoted client, particularly if the client's attitudes are disruptive to group living. Having the confidence to be able to challenge these activities can stem from having built a relationship. However, challenges of this kind will also require teamwork and team strategies. Workers should not be expected to undertake such challenges on their own, but with other workers as part of a plan worked out together.

It can also be important to be aware of one's own values and how they may impact on others. Asserting values which relate to the way in which people deal with others, when those values are held by the organisation providing care, is legitimate; simply seeking to impose our own views on others who may be vulnerable is not. This may sometimes present workers with real dilemmas when clients seek to do something that conflicts with their own values but not with the values of their organisation.

Skills

Health and social care workers need good language skills: both speech and comprehension. They need language and listening skills for communicating effectively when:

- talking one-to-one with a client, a colleague, or on the telephone
- talking to a group and perhaps giving a presentation to a group
- participating in group discussions.

Good communication demonstrates:

- clarity (are you being understood?)
- pace (are you talking too fast or slow, are new ideas being introduced too quickly?)
- tone of speech (a tone appropriate for a child will be patronising if used with an older person)
- appropriate prompts (to encourage the client)
- open questioning
- checking on understanding of content
- empathy
- respecting the client's silence
- responding firmly, authoritatively and assertively.

A poor communicator:

- uses inappropriate language (such as jargon, dialect or slang)
- asks closed questions (which limit the response)

- interrogates rather than questions
- parrots rather than reflects
- is aggressive or submissive.

In choosing the right word, it's not enough to be technically correct or to meet a precise dictionary definition; the important thing is to be unequivocally understood. In face-to-face interactions, one can check the other person's reactions as one indicator of this, and use demonstrations to explain more clearly and to help confirm that communications are understood.

As well as spoken language, the ability to use written language is a vital part of effective communication, to inform and to ensure that others can understand. Legible, comprehensive, easily understood written records require effective communication skills.

66 *The complainant said she was in pain and had told the nurse, but nothing was done. The nurse said this was not true; she had done a number of things to help relieve the pain. Unfortunately there was no evidence in the notes that the nurse had done anything.* 99

anonymous

ACTIVITY

Work in pairs or threes. Think how many meanings you can convey by placing different emphasis, pitch and volume on the single word 'really'. It can be a statement, an exclamation, a question, a confirmation, a prompt, an affirmation, an expression of doubt, disbelief, emphasis or cynicism. Now imagine how much more room there is for confusing messages when you add facial expression, body posture and gestures that might further confuse communication.

More than words

Sensitivity to language includes more than the words that we use; it's also the way that we say them. How something is said is often far more important than what is said. Consider the simple four words 'Do you like swimming?' Think about the different messages these four words can convey depending on where the emphasis is placed:

- '**Do** you like swimming?' (i.e. is it something you like doing?)
- 'Do **you** like swimming?' (i.e. you rather than someone else)
- 'Do you **like** swimming?' (i.e. do you actually enjoy it?)
- 'Do you like **swimming**?' (i.e. rather than some other activity).

Placing the emphasis on a particular word conveys different messages. Even more variations can be created by a tone – questioning neutrally or questioning in anticipation of a positive or negative answer by the intonation or by suggesting disbelief, encouraging support or sarcasm. You can even make the same four words into an exclamation! Try it using other examples.

Effective questioning

Interaction frequently involves workers gathering information. To do this, they need to develop skills in asking questions. There are five main types of question, all of which most people use automatically in the course of a conversation.

Type of question	What is it? When is it used?	Examples
Closed question	Can be answered in one or two words, often Yes or No. Useful for collecting factual information quickly.	■ Do you take sugar? ■ How old are you? ■ Can you make an appointment next Friday at 3?
Open question	Encourages a longer answer, giving an opportunity to explore detail. Useful for collecting information about feelings and emotions. Open questions usually begin with How . . . ?, What . . . ?, Why . . . ?, Where . . . ?, When . . . ?	■ How do you manage to make a cup of tea? ■ What are your views on that? ■ Why don't you want to move into sheltered accommodation?
Probe	Develops the response to another question. Useful for collecting more detail on a subject.	■ Open question: How are you feeling at the moment? ■ Response: I've got an awful headache, and I'm not coping too well with John. ■ Probe: How has John been the last week or so?
Prompt	Useful for collecting more information on a subject and keeping someone talking.	■ Open question: How are you feeling at the moment? ■ Response: I'm having a bad day today. Actually I'm feeling quite depressed. ■ Prompt: So you're feeling down at the moment?
Leading question	Gives help with the expected answer. Can be useful if a client is shy or lacks confidence.	■ You probably find it hard to get upstairs now, do you? ■ It's getting late – perhaps you'd like to stop now and come back next week?

At the start of a conversation and on first meeting a client, a worker may use closed questions to collect factual information quickly. As closed questions are usually easy to answer, they can help to put people at ease.

Once the interaction is under way, open questions, probes and prompts can be used to encourage someone to express their feelings and expand on particular subjects. Used sensitively, they show that the worker is listening to the client and interested in what they're saying. Leading questions can be particularly helpful if someone is distressed or lacks self-esteem.

Special needs

The worker must be aware that many clients have special needs such as:
- a different language from the worker's
- hearing disability
- visual disability which limits their ability to understand non-verbal signals
- a disability which may impair their ability to communicate clearly
- mental health difficulties which impair confidence
- anxiety or stress which might affect concentration and understanding
- poor literacy
- physical disabilities which might affect where the interaction can take place.

ACTIVITY

Languages and systems have been developed to communicate with people with special communication needs, including British Sign, Makaton and Braille. Find information about one of these and put together a report that explains:

■ who the language or system is for

■ how it works

■ how workers can learn to use the system.

Disability etiquette

- In conversation: When talking to a person with a disability, look at and speak directly to that person, rather than through a companion who may be present. Be prepared to offer a visual cue to a hearing-impaired person or an audible cue to a vision-impaired person, especially when more than one person is speaking.

- Relax. Don't be embarrassed if you happen to use accepted common expressions such as 'See you later' or 'Got to be running along' that seem to relate to the person's disability. When introduced to a person with a disability, it is appropriate to offer to shake hands. People with limited hand use or who wear an artificial limb can usually shake hands. Shaking hands with the left hand is acceptable. For those who can't shake hands, touch the person on the shoulder or arm to welcome and acknowledge their presence.

- When greeting a person with a severe loss of vision, always identify yourself and others who may be with you, e.g. 'On my right is Mary Smith.' If the person does not extend their hand to shake hands, verbally extend a welcome. When offering seating, place the person's hand on the back or arm of the seat. A verbal cue is helpful as well. Let the person know if you move or need to end the conversation. In a group, give a vocal cue by announcing the name of the person you're speaking to. Speak in a normal tone of voice.

- To get the attention of a person with a hearing impairment, tap the person on the shoulder or wave your hand. Look directly at the person and speak clearly, naturally and slowly to establish if the person can read lips. Not all people with hearing impairments can lip-read. Those who can will rely on facial expression and other body language to help in understanding. (Note: It's estimated that only four out of ten spoken words are visible on the lips.) Show consideration by placing yourself facing the light source and keeping your hands, cigarettes and food away from your mouth when speaking. Keep moustaches well trimmed. Shouting distorts sounds accepted through hearing aids and inhibits lip reading. Only raise your voice when requested. Brief, concise written notes may be helpful.

- When talking with a person in a wheelchair for more than a few minutes, use a chair, whenever possible, in order to place yourself at the person's eye level. Never lean on the person's wheelchair – it's part of the space that belongs to the person who uses it. Enable people who use crutches, canes or wheelchairs to keep them within reach. Be aware that some wheelchair users may choose to transfer themselves out of their wheelchairs (into an office chair, for example) during an interview/conversation.

- Listen attentively when you're talking to a person who has a speech impairment. Keep your manner encouraging rather than correcting. Exercise patience rather than attempting to speak for a person with speech difficulty. When necessary, ask short questions that require short answers or a nod or a shake of the head. Never pretend to understand if you are having difficulty doing so. Repeat what you understand, or incorporate the interviewee's statements into each of the following questions. The person's reactions will clue you in and guide you to understanding. Do not raise your voice. Most speech-impaired people can hear and understand.

- Treat adults in a manner befitting adults: Call a person by his or her first name only when extending that familiarity to all others present. Never patronise people using wheelchairs by patting them on the head or shoulder.

- Offer assistance in a dignified manner with sensitivity and respect. Be prepared to have the offer declined. Do not proceed to assist if your offer to assist is declined. If the offer is accepted, listen to or accept instructions. Allow a person with a visual impairment to take your arm (at or about the elbow). This will enable you to guide rather than propel or lead the person. Offer to hold or carry packages in a welcoming manner: 'May I help you with your packages?' When offering to hand a coat or umbrella, do not offer to hand a walking stick or crutches unless the individual requests otherwise.

adapted from detailed web site on Disability etiquette by City of San Antonio Disability Access Office
(*http://www.ci.sat.tx.us/planning/handbook/*)

DISCUSSION POINT

What would you need to consider when communicating with the following people for the first time? How would you go about establishing their preferred form of interaction?

■ an older man who is hard of hearing but refuses to wear a hearing aid

■ a family (mother, father and two children) who have recently arrived in the UK from India, Romania or Ethiopia

■ an adolescent girl with severe physical disabilities which prevent her communicating in spoken language

The need for an interpreter

Interpreting involves explaining the meaning of a piece of information in a way that an individual can understand. This may be necessary when:

■ someone doesn't speak English as their first language (many local authorities and hospitals have lists of interpreters for health and social care workers to use)

■ someone is deaf or hard of hearing, and needs information interpreted in sign language

■ information is complex or involves a lot of specialist terms, and needs interpreting in a simple way for a member of the general public; this is particularly important for medical workers.

Care organisations need to be aware of the language needs of clients, and provide interpretation services when necessary. These may include:

■ language interpreters for people who don't speak English as their first language

■ sign language interpreters for clients who are deaf or hard of hearing

■ leaflets, posters and booklets translated into different languages, or produced in Braille for people with visual impairments

■ staff who are trained in explaining complicated, specialist information to members of the general public.

In areas where there are relatively large minority groups who do not speak English, health providers may employ link workers from those groups. These workers not only understand the cultural norms and language of the group but also are trained in medical and nursing interpretation. Sometime using a family member as an interpreter has to be considered sensitively; for example, it may not be appropriate to communicate a mother's intimate medical details to her son; or a parent's poor prognosis to a young daughter or son. It may be better to seek out local interpreters with professional experience of interpretation and who understand and respect the need for confidentiality. However, this too may not be suitable for every client and if it is planned to use an interpreter, make certain that the client and the carers are happy with the person selected. If they aren't, someone else, or a different method of communicating with them, will need to be sought.

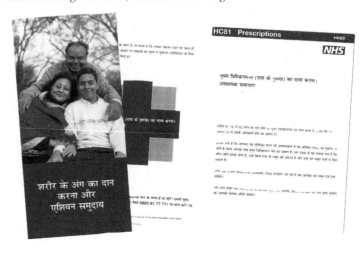

Empowerment and assertiveness

People can only make sound decisions about their care and treatment if they have information. Therefore giving clients information is an important part of empowering them – increasing their independence and ability to make choices.

Many different types of information can empower clients. For example:
- someone arriving at a clinic feels in control of the situation if they are given clear information on where to wait and where to go
- a patient in hospital with a serious illness can be involved in decision-making about treatment if they are given clear information on the different options
- an older person in a residential home can structure their own day if they know when different activities take place.

In the past, care settings tended to reinforce the notion of clients as passive recipients of care. Workers were the experts, and knew what was best – individuals had little control over, or involvement in, the care they received. This has changed as most care settings take steps to involve people in making decisions about their own care. This means giving people the information they need to make sound decisions, and respecting their needs and wishes as individuals. In some cases, their choices will be limited by their specific needs, in particular for medical care. However, workers can still ensure that people understand the situation and are aware of possible alternatives, so that they feel involved in the decision-making process.

Advocacy

Advocates can provide representation and information on behalf of the client. Where the client is unable to handle knowledge himself or herself, an advocate can become the holder and user of knowledge for them.

Clients may find it difficult or impossible to express and assert their needs, wishes and rights effectively. Sometimes this is because illness or disability prevents them communicating clearly. In other cases language differences may create problems, or they may simply be too shy or frightened to speak up for themselves.

The advocate is usually a carer, friend or relative – someone who understands the client's beliefs, values and feelings, and is able to communicate them to workers.

As far as possible, workers aim to promote self-advocacy, encouraging clients to develop skills in expressing themselves, making decisions and asserting their own rights. Whether self-advocacy is possible depends on the needs and disabilities of the individual.

> 66 *It's the first time anyone asked me what I want . . . the advocacy service has a totally different attitude. The people there are on the side of reason rather than just trying to get away with things or pass the buck. I'm often treated as a 'disabled person' but the advocacy service treats you as a 'person with a disability'.* 99

> *client who took advantage of an advocacy service*

DISCUSSION POINT

Should children have the same rights to be involved in their own care as adults? When might workers have to treat children differently?

If a hospital patient is under 16, parents are responsible for signing a consent form for an operation to go ahead. Do you think this is fair? If you were a nurse or doctor, how could you involve the child in making the decision?

An **advocate** is someone who speaks on behalf of another and has the faith, confidence, and trust of the person they are representing.

DISCUSSION POINT

If you were unable to communicate your own beliefs and feelings, who would you want to act as your advocate and why? What factors do you think workers should consider when arranging advocacy?

93

ACTIVITY

Imagine that you are an advocate for an elderly person or someone with mental health problems. Write down what kinds of information you would need to have in order to meet with the social worker who is coming to talk about changing their existing services. What help would you be able to give? Where might you speak on their behalf?

By using their knowledge of the system, advocates can represent users at case conferences, assessment meetings or in the care plan reviews. They have only one interest to represent and argue for – that of the user.

Some workers encourage selected clients to attend a training programme or college course as part of their route to independence. Training can offer opportunities to learn new skills, acquire information and knowledge and, for young people or adults of working age, a chance to become qualified.

2.2.3 Influences of interaction on health and social wellbeing

Human beings are social creatures. People learn in groups, play with friends, live in families and work with colleagues. Most depend on interacting with others, and find living alone or being isolated from society depressing and disturbing.

Yet interacting with other people can be both positive and negative – people don't automatically come away feeling satisfied and happy.

Mrs Hargreaves, an 86-year-old woman, explains how she misses the positive effects of interacting with other people:

ACTIVITY

Read through what Mrs Hargreaves said again. List the positive influences that interpersonal interaction had on her life when she was younger, and the negative influences that lack of interaction is having on her life now.

Talk to a care worker who has regular contact with older people, and ask whether Mrs Hargreaves' feelings are common.

- What practical steps could be taken to increase an isolated older person's contact with people?

- What factors would a care worker need to bear in mind when suggesting these measures?

66 *When I was younger, I had lots of friends. I came from a large family, my husband and I had two children of our own, and our house was always full of people laughing, talking and joking. I loved being around people, sharing stories and secrets, helping them out in the bad times and enjoying the good times. I was always the life and soul, and knew I was important to people. And I knew that someone was there for me if I needed help.*

Today my life's very different. My husband, brothers and sisters, and almost all my friends have died. My children are living abroad, and I'm left living alone and feeling very isolated. It's funny, but without people to talk to you start thinking you're going mad. I get myself into a state over the silliest things, like the radiators making a funny noise, just because I haven't got anyone to talk to about it. When I get a cold it seems to drag on and on – it's almost as if there's no point in getting better. I can't stand feeling I'm of no use to anyone. When I think how confident and happy I used to be, it's hard to believe I'm the same person. 99

If an individual is forced to interact with people who make them feel uncomfortable, or to join in with a group in which they feel they don't belong, this can increase their feeling of loneliness. Failing to succeed in interaction tends to make people feel inadequate, which in turn can lower their self-esteem, and in the long term lead to depression and loss of self-esteem.

Interaction can also have a negative influence if people don't understand an individual's needs and feelings, and say things that upset or threaten them. Health and social care workers must be particularly aware of this, as many clients may feel vulnerable and react badly to insensitive communication.

ACTIVITY

Read through the following conversation between Moira, a family care worker, and Emma, a young mother who is struggling to cope with her baby.

Moira: Hi, Emma. How are you feeling today? And how's this little one? (picking up the baby, who is crying)

Emma: Not too great actually. She won't stop crying and I just can't cope with her. Sometimes I have to walk out of the room because I'm afraid what I might do.

Moira: Look, we all feel like that sometimes. I know I did when my Darren was born and he was a real terror. Don't worry. We were fine in the end.

Emma: But I'm really worried we won't be.

Moira: Now don't get all upset, it's not going to help the baby, is it? Look, she's quietening down already with me. She's a lovely little thing. Have you been to the mother and baby group again?

Emma: No, it's not for me. They were really cliquey and all seemed to be such perfect mothers it made me feel even worse.

Moira: I'm sure it's in your imagination. You've really got to make the effort, you know. This should be the most wonderful time of your life.

By the end of this conversation, Emma felt more miserable and inadequate than she had before Moira arrived. In small groups, discuss why you think this is. What did Moira say and do that upset Emma? Talk about what you think she should have said and done to have a more positive effect.

Key questions

1 Identify at least five characteristics of a good listener.

2 Give five different types of body language.

3 How may cultural differences affect communication?

4 What is mirroring?

5 Describe and give examples of four different types of question that can be used to seek information.

6 Give three situations where language and listening skills need to be effective.

7 What is empathy?

8 Name five different types of client who may have special communication needs.

9 Describe how you would communicate with a person in a wheelchair.

10 Give two examples of optimising interaction by using interpretation.

11 What contribution does advocacy make to empowerment?

SECTION **2.3**

Communication skills in groups

In this section you will find out about the many types of group, both formal and informal, that can form in a health and social care environment, how they work (their dynamics), and how to communicate effectively in a group context to improve the group's performance.

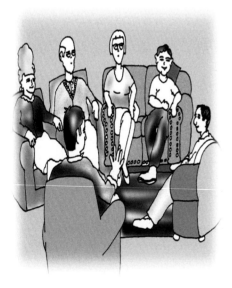

2.3.1 Types of group

Groups can be informal, coming together casually with no specific purpose or organisation. These tend to be social in nature but can be important for both helping with the wellbeing of members and encouraging social cohesion.

Formal groups occur at specified times, follow particular rules and have specified goals. Examples are:

- case conferences
- ward rounds
- staff meetings
- committee meetings
- formal teaching
- organised recreational activities (such as a quiz).

A group is not just a random collection of people. What distinguishes it is some kind of shared purpose, perhaps an interest, or a task which can't be done or done so well by one person alone: an activity which is more practical and economical when done by a number of individuals – a team – at the same time. Groups share something in common. They may share any or all of the following:

- aspirations
- qualities
- interests

- goals
- values and beliefs
- activities.

Sometimes the group's purpose is imposed or defined by the members who have been gathered because they represent other groups and purposes. Then the tensions of torn loyalties and different agendas can present risks and challenges to group members. Their individual differences and personal agendas can be just as divisive – and sometimes more dangerous – if they are unseen or unsuspected. One of the skills of effective group interaction is to identify these differences and the impact they may have on:

- individual group members
- the achievement of objectives.

Appropriate communication strategies need to be used to harness energies and keep members focused on the common purpose.

2.3.2 Running a group

The power or potential of a group is more than the sum of the individuals. In the time the group is together, it can show a unique 'personality' of:

- anticipation and uncertainty
- a settling-in phase as they take stock of what is happening and relate it to previous experience
- expectation
- different responses.

Effective group interaction is more likely if the group interactions are skilfully managed. If ten people chosen at random were put in a room and asked to solve a problem within a certain timescale, they may be unproductive unless a leader emerged. To ensure that the group achieves its outcomes, participants need a range of support before and during the interaction. It is usually the responsibility of the person organising the meeting to:

- make the environment comfortable and relaxing
- reduce stress as much as possible
- make sure that individuals can play a full part in the discussion.

This involves establishing participants' needs, and being sensitive to their feelings throughout the discussion.

Planning

Before the interaction

Managing effective group interaction begins with planning, for instance:

- What are the intended aims of the group? What will be discussed?
- What do individual participants hope to achieve?
- Do participants know what they will be discussing, and what the aims of the interaction are?
- When will it be held? How many people will be involved? Who will they be?
- Do participants have any other special needs (for example, wheelchair access, sign language interpreter, other language interpreter)?
- How long will the interaction last?

A volunteer counsellor who leads groups for an organisation for people with eating disorders explains why it is important to establish the support people need before the group meets:

66 *Careful planning is the key to good interaction. Many people who take part in our group sessions feel vulnerable, upset and depressed. As a result, it's vital to put them at ease right from the start by making sure that everything is exactly right. I begin planning a series of group sessions well in advance to make sure I'm absolutely clear about what we're trying to achieve. I find out how many people will be attending, then book a room which is big enough, but not so big that participants will feel lost. I make sure that it has comfy chairs, toilets nearby, and facilities for making tea and coffee. I also check that I'll be able to borrow any equipment I'm likely to need, such as an overhead projector or flipchart.*

Once I've booked the room, I write to all the participants. I introduce myself, explain how many people will be in the group and what we will try to achieve, give them an outline of what we will cover in each session, and then tell them where to be, when, and how to get there. At the bottom of the letter I include a tear-off slip for them to fill in and return to me, so I know whether they have any specific needs such as language difficulties or dietary preferences. I also ask them to summarise in one sentence what they hope to achieve from the day – this gives me a good idea of the areas to cover.

On the day of the group, I arrive early, make sure I have all the information and equipment I need, and that the room is set up well. Participants arrive to a warm and comfortable environment, already have an idea of what to expect because they've seen my introductory letter, and tend to settle down into a useful discussion very quickly. On the whole, I find that time and effort invested at an early stage is well spent. 99

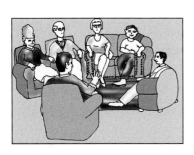

Optimising the environment

It is easy to underestimate the importance of the environment in which group interactions take place. Many potentially useful discussions have been disrupted because participants were cold and uncomfortable, or unable to hear what was being said.

People organising groups can take steps to optimise the environment both before and during a discussion:

■ Check that the room is at a suitable temperature.
■ Make sure that there are enough chairs (comfortable ones, if possible); chairs should all be the same height, so no one appears to be in a position of power.
■ Think about how to position group members so that they can all be seen – arranging chairs in a circle or a horseshoe can encourage an open discussion in which everyone joins in; rows tend to look intimidating, mean that people can't be seen, and can remind people of being at school!
■ Leave space between chairs, so people don't feel their personal space is threatened.
■ If there is a group leader, think about where they will sit; if they are behind a desk or on the other side of a table, this can create a barrier and suggest that they are going to dominate the discussion.
■ Make sure that any equipment and furniture needed (tables, blackboard, flipchart, OHP and so on) is available.
■ Check the lighting in the room – if participants don't need to write and the lighting seems harsh and glaring, consider bringing in small lamps to put around the room.
■ Try to arrange for facilities for making tea or coffee – chatting over refreshments can help to put people at ease.
■ Deal with potential disruptions – such as a noise outside the room, or a flickering light.

Managing the discussion

Once the group is under way, someone needs to take responsibility for supporting and guiding the discussion. It's often useful to appoint a leader to do this.

The leader's role is not to dominate the discussion, but to create a positive atmosphere and enable everyone to participate. This may involve:

■ giving everyone an opportunity to introduce themselves
■ introducing the subject and explaining the aims of the interaction
■ arranging for someone to take notes, if appropriate, so that decisions and opinions are recorded
■ using questioning and listening techniques to encourage people to talk (especially those who are quiet)
■ preventing everyone from speaking at once

- checking meaning and clarifying what participants say, often by using reflective listening
- using body language well to promote an open and relaxed discussion
- moving the discussion in new directions where appropriate
- asking for people's views at the end of the meeting and summarising key points
- making sure that the discussion doesn't go on for too long.

Concluding the discussion

Concluding a group effectively is part of group management. The group leader needs to ensure that matters come to a satisfactory conclusion, with objectives achieved and individuals:

- feeling they have had their say
- being clear about the outcomes
- knowing what comes next.

Effective managers round off the group interaction decisively before people start looking at their watches or drifting away. They may provide a brief concluding summary of what has been done, what action if any has been agreed and, if appropriate, what will be done at the next gathering and how and when that will be arranged. They should check that participants have understood and are agreeable.

The organiser also needs to thank hosts or speakers (remember, you may want their services again in future) and everyone else for their participation. The aim is for everyone to leave on a positive and committed note.

Depending on the nature and purpose of the group you may have additional final tasks after the meeting. For instance, you may need to ensure that:

- minutes are produced and circulated
- follow-up actions are carried out
- organisational records are produced and filed.

2.3.3 **Group stages**

From its first tentative and innovative stages, a group will establish its own norms and patterns. It will then tend, if it survives and succeeds, to go through a relatively steady state of delivering its objectives. Eventually it may encounter change from inside or outside. The shared purpose has become obscure or irrelevant. Then the group may disband, new members may arrive and set a new direction or the group may reform with changed objectives.

B. Tuckman suggests that there are four stages in the development of a group ('Development sequence in small groups', *Psychological Bulletin*, LXIII (6) 1965).

Stage	Structures	Activity
Forming	The group gathers, often with anxiety, and a strong leader emerges. There may be scapegoating.	Members identify the task, roles and appropriate methods.
Storming	Leadership challenges, conflict between sub-groups, opinions are polarised.	Emotional resistance to the task.
Norming	Group cohesion develops, norms emerge, conflict is replaced by mutual support and development of trust.	Open exchange of views and feelings, cooperation develops.
Performing	Interpersonal problems are resolved and roles become more relaxed and flexible.	Solutions emerge and there are constructive attempts at task completion – the major work period.

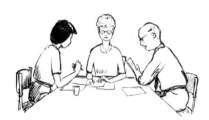

2.3.4 **Dynamics in groups**

Group dynamics relate to the way the individuals in the group form positive and negative patterns of behaviour and relationships. These include alliances, pairings, protectiveness, hostilities, and also domineering, blocking, ignoring and other collusive behaviours.

As well as recognising and accommodating individual needs and differences in group members, you should be aware of the effect of various behaviours within groups. The behaviours may not necessarily be evident or have such impact when the same individuals are outside the group.

Sometimes a combination of members or a personality clash within the group, or the purpose and circumstances of the group, can stimulate or exacerbate behaviour outside an individual's familiar repertoire. In many cases where a group meets regularly, the leader and individual members recognise and come to expect certain behaviour patterns from various members and can plan how to deal with them.

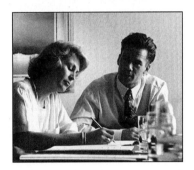

Managing group dynamics

Group dynamics need awareness and managing. Some communication skills are effective with many potentially difficult or disrupting dynamics.

The choice and layout of a meeting venue can inhibit or enhance group attitudes and behaviours. In round-table meetings, for example, having people with opposing views opposite each other increases the confrontation. If they are sitting side by side, conflicts are less likely to be inflammatory, get out of control and disrupt the meeting. Similarly it may be as well to avoid placing known cliques together, especially if they are at one end of the table or corner of the room where they may tend to have a separate sub-group meeting.

If one group member is known to be distracting, disruptive or prone to go off at tangents, the leader might delegate the person the task of note-taking. It's usually counter-productive for the leader to have sole responsibility for note-taking – to be sure of doing that well usually means they can't devote enough attention to the content and process of the meeting and the dynamics within the group.

2.3.5 **Group behaviours**

Groups can operate in many ways and this will depend on an interaction between two factors:
- the nature and purpose of the group
- the personality of the group members.

Group task roles	Building and maintenance roles	Self-centred roles
■ initiator-contributor	■ encourager	■ aggressor
■ information-seeker	■ harmoniser	■ blocker
■ information-giver	■ compromiser	■ self-confessor
■ energiser	■ group observer	■ dominator
■ recorder	■ follower	■ special-interest pleader

Roles are not static and, during the course of a single session, roles will switch around with individuals being both dynamic and negative at different times. Whether the group becomes a 'performing' one will depend very much on how the conflicts of the 'storming' stage are resolved. This will depend both on the skills of the group leader and the motivation and contributions of the group members.

UNIT

2

SECTION **2.3**

> ### ACTIVITY
>
> To increase your sensitivity to the effects of certain behaviours in a group, organise a group or 'fishbowl' exercise. Group members (no more than five or six around a table) each draw from a hat a slip on which various 'behaviours' have been written – some inhibiting, some enhancing, some just saying 'be yourself'! Don't show the leader or other group members/observers your slip. In a ten-minute discussion on a general, study-related topic (perhaps your GNVQ), make an effort to demonstrate that behaviour.
>
> Afterwards discuss the activity:
>
> ■ Did you stick to 'your' behaviour?
>
> ■ How accurately can you state the behaviours of other group members?
>
> ■ What were the effects the behaviour had on the content and process of the group?
>
> ■ How effectively did the leader deal with the group?
>
> ■ How did the process feel to both the leader and group members?

2.3.6 Styles of groups

Groups vary in their structure and formality. These affect the individuals in the group and life in the group. Some group interactions, topics and goals require a formal approach, others a less formal structure and interaction.

Some groups require specific conventions:
■ committee meetings
■ disciplinary or investigation enquiries
■ trust or board meetings
■ juries
■ health or social care case conferences.

The formality and strictness of the procedures helps to ensure that business is fully and systematically dealt with. The structure imposes a certain impartiality and is often appropriate to the seriousness of issues and outcomes involved. These are not the occasions for brainstorming, creativity and experimentation – and the formal style tends not to encourage these processes.

With other groups, such as a playgroup or residential care home, a highly structured style may not be effective – although structure can be comforting, reassuring, safe and efficient. Some clients, such as those with sensory impairment or dementia, prefer clear and unvaried routines. However, for a newcomer to the group, rigidity and uncertainty about what the 'rules' are, can be intimidating. Free, informal, unstructured groups can be uncomfortable for other individuals, but they may be an ideal format for stimulating a free flow of ideas and imagination.

ACTIVITY

Examine various groups. List a few different groups with which you are familiar. Designate a number or name to each group. Create a grid with the groups along one axis, and the following along the other:

- purpose
- number of individuals
- type of people
- frequency of meeting
- venue
- degree of formality/structure
- leader (if there is one)
- documentation and reporting.

Include any other factors that you feel are relevant. Rate the effectiveness of each group. Identify the factors contributing to this and your ideas for possible improvements.

2.3.7 **Enhancing the group experience**

DISCUSSION POINT

Think of an occasion recently when you have felt under stress during a group interaction. How did it affect your participation? What could other participants have done to help reduce the stress?

Reducing stress

If people are feeling worried and under stress, they're less likely to take part in a group openly and honestly. An important part of managing the interaction is helping to reduce this stress, and put participants at ease.

Addressing individual needs

The people who take part in an interaction are individuals with their own needs and preferences. Sometimes these may have a direct impact on the success of the group, and need to be supported through specific measures. If a participant:

- uses a first language that is not English, an interpreter may be needed
- is hard of hearing, an induction loop or sign language interpreter may be needed

- has a different level of knowledge and understanding from most group members (for example, if a group includes children and adults), the leader needs to be aware of this and make sure everyone understands the views being expressed
- is in a wheelchair, they may need access to a toilet designed for disabled people.

If refreshments are provided, the organiser needs to be aware of any special dietary needs.

The person organising a group interaction should try to find out about individuals' needs in advance so there is time to make any special arrangements necessary. If the group isn't large, they may be able to do this by talking to participants. However, if the group involves a large number of people, it's often easier to find out about their needs by sending a short questionnaire in advance.

Key questions

1 Name and describe one model of the stages of groups.

2 List six factors to consider when planning a group interaction.

3 What factors would you consider when planning the degree of formality and structure of the group?

4 What are the features of structured groups? Explain the pros and cons of structured, more formal groups.

5 How would you identify an informal group? In what health and care situations might an informal group be preferable to a more structured group interaction?

6 Name and describe behaviours that enhance group interaction.

7 Name and describe some barriers to effective group interaction.

8 How can you support individuals during a group interaction?

9 How can you make the most of the environment for a group interaction?

10 Name four roles which group members play in order to build and maintain the group.

SECTION **2.4**

Evaluating communication skills

To be an effective worker, you will need to learn how to analyse one-to-one and group interactions. You will need to observe and reflect on your own interactions as well as those of others, and you will need to be open to feedback from others and prepared to change how you go about communicating with people. In this section you will learn about the various ways in which communication can be evaluated.

66 *Know your reputation. How other people see you influences how they approach you in conversation. If there are negative sides to your reputation as a communicator, work hard to change them.*

Accept responsibly. Blaming the other person for not understanding you – or for you not understanding them – is pointless. While you can't be responsible for the other person's efforts, you can for your own.

Base your feedback on facts. Offer helpful feedback based on a simple description of the behaviour and its impact. Before you offer advice or guidance, make sure you have enough information. **99**

from BT TalkWorks

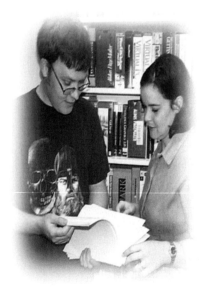

2.4.1 Why evaluate?

Workers in health and social care communicate in three contexts:

- one-to-one (whether face-to-face or by telephone)
- groups (formal or informal)
- by writing (through recording or writing letters or memoranda).

Each of these has its peculiarities. In one-to-one communication the worker is very much on his or her own with one other. Fellow workers (a colleague or supervisor) can give feedback in a way which is neither challenging nor undermining. With clients, less direct methods of seeking feedback may be needed, particularly where there are communication difficulties. In the case of a senior manager, or someone from another agency, it may be too threatening to seek feedback.

Group situations have many more actors in them, but seeking feedback can still be threatening, particularly if you are junior or not very confident of your skills. An insensitive or misplaced word may be positively undermining and the person who gives it is unlikely to seek or receive feedback themselves!

Even when writing reports or letters, workers are not in the position that you, as a student, are – they're unlikely to find marginal notes on their reports or a scoring system that allows them to measure current performance against past.

Finally, what can you do to analyse the effectiveness of your own and other people's communication skills?

With all these problems, why try to evaluate the effectiveness of communication? There are many reasons:

- to try to ensure the optimum outcome for the participants
- to check that there have not been negative outcomes
- to consider the learning process for the participants
- to develop skills and techniques
- to learn from mistakes
- to make improvements in the future.

To understand why this is necessary, it may be worth considering the way in which we learn from our experience. There is a four-stage process which, if we are to benefit from our learning, we go through:

- Experience (N) – what happens to us or what we have caused to happen
- Reflect (E) – we think about what has happened
- Conclude (S) – what lessons are to be learned from our reflections
- Plan (W) – we decide how to apply the conclusions to the next experience.

All of us have different learning styles which relate to the type of person we are:

- **Activists** learn from constant exposure to new experience – they immerse themselves in experience and are enthusiastic about anything new – 'act first and think about the consequences later'.
- **Reflectors** learn best from activities that allow them space to think about experience; cautious and thoughtful, they consider all the angles before making a decision – listeners and observers.

- **Theorists** learn best from activities that allow them to integrate observation into logically sound theories – they think through problems in a step-by-step way.
- **Pragmatists** learn best from activities that have clear practical value and that allow ideas to be tested in practical settings – they are down-to-earth people who like to get on with things rather than talk about them.

Few people reflect just one of these types, most of us are a mixture of two or more. Ideally we should have some aspects of all four.

2.4.2 How are communication skills analysed?

No matter what the nature of the interaction, there are certain criteria that you can always apply:
- Was there participation by all those involved?
- What was the quality of each person's participation?
- What understanding of what happened did the participants have?
- Did the interaction achieve something for some or all of the participants?
- Was the interaction more effective than previous interactions?

2.4.3 Feedback

Feedback is a response to what someone says. Giving and seeking feedback optimises interaction by showing that the listener is listening to, and has understood, what the speaker says.

When talking to clients, health and social care workers will give feedback to show that they are listening and have taken in what the person has said by:
- saying things like 'Go on' and 'Yes', and nodding while the person is speaking
- summarising what the person has just said
- asking prompt and probe questions about what the person has just said
- repeating important points
- seeking feedback to check that the person has understood
- observing their body language as they listen
- asking open questions related to a subject they have just explained.

Feedback from clients or carers will usually be verbal. The health and social care worker may ask for their views on how a discussion went, what they felt they gained from the interaction, and how similar sessions could be improved in the future.

An observer may give either oral or written feedback. Assessment sheets and evaluation forms can be a good way to assess someone's performance while an interaction is taking place. This makes feedback more immediate, and often

'IT'S GOOD TO TALK'

BT, in a noted series of advertisements in the 1990s, coined a slogan 'It's good to talk' and backed it up with suggestions about how to get more out of life through better conversations under the heading *TalkWorks* (*http://www.talkworks.co.uk*).

As part of this they asked hundreds of people about what distinguished a good conversation from a bad one. They boiled it down to four key factors. In good conversations:

- it feels like a genuine two-way experience, with both of you equally involved and interested
- you both feel you're being heard and understood – there's a willingness on both sides to be open
- the atmosphere feels comfortable so even if what you're talking about is difficult, the most important things get said
- the conversation makes a difference – something useful or satisfying happens as a result.

DISCUSSION POINT

You may have experience of evaluating your own and other people's work as part of your GNVQ or other courses. From your own experience, what are the important things to remember when giving someone else feedback on their performance? What should you avoid?

more relevant. Whether feedback is verbal or written, it should be given in a constructive, supportive way, so that workers can build on their skills in the future.

66 *Our tutor usually gives us verbal feedback on our contribution to an interaction as well as written feedback. She chats with each of us for five minutes or so individually. She usually begins by picking up on good points about my contribution – perhaps my body language was good, or I used language well. Then she makes some constructive criticisms and suggests how I could improve in the future. Doing this face-to-face gives me a chance to respond, disagree or ask questions. If there's anything I don't understand, we can talk about it in greater depth. Sometimes when you just read something on paper, it can seem harsh and doesn't give you a chance to find out more.* 99

student

When inviting verbal feedback from other participants – in particular, fellow students – it is worth remembering that people's opinions are often subjective.

If you're concerned that you may not like what you hear, or may become defensive, you may find it more constructive to seek feedback in other ways such as:
- by watching a video of your participation
- inviting an independent observer to offer feedback privately
- inviting written feedback which you may read in your own time.

There are three main responses to verbal feedback:
- 'Oh no, that's not me.'
- 'That's interesting.'
- 'Yes, that's me.'

Aim not to be defensive. Instead, be thoughtful. If you're unsure that the feedback is correct, try not to reject it straight away. Reflect on it a while. It may not be wholly accurate, but often there is something to learn in all feedback.

Written feedback on your own contribution to an interaction is useful because it acts as a permanent record. It can be collected from independent observers and other participants in an interaction.

Written feedback is usually collected on evaluation forms or assessment sheets. These may be completed during, at the end of or after an interaction. As with verbal feedback, it is important to:
- be sensitive when commenting on someone else's contribution – don't get personal
- take written feedback from others seriously – don't dismiss something because it's not what you want to hear.

DISCUSSION POINT

Discuss your responses to feedback, both positive and critical, in the past. Are you good at receiving feedback?

Then discuss the components of effective feedback.

109

ACTIVITY

ACTIVITY

Working in pairs, roleplay one of the following situations:

- a patient and a doctor
- a client and a social worker
- a customer and a shop assistant.

In the interaction the first person is seeking a particular service, the second person is trying to persuade them that they want something different. It doesn't matter what the things are – you can decide that for yourselves.

After five minutes evaluate your own performance and your colleague's. How do the two views compare?

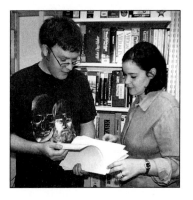

DISCUSSION POINT

Having read this extract from Susan's diary, what problems can you see with using self-reflection to evaluate the perception of other participants?

Throughout this unit, and in other parts of the book, you'll find activities that ask you to do something and then think about:

- what you did
- why you did it
- how well you did it
- what you achieved by it
- what the implications were.

This process is called 'self-reflection'.

Self assessment is a process that you will already be familiar with from school or college reports where you're asked to comment on your performance and the things that you could do better at. Self-reflection involves mentally standing back to review effectiveness during an interaction. You use it to:

- analyse and try to understand what you and others have done
- deal with your feelings
- develop self-awareness and become more sensitive to others
- improve your performance for future occasions.

The important point about self-reflection is to make it as honest as possible. It is often hard to be objective – some people tend to think they've done worse than they actually have, while others think they've done better. Sometimes generalisations and personal preferences stop us from assessing others' participation objectively.

Self-reflection – for example, by keeping a diary of an interaction – is most useful when evaluating your own performance. But it can also be a helpful source of data when evaluating the feelings and contributions of other participants.

Other ways you can assess your own performance are by keeping a journal or writing a regular report on your performance.

Susan Brown kept a detailed record of her actions and feelings when organising discussion groups on equal opportunities and then made notes during the interaction which she later wrote up as a diary of the afternoon. As well as covering her own contribution to the session, this provided useful insight into how other participants did, as the following extract shows.

Began general discussion about sex discrimination in health and social care. I set the ball rolling by giving figures on men and women working in different roles in health and social care. Jo immediately stepped in and started talking about her own experiences, which was a good way to get more people involved. Anna, Natalie, Soraya and Tim all made good contributions and got a lively discussion going. All seemed interested in the issues, and everyone seemed to be listening, even if they weren't participating. Jake got bolshy and started saying he doesn't think there's any such thing as sex discrimination. He didn't seem to have taken in what the speakers had said.

ACTIVITY

Carry out a SWOT analysis of your communication skills (S = Strengths, W = Weaknesses, O = Opportunities and T = Threats). Think of how you have performed in recent interactions and jot down, as honestly as you can, your views under each heading.

The objectives are to explore:

■ how any weaknesses can be overcome or turned into mere threats about which to be more aware

■ how opportunities can be maximised and consolidated into strengths.

This is for your own benefit – there is no point in being anything other than honest with yourself!

Susan could have used four different sources of data to evaluate how effective the interaction was from the point of view of the other participants:

■ oral feedback – by allocating five minutes at the end of the session for people to give their views on the interaction, and by talking to participants individually after the session

■ written feedback – by giving people a short evaluation form to fill in at the end of the session

■ observation – by watching a video recording of the interaction

■ self-reflection – by keeping a diary of the session.

2.4.5 **Peer assessment**

ACTIVITY

Can you see yourself as others see you? Working as a group, anonymously circulate sheets of paper which name all group members. In two columns against each name, each participant in the group should anonymously jot down the two or three strong points they have appreciated about that person's interactions and one point for improvement. The papers should be sorted out and returned to their owners to read and reflect on. A group discussion could be held afterwards on how to develop and practise the points raised.

Peer assessment means seeking feedback or evaluation from your colleagues. This can be done by seeking:

■ oral feedback – from the other participant or participants

■ written feedback

■ written evaluation on forms

■ a colleague to be an observer who can report on the process.

The last three can be particularly helpful when working with groups.

Your peers are your equals in terms of status, hierarchy, power and general ability. Feedback from peers can be gained by asking participants what they thought of an interaction, including your own participation and effectiveness. This can be done:

■ at the end of the interaction, during a general summing up of the session – this can be an efficient way to collect information from everyone involved, but participants may be constrained in what they say because of the other people present

■ after the interaction, by approaching participants individually and asking for their views – feedback gained in this way is more likely to be honest and constructive, but can be time-consuming.

ACTIVITY

Design a short evaluation form that you could give to fellow students for obtaining written feedback on your participation during a GNVQ lesson, discussion group or other group activity. Plan your evaluation criteria using the examples of criteria listed in section 2.4.2.

DISCUSSION POINT

Have you ever watched yourself on video, or listened to yourself on audio tape? What did it show you about the way you communicate with people?

Making a video or audio recording of the interaction – with the client's permission if they are involved – can be an effective way for workers to evaluate the interaction, including their own performance. Replaying and analysing a tape, either alone or with other people, provides an opportunity to focus on particular skills.

How might watching a video of the interaction in which you participated help to ensure that your reflection on your performance is fair and objective?

Written feedback offers a more formal record of your peers' views on your effectiveness during an interaction. You could distribute evaluation forms for participants to fill in, either:

- at the end of the session, before they go home – this has the advantage of the interaction still being fresh in people's minds; it's also easy to collect the responses
- after the session, once they've had time to reflect on the experience – however, this results in a less reliable response rate, and may mean that people forget how they felt during the interaction.

ACTIVITY

Choose an interaction for which you can carry out a detailed evaluation. You may decide to focus on a class discussion, a roleplay, or a meeting you attend while on work experience.

Your evaluation could be based on the following criteria:

- participation
- quality of contribution
- improvements from previous occasions
- knowledge and understanding of participants.

Using these criteria, invite an evaluation of:

- how effective the interaction was in terms of the other participants
- your own contribution to the interaction.

Your evaluation should include information from:

- verbal feedback
- written feedback
- observation
- self-reflection.

Based on your findings, make notes for a report evaluating other participants' views on the interaction, and your own contribution to the interaction.

Audio tape and video tape records

If you've used closed circuit video to record classroom sessions, in particular roleplays, you'll have experienced a degree of disorientation. 'That wasn't me, was it?' 'I don't sound like that, do I?' 'I don't have all those irritating mannerisms, do I?'

This is the early part of learning what you're really like to others. TV also has a slightly distancing effect and allows you to view what goes on in a much more objective way, even when you've been one of the participants. It can be particularly helpful when assessing your body language and other non-verbal communications. It can also be stopped or run back in order to check or highlight a particular point.

By careful study of video tape you can ask:

- what do people's facial expressions show?
- what does people's body language show?
- how well are different people contributing?
- is everyone participating?
- do participants seem to be developing knowledge and understanding?

Audio tape, while being able to illustrate less, can be used in a wider range of settings. It can be particularly helpful in monitoring the balance of contribution to a discussion and whether one person is dominating or another being excluded.

Key questions

1 Why is it important to evaluate the effectiveness of interpersonal interactions in health and social care?

2 What are the four stages of the learning process?

3 What are 'evaluation criteria'? Why are criteria necessary in the evaluation of performance?

4 What criteria might you use to evaluate your own contribution during an interaction?

5 List some sources of information you might use for evaluation.

6 What is the role of feedback in evaluation?

7 Explain factors that enable feedback to be effective.

8 How can you collect written feedback?

9 What is 'peer assessment'?

10 Explain the purpose of self-assessment, and how you can assess yourself.

11 Explain methods of evaluating interaction by observation.

12 How could you observe your own skills and contribution?

13 List ways you might recommend of improving a group interaction for participants.

14 What are the pros and cons of getting verbal feedback at the end of an interaction compared with waiting a short time after the interaction?

SECTION **2.5**

Maintaining client confidentiality

In this section you will find out about the importance of confidentiality in establishing trust with clients, possible dilemmas that could arise, how to ensure confidentiality, and legislation governing who may or may not have access to confidential information.

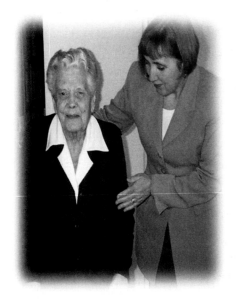

“ No one shall be subjected to the arbitrary interference with his privacy, family, home or correspondence, nor to attacks upon his honour and reputation. Everyone has the right to the protection of the law against such interference or attacks. ”

Article 12 of the Universal Declaration of Human Rights

“ Confidentiality means different things to different people and no consensus about definition or practice has ever been reached. I have been horrified on occasions at how confidentiality has been breached by staff, but this is mainly due to lack of training and supervision. ”

Jacki Pritchard, a trainer, in Good Practice in Supervision *(Jessica Kingsley, 1995)*

“ When a new resident joins us, I explain to them how we keep information about them. We give them a leaflet which tells them about our confidentiality policy. This includes how they can see their own file and make their own contributions to it. I show them the filing cabinet in the office so that they can see that it's kept securely locked. All this is aimed at reassuring them that we will keep their affairs private. ”

senior care officer at a residential home for elders

2.5.1 **Promoting good interactions through confidentiality**

Preserving confidentiality and establishing trust is the key to promoting good relationships and interaction. Without this trust, workers would not be able to offer the care and support needed by clients. The client must feel confident that they can talk to the worker and know that the information they've given:

- will be kept private
- will be passed on only with their consent
- will be passed only to a person who needs to know
- can be corrected if it is recorded or passed on inaccurately.

The relationship between the client and worker must be based on trust so that the client will feel able to disclose sensitive information and feel confident that it will not be misused. There are many situations where such disclosure may be central to understanding a client's needs and how best to help them. Examples of such information are:

- an embarrassing medical condition
- a history of mental illness
- details of financial resources or needs
- disclosure of abuse.

Confidentiality also governs the way that workers, either within the same organisation or in different agencies, seek information from or share information with each other. This communication is essential if clients are to receive the care and support they need. Information will include personal details, the reason they need the service, the assessment of their needs and details of the service or help they are being given.

Essential patient information must be able to pass between the NHS, local authority social services and other services where those agencies are contributing to or planning a programme of care, or where one may need to be initiated. The client needs to be aware that some information will be shared; this can usually be discussed during the care planning process. Where a patient's information is shared with another agency, there should be agreements on how it will be treated and stored according to specified security standards.

If the client raises objections, the possible consequences for a coordinated care programme should be explained and assurances given that other agencies would receive only information that they really need to know. However, the client's ultimate decision should be respected unless there are overriding considerations to the contrary, as discussed in section 2.5.2.

Even within organisations, a great deal of information passes between workers. This should be done on the basis of the 'need to know'. For example, when staff on a ward or a residential care home change shift, information about what has happened to the clients and details about their future care are reported. This could include explaining why one person is particularly upset.

Although health and social care organisations have policies and procedures for dealing with the collection, recording and passing of information, workers are themselves responsible for implementing them.

ACTIVITY

Mrs Jones, a resident of a home, is upset because her daughter is unwell. Which of the following would it be a breach of confidentiality to give information to?

- another care worker when handing over at the end of the shift
- the line manager in supervision
- Mrs Jones' former neighbour when she telephones to ask about her
- another care worker while waiting for the bus after work.

Can you give reasons why, in some of these instances, it would be necessary to give this information to another person? What action could the worker take to reassure Mrs Jones?

Workers are accountable to their agencies and their management. This means that they can't give a complete guarantee that information will not be given to others within the agency. Workers will need to record and pass on information about the health and wellbeing of the client to other carers – perhaps at changes in shifts in residential care or where responsibility for care is shared.

Because all workers are supervised by a more experienced person, they will need to discuss clients in order to develop their own skills and practice. This is a safeguard for clients because it ensures that workers are subject to oversight and advice in how they carry out their work. There should be no problem about this if workers are open with their clients about this relationship.

There will be occasions when the agency or workers from several agencies will be required to make decisions about the client or their care. It may be that a court may require a report.

On most day-to-day occasions, the worker is able to deal with this dual responsibility by explaining to a client:
- the reason why the information is being sought
- whether it will be recorded and held on file
- who else will be told the information.

Normally, the worker will also gain the client's consent for passing the information to someone else.

Finally, workers cannot keep to themselves information that might concern action that would harm the client or others, or is criminal. This is not a matter of client choice but an obligation that the worker is under. If, for example, a parent were to tell their social worker that they had severely beaten their child, the social worker would have to explain to them that this information would have to be shared with others, including the police, and could result in court proceedings. They will be seeking to gain the client's agreement that this information should be shared.

What dilemmas are there in maintaining confidentiality?

Agency rules do not always help care workers avoid dilemmas. When the client/worker relationship is close, the client will give the worker a lot of personal information. Much of this may not be recorded. One of the hardest situations for a care worker is: 'I'm telling you this but I don't want anyone else to know.' This is difficult because a worker will want to respect a confidence since breaking this trust could affect the relationship between the two. However, nearly all agencies would agree that such a confidence should be broken if someone's welfare was at risk. The best way for workers to handle this situation is for the worker to explain that they cannot give such a blanket guarantee.

Myra has epilepsy and is on daily medication to manage her condition. She attends a further education college and has been talking with the student welfare officer about problems with studying. She tells him that because she doesn't like the side effects of the medicine, she occasionally 'forgets' to take it.

He is concerned and asks Myra what could happen if she didn't have the proper amount of medicine. Myra is very clear about the consequences. The welfare officer reinforces this and explains that other students could be upset if she had a fit at college. It's clear that Myra is not going to talk to her doctor about the side effects, and so he offers to tell the doctor on her behalf.

What should he do if Myra disagrees?

What is the client's right to know?

This principle of the right to know is usually extended to mean that clients have a right to have the information explained in a way that they can understand. It also means that organisations expect records to be compiled with client access in mind. However, there still remains a problem where records were compiled before this change in practice. Organisations usually ask for these older records to be summarised before being seen by the client. Workers need to refer to the organisation's policy and seek guidance from responsible officers.

There are exceptions when clients will not be able to see all information on their files. This is usually where that information is about another person or could cause harm to the client. Some of the reasons are to protect:

- sources of information (e.g. informers, relatives, police, teachers or specialists)
- other parties (e.g. a parent placing a child for adoption)
- the rights and confidentiality of others
- the worker themselves where the information could place them in danger or hinder the achievement of the case objectives.

Withholding information on the grounds that it might be uncomfortable or inconvenient to the organisation or the workers, or it is easier not to do so, is not justifiable.

SEEING THE RECORDS

Bob is 17. He had been 'in care' since his mother died when he was only three, apart from six months in a children's home when he was twelve. Now he plans to go to college and wants to see his records so that he can begin his adult life with a clear picture of his past. Myrtle, his social worker, has talked to him about doing this and is certain that he understands that he might be unsettled by some of the things in his file. He's accepted her offer to support him through the process.

Bob wrote to the appropriate manager in the Social Services Department to ask to see his files and was given an appointment to go into the Area Office 25 days after his letter was received. He knew that he would not see everything in his file because material by or about third parties can be withheld where that person has not given their consent. In addition, the manager might decide that some of the material would seriously damage his mental or physical health.

Myrtle prepared Bob for his appointment. She then checked that the file was complete and up to date and that she could answer any questions Bob might ask. She explained that he would not be able to take anything out of the file but that he could have extracts from any of the records.

When Bob looked through his records, he noticed a note from his time at the children's home that he thought untrue. He queried it with Myrtle, who spoke with the manager. Together it was decided that Bob was right and it was agreed to correct the record. At the end, Bob signed that he had had access to the file.

Ensuring confidentiality

The need for confidentiality is underpinned by legislation, the requirements of the Department of Health, professional codes of practice and organisational procedures. These clearly state what is expected of the worker in relation to:

- conversation
- records
- exchanging information
- resolving dilemmas and conflicts.

Organisational confidentiality

The *Code of Practice on Openness in the NHS* was published in April 1995. It sets out basic principles of public access to information about the NHS. The code covers NHS organisations as well as family doctors, dentists, opticians and community pharmacists. Its aims are to ensure that people:

- have access to information about the services provided by the NHS, their costs, quality standards, and performance against targets
- are provided with explanations about proposed service changes and have the opportunity to influence decisions on such changes
- are aware of the reasons for decisions and actions affecting their treatment
- know what information is available and where they can get it from.

Information available under the Code of Openness

Apart from some exemptions, NHS trusts and authorities must make available the following information:

- what services are provided, the targets and standards set and the results achieved, as well as the cost and effectiveness of services
- details about important proposals on health policies or proposed changes in service delivery
- how health services are managed and provided, and who is responsible
- how the NHS communicates with the public, including details of public meetings, consultations, suggestions and complaints procedures
- how to contact the Community Health Council and the Health Service Commissioner
- how people can have access to their personal health records.

The code recommends that no charge should be made for information in the majority of cases.

Information that may be withheld

NHS trusts and authorities must provide information unless it falls into one of the following categories:

- personal information – people have a right of access to their own health records but not normally to information about other people
- requests for information which are 'manifestly unreasonable', too general, or would require unreasonable resources to answer
- information about internal discussion and advice, where disclosure would harm frank internal debate (except where this would be outweighed by the public interest)
- management information, where disclosure would harm the proper and effective management of the NHS

- information about legal matters and proceedings, where disclosure would prejudice the administration of justice and the law
- information which could prejudice negotiations or the effective conduct of personnel management, or commercial or contractual activities
- information given in confidence – the NHS has a common law duty to respect confidences except where this is clearly outweighed by the public interest
- information that would soon be published or where disclosure would be premature in relation to a planned announcement or publication
- information relating to incomplete analysis, research or statistics where disclosure could be misleading or prevent the holder from publishing it first.

The Caldicott committee's report of December 1997 made recommendations aimed at improving the way the NHS handles and protects confidential patient information. These include:

- protocols to govern the sharing of information between NHS organisations and its partner organisations
- training and awareness-raising of confidentiality security issues among NHS staff at all levels
- the appointment of a local guardian of patient information in each NHS organisation.

In January 1999 chief executives of NHS organisations were required to appoint a guardian, who should be a senior health official.

ACTIVITY

Contact your local NHS trust to find out who is their guardian and write a short report on their role.

2.5.4 **Openness**

All health and social care organisations, whether the NHS, local authorities, voluntary organisations or private agencies, should have an active policy for informing clients of the purposes for which information about them is collected, and the categories of people or organisations to which information may need to be passed. For example, where other bodies are providing services for, or in conjunction with, the NHS, those concerned must be aware of each others' information policies.

In the NHS, subject to important common elements the precise arrangements for informing patients are for local decision, taking account of views expressed by community health councils, local patient groups, staff, and agencies with which the NHS body is in close contact. However, those concerned should bear in mind that:

- as a general rule, patients should be told how information would be used before they are asked to provide it and must have the opportunity to discuss any aspects that are special to their treatment or circumstances
- advice must be presented in a convenient form and be available both for general purposes and before a particular programme begins.

Methods of providing information to clients include:

- leaflets enclosed with patients' appointment letters or provided when prescriptions are dispensed
- GP practice leaflets and/or notification on initial registration with a GP
- routinely providing patients with necessary information as a part of care planning
- identifying someone to provide further information if patients want it.

Patients registering with a GP should be made aware that certain basic personal information will be kept on a central register.

Clients' rights of access to their own records

Individuals also have rights of access under:

- the Data Protection Act 1999 which, with some exemptions, entitles individuals to a copy of computerised information held about them
- the Access to Personal Files Act 1987 which concerns personal information held by local authority social services and may therefore be relevant in cases of joint care
- the Access to Medical Reports Act 1988 in respect of reports for employers and insurance companies.

The Patient's Charter includes 'the right to have access to your health records':

- Subject to certain safeguards, patients may see their own manual health records made after 1 November 1991 and earlier records if they are necessary to understand the later ones. Patients do not have to give reasons for seeking access.
- Although there is no general statutory right to see manual records made before November 1991, access should be given whenever possible, subject to the judgement of the health professionals responsible for the patient's care and safeguards for other people who may have provided information about the patient.
- There is specific guidance on access to records made at any time sought in connection with legal proceedings.

Social services departments and voluntary organisations will offer the same rights to their clients. Some services operate an open file policy that will encourage clients to see their files, make alterations and share responsibility for making records.

Giving medical records to patients to keep at home is being introduced in some GP practices or hospital services. Pregnant women, for instance, have their own records so that they can take them to the different clinics and specialists they have to see.

Security and accuracy

Ensuring the security and accuracy of client information is a responsibility of management and staff at all levels. In particular:

- arrangements for the storage and disposal of all client information (both manually recorded and computer-based) must protect confidentiality

- security measures must be in place to protect information, including information on the networking systems
- care should be taken to ensure that unintentional breaches of confidence do not occur (e.g. by not leaving files, fax machines or computer terminals unattended, double-checking to avoid transmitting information to the wrong person, not allowing sensitive conversations to be overheard, guarding against people seeking information by deception).

Individual workers

❝ *While visiting my mum in a nursing home one evening, I overheard two nurses writing up patient records asking, 'What's that word for patients passing a lot of urine at night? Is it "nocturia"? Let's look it up in the dictionary.' I thought, if they have to look it up, the other nurses probably won't understand it either.* **❞**

carer

A simple remedy to this situation is the 'Right' rule. Avoid using words unless you're comfortable with them, and know that they are the right words. Then use:
- the right word
- at the right time
- for the right thing
- knowing that the meaning is right too.

Written records

Written communications are effectively delayed and indirect interactions. They involve important skills that have much in common with verbal interactions. The written word may be more distant and impersonal (but can also be very personal – e-mails from loved ones, love letters, poetry). Certainly there is a permanence that a telephone call lacks.

When writing official documents, health and social workers are often faced with the problem of knowing what to write, and how to write it. Sometimes we literally can't remember a word, or more often we try to use words we don't fully understand.

It is important, therefore, that written records are clear, accurate, comprehensive and informative. Records need to:
- be factual, consistent and accurate
- be written as soon as possible after an event has occurred, providing current information on the care and condition of the patient
- be written clearly and in such a manner that any alterations or additions are dated, timed and signed so that the original entry can still be read clearly
- be accurately dated, timed and signed, with the signature printed alongside the first entry
- avoid abbreviations, jargon, meaningless phrases
- exclude irrelevant speculation and offensive subjective statements
- be readable as a photocopy
- be written wherever possible with the involvement of the client or their carer
- be written in terms that the client can understand

ACTIVITY

Examine the various forms involved in care plans, for example those used for looking after children. See how the forms relate to each other and will provide long-term, working documents as well as essential basic information for use in emergency.

- be consecutive
- identify problems that have arisen and the action taken to rectify them
- provide clear evidence of the care planned, the decisions made, the care delivered and the information shared.

Much written communication in health and social care involves the completion of standard forms and reports. These have been designed to:
- contain all the information required in a consistent format
- meet quality standards (relating to equal opportunities and other legislation)
- enable processing, storage and retrieval.

2.5.5 Legislation

Although equal opportunities legislation, and the Acts which determine how health and social services are organised, support confidentiality, the major pieces of legislation which cover confidentiality are the:
- Access to Personal Files Act 1987
- Access to Medical Reports Act 1988
- Data Protection Act 1998.

Individual rights to privacy have been strengthened further through the Human Rights Act 1998 (coming into force from October 2000). This will extend protection in relation to people caught on closed-circuit television (CCTV). The Freedom of Information Act 2000 is likely to extend the rights of individuals to have access to information about them held in official records.

Access to Personal Files 1987
This extended the right of individuals to see personal information on their housing and social services files. Not all information is available, as information concerning third parties is excluded.

Access to Medical Reports Act 1988
This gives individual rights of access to medical reports in certain circumstances, supplied by a medical worker and prepared for employment or insurance purposes.

Data Protection Act 1998
This Act replaces and updates the Data Protection Act 1984. This earlier legislation gave individuals rights in relation to the growing computerisation of information. Individuals were given the right to know what data was held on them and the right to compensation where the data was incorrect. It placed on organisations the requirement to register with the Data Protection Registrar (now called Data Protection Commissioner) the type, purpose and recipient of their data kept on computers. It required organisations to hold only information that is appropriate to their registration.

The eight principles of the Data Protection Act 1998

1 Data must be processed fairly and lawfully.

2 Data must be processed for a specified purpose.

3 Data must be adequate, relevant and not excessive.

4 Data must be accurate and up to date.

5 Data must not be kept longer than necessary.

6 Data must be processed in accordance with the rights of the individual.

7 Appropriate technical and organisational measures are taken.

8 Personal data transferred outside the European Community must have a level of protection similar to the UK or EC.

The 1998 Act makes changes to eight principles set out in the 1984 Act and strengthens the rights of individuals so that in relation to information held on them, they are entitled to:

- be given a description of the data
- be given any information concerning the source of the data
- know the purpose for which the data is being processed
- know the type of individual or organisation to whom the data may be disclosed
- be informed of the logic behind any automated decision-making process
- prevent the processing of data where this may cause damage or distress
- prevent processing of data for direct marketing purposes
- seek compensation for damages caused by failure to comply with the Act
- information in a format intelligible to the individual who is subject to the data.

Protection has been extended to cover manual (paper) structured files so that data subjects can see information held about them in paper record-keeping systems. There are some exemptions; for example employees will not be able to see employment references about them supplied in confidence.

Implementation dates

The provisions of the Act are being introduced over a number of years:

- organisations registered under the 1984 Act are valid until October 2001
- manual files will come into the scheme in October 2001
- manual files are exempt from the requirement to be kept for a specified purpose and not being kept for too long until October 2007.

Under the Act individual employees can be held liable for breaches if it can be proved that they have acted wilfully or with neglect.

One consequence of the Act is that any organisation collecting personal data on forms must provide a statement that has three elements:

- identification of the organisation collecting the data
- statement of purpose for which data will be used
- identification of organisations and individuals to whom the data will be disclosed.

Much stricter conditions apply to the processing of sensitive data, which includes information relating to racial or ethnic origin, political opinions, religious or other beliefs, trade union membership, health, sex life and criminal convictions. Where this information is being collected and processed, the data subject generally has to give explicit consent.

Health and social care organisations need to take reasonable safeguards to protect personal data held on computer or in their files. There should be procedures for staff dealing with:

- collecting information from clients
- keeping information on computer or files
- giving this information to third parties.

ACTIVITY

Find out and note down the *original* eight principles of the Data Protection Act and the implications for health and social care organisations of implementing them. What are the implications of implementing the new provisions? What problems might be envisaged in care settings and how can they be overcome? Detailed information and guidance are available on the Internet: *http://www.dti.open.uk/ dpr/dprhome.htm* and *http://www.open.gov.uk/ dpr/prepare.htm* or from the New Law Section, Office of the Data Protection Registrar, Wycliffe House, Water Lane, Wilmslow, Cheshire SK9 5AF.

Key questions

1 What information may a client tell a worker, if they can trust that worker?

2 Who is covered by the NHS *Code of Practice on Openness*?

3 Name three Acts of Parliament that affect clients' rights regarding confidentiality.

4 In what circumstances will a worker pass on information without the client's consent?

5 What types of information are covered by the Data Protection Act 1998?

6 How can a worker ensure that written material is secure?

7 Explain the grounds on which NHS trusts and authorities may withhold information from clients.

8 Who do organisations register with under the Data Protection Act?

9 What is the 'Right' rule about using words in written communications?

10 List up to five characteristics of well-completed client records.

Assignment

Produce a report examining communication skills within either a health, social care or early years setting. You will also need to produce records that show your effective communication skills in one one-to-one interaction and one group interaction. The client group must be different for each interaction.

Key skills

You can use the work you are doing for this part of your GNVQ to collect and develop evidence for the following key skills at level 3.

when you	you can collect evidence for
	communication
take part in fish bowl exercises, decision-making forums and team-building, roleplay communication skills, take part in counselling-type training, use communication skills in real-life interactions, and take part in task-orientated group work	key skill C3.1a contribute to a group discussion about a complex subject
present communication skills using audio and video recordings	key skill C3.1b make a presentation about a complex subject, using at least one image to illustrate complex points
research appropriate legislation	key skill C3.2 read and synthesise information from two extended documents about a complex subject; one of these documents should include a least one image
explain the factors that influence communication, and write scripts	key skill C3.3 write two different types of document about complex subjects; one piece of writing should be an extended document and include at least one image
	improving own learning and performance
assess your own communication skills	key skill LP3.1 agree targets and plan how these will be met, using support from appropriate others
develop your communication skills	key skill LP3.2 use the plan, seeking and using feedback and support from relevant sources to help meet the targets, and use different ways of learning to meet new demands
demonstrate your communication skills and review your progress	key skill LP3.3 review progress in meeting targets, establishing evidence of achievements, and agree action for improving
	working with others
plan team-building and task-oriented group work	key skill WO3.1 plan the activity with others, agreeing objectives, responsibilities and working arrangements
take part in team-building and task-oriented group work	key skill WO3.2 work towards achieving the agreed objectives seeking to establish and maintain cooperative working relationships in meeting responsibilities
review the group activities	key skill WO3.3 review the activity with others against the agreed objective and agree ways of enhancing collaborative work

UNIT 3

Physical aspects of health

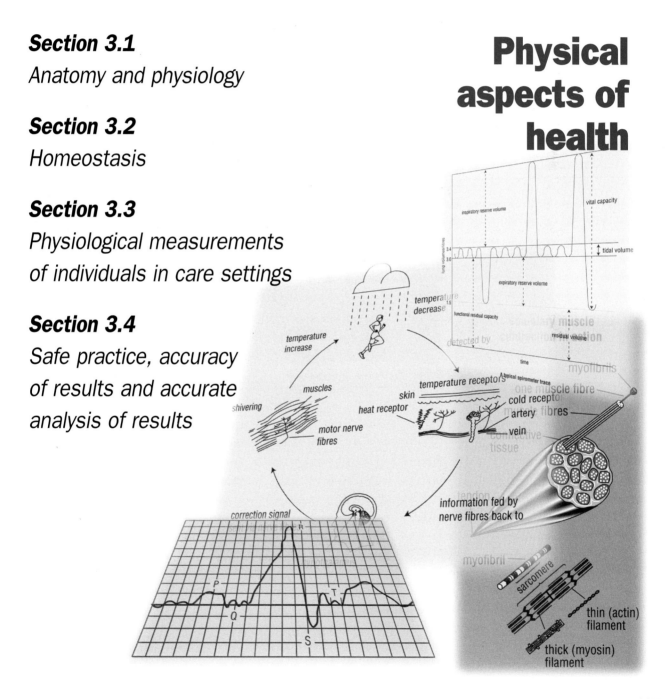

About this unit

This unit explains the basic anatomy and physiology of the major systems of the body. You will observe and record the physiological measurements of individuals in care settings.

You will learn:

- about human body systems
- how body systems depend on one another to function effectively
- to recognise measurements that fall outside the expected range
- to apply science in a care context

The unit complements unit 4 Factors affecting human growth and development. The work you carry out for these units will help you understand the science of some aspects of health promotion. It will also provide a firm basis for the science-based optional units such as unit 13 Physiology for health care.

66 *Although it is important to seek to understand the intricate internal workings of the body using a range of scientific methods, you need to remember that the body is not simply a machine. A range of influences on the body, such as heredity, developmental defects, environmental, cultural and lifestyle choices all contribute to an individual's experience and perception of their own health.* **99**

health promotion specialist

Anatomy and physiology

To understand control mechanisms in the body you must know about the structures and systems within the body and how they work. Control mechanisms help to maintain the normal functions of the body. People working in health, social care and early years need to understand the ways in which the human body works normally and how to recognise the abnormal.

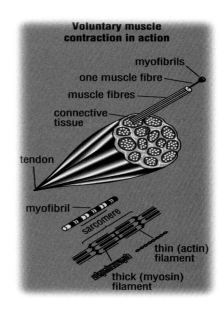

Voluntary muscle contraction in action

myofibrils
one muscle fibre
muscle fibres
connective tissue
tendon
myofibril
sarcomere
thin (actin) filament
thick (myosin) filament

The major cell components

You need to be aware of the roles of cells and tissues in order to understand the disease processes which clients may display. Cells are the simplest structural and functional units from which organisms – including human beings – are made.

Cells are too small to be seen with the naked eye – human body cells are between about one-hundredth of a millimetre and one-tenth of a millimetre in size. (The largest human cell is the female ovum.) Since the development of the electron microscope biologists have developed much greater understanding of the structure of cells.

There are many different types of cell in the human body; they vary in size, shape, composition and function, but they all have certain similar characteristics in structure and activity.

As cells develop, their structure changes to allow them to fulfil special functions efficiently. Specialised cells act together to form tissues, which are then used in making organs. In turn, organs work together to form body systems with a particular function.

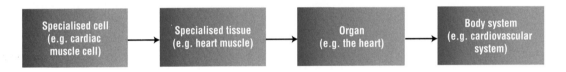

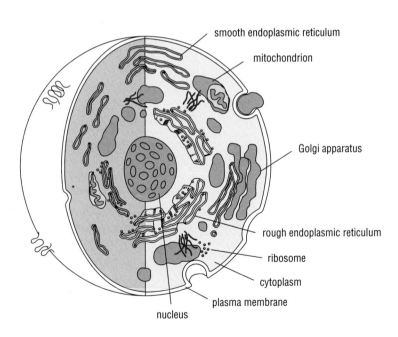

Look at a micrograph of a human body cell, and identify:

- plasma membrane
- endoplasmic reticulum
- mitochondria
- ribosomes
- nucleus.

Calculate the distance across the middle of the nucleus using the information given about magnification.

Based on your observations, draw a diagram showing the main parts of a cell. To go with your diagram, write a short paragraph explaining the structure and function of each part.

The cell is held together by a thin boundary, often called the plasma membrane. Inside this membrane is the cytoplasm, which contains the different components of the cell suspended in a fluid called cytosol. These components – known as organelles – have their own structures and purposes. They include:

- endoplasmic reticulum
- ribosomes
- mitochondria
- nucleus.

Cell membrane

The cell or plasma membrane is the outer boundary of the cell. It:

- holds together the cell's contents
- stops the cell's contents mixing with substances outside the cell or in neighbouring cells
- controls what substances enter and leave the cell.

Features of the main tissue types

Most cells don't function on their own in the body. Instead, cells with a similar form or function join together to make tissues. The study of tissues is called histology.

Just as the cells of one type vary in composition, size, shape and arrangement from those of another, the intercellular substance varies in its nature and amount. It may be dense and hard, fluid or gel, or may exist as fibres. It may be rigid or pliable, elastic or non-elastic, tough or fragile. The ratio of cells to intercellular substance also varies according to the type of tissue.

Tissues consist of several different types of cell. The cells in tissue are surrounded by tissue fluid, which carries materials in to and out of the cells. This tissue is also known as extracellular fluid and constitutes about half of our total body fluid. Intracellular and extracellular fluid have to be kept at a constant composition, chemical reaction and temperature (homeostasis) in order to maintain function and health.

Types of tissue

The four main types of tissue in the human body are:

- epithelial – provides protection and secretes substances
- connective – supports the body
- muscular – controls movement
- nervous – communicates messages around the body.

Variations exist in the tissues of these major categories as the cells are adapted to meet the various needs of the body. Within each main type of tissue there are also several specialised sub-types.

Epithelial tissue

Epithelial tissues function in protection, secretion, absorption and filtration. They cover all external and internal surfaces, and are found as well in secreting structures. They consist mainly of cells with a minimal amount of intercellular substance. Epithelial cells reproduce frequently, which is essential to maintain the surface and lining tissues.

Examples of epithelial tissues include:

- the skin
- mucous and serous membranes
- the endothelial lining of the blood and lymph vessels and heart chambers.

Simple squamous

This is simple epithelial tissue, consisting of one layer of flat, thin, irregularly shaped cells, each with a nucleus in the middle. The bottom of each cell sits on the basement membrane; the top surface is free. Cells are packed together closely, with little fluid between them. (Simple squamous tissue is sometimes called pavement epithelium.) This sort of tissue is found in, for example:

- blood vessels
- lymphatic vessels
- lung alveoli.

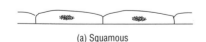

(a) Squamous

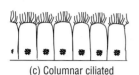
(b) Cuboidal

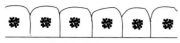
(c) Columnar ciliated

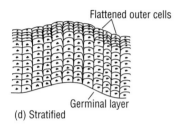
Flattened outer cells

Germinal layer
(d) Stratified

Cuboidal
This is simple epithelial tissue, consisting of one layer of cube-shaped cells. They are found in kidney tubules and they cover the ovaries.

Columnar
These are also simple epithelial tissue, consisting of one layer of elongated, column-shaped cells. They often have cilia (small hairs) on the top surface. This type of tissue can be found in the lining of the digestive system.

Stratified squamous epithelium
This is compound epithelial tissue, consisting of many layers of cells. The lower layers are cuboidal or columnar, the top layers are flatter (squamous). The lowest layer of cells sits on the basement membrane. Examples can be found in the lining of the:

- mouth
- tongue
- vagina
- oesophagus
- rectum.

They are also contained in the skin (with an extra layer of dead cells for protection).

Connective tissue
Connective tissues are mainly concerned with the physical form and mechanical activities of the body as opposed to its physiological activities. They are the most common types of tissue in the body. They provide an internal supporting framework, protection for other structures and connections between parts of the body in order to make them a functional unit. The intercellular substance has a vital role in connective tissue, and gives these tissues their special characteristics. Examples include:

- bones
- tendons
- ligaments
- cartilage
- fascia
- adipose tissue.

Blood is also classified as a connective tissue, although in this instance the cells have an equally significant role as the intercellular substance, the plasma.

Blood
Blood is a vital connective tissue, which:
- carries oxygen to every part of the body
- plays an important role in the body's immune system
- supplies glucose to tissues and organs
- carries away waste products.

ACTIVITY

Carry out research to find out the proportion of white blood cells (leucocytes) you would expect to find in:

- a healthy adult
- someone with an infection
- someone with lymphatic leukaemia
- someone suffering an allergic reaction.

Explain your findings.

A fluid matrix called plasma, which comprises over half the total volume of blood, surrounds blood cells. The following table shows the structure and function of different types of blood cells contained within this matrix.

Cell	Structure	Function

Red blood cells (erythrocytes)

Red blood cells (erythrocytes)

2.5µm
(a) 7µm (b)
(a) = plan
(b) = section

- no nucleus
- contain the red pigment haemoglobin
- don't contain ribosomes, so can't produce proteins, grow or repair
- survive in the blood for about four months

Collect oxygen from the lungs and deliver it to the body's tissues. There are over a thousand times as many red cells as white cells.

White blood cells (leucocytes)

Lymphocytes

10µm

- no granules in cytoplasm
- relatively large nucleus
- appear spherical

Produce and may carry antibodies, and play an important part in the body's immune system in response to infection.

Monocytes

16µm

- no granules in cytoplasm
- large cell
- kidney-shaped nucleus

Detect chemical substances produced by bacteria, move towards the bacteria, and engulf them in a process called phagocytosis.

Neutrophils

12µm

- granules in cytoplasm
- irregular nucleus, usually with three to five bumps

Locate and engulf bacteria (as monocytes, above).

Basophils

10µm

- spherical granules in cytoplasm
- kidney-shaped nucleus

Produce histamine.

Eosinophils

12µm

- granules in cytoplasm
- c-shaped nucleus

Involved in responding to allergic reactions. The number of eosinophils in the blood increases rapidly during an allergic reaction.

Muscle tissue

The three types of muscle tissue are:

■ skeletal muscular tissue (also known as 'voluntary' or 'striated' muscle tissue)

■ smooth muscular tissue (also known as 'involuntary' or 'unstriated' muscle tissue)

■ cardiac muscular tissue (only found in the walls of the heart).

Skeletal muscular tissue

As its name suggests, skeletal muscular tissue is attached to the body's skeleton (bones), and controls its movement. It is made up of long cylindrical muscle fibres, which are controlled voluntarily. This means that an individual can decide to walk, chew, smile, talk and so on, and control the contraction of the appropriate muscles.

Some muscles contain up to a thousand muscle fibres, each of which is a single muscle cell and may be as long as 30 cm. These are held together in a bundle by collagen (a protein which forms the basis of bones). In turn, each muscle fibre contains a bundle of smaller sub-fibres called myofibrils, made of tiny protein filaments. These lie in line with one another, and make skeletal muscular tissue look striped (striated) when it is viewed under a microscope.

Smooth muscular tissue

Smooth muscular tissue is also known as involuntary muscle, because it isn't usually controlled consciously by the individual. Unlike skeletal muscular tissue, it doesn't have a striped appearance when viewed under a microscope. (It is unstriated.)

Voluntary muscle contraction in action

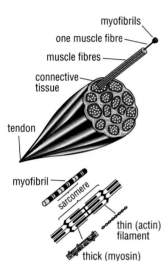

Smooth muscular tissue

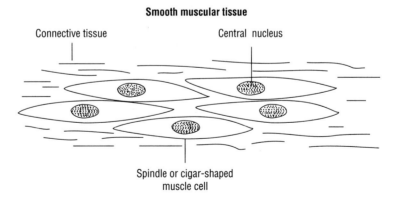

Smooth muscular tissue is made up of spindle-shaped muscle cells containing one nucleus, joined together in sheets. These sheets run in muscle layers around and down cylindrical organs such as blood vessels, the intestines, the bladder, the respiratory tract and the uterus. The muscular tissue enables the organ to contract and relax rhythmically on its own:

- contraction of the muscle cells running around the organ causes it to become narrower
- contraction of the muscle cells running down the organ cause it to become longer (and sometimes wider).

Cardiac muscular tissue

Cardiac muscular tissue is only found in the walls of the heart. Like skeletal muscle, it has a striped (striated) appearance, but like smooth muscle it can't be controlled consciously. (Movement is involuntary.)

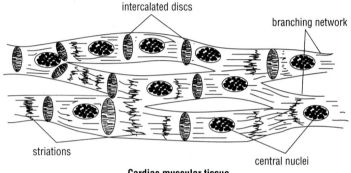

Cardiac muscular tissue

Cardiac muscular tissue is made up of branching muscle fibres that are interconnected and spread in a network across the heart. The fibres are divided into individual muscle cells by intercalated discs, made of several layers of membranes. These discs strengthen the muscle fibres, and help to conduct the electrical stimulus called the cardiac impulse, which causes the whole heart muscle to contract and relax rhythmically. Each individual muscle cell has a central nucleus, and many mitochondria that provide the energy needed for contraction.

Compact bone

Compact bone is the most dense and rigid tissue found in the body, and is opaque on an X-ray. It is found on the outside of all bones, and inside long bones of the skeleton (such as the femur). Its function is to:

- bear the weight of the body
- protect and support other tissues
- withstand the stresses of movement.

The inter-cellular matrix of compact bone contains:

- a network of collagen fibres, which enable the bone to bear strain and ensure that it is not too brittle
- mineral salts (in particular, complex phosphates of calcium), which impregnate the collagen; these give the bone great strength and hardness.

Compact bone tissue is made up of Haversian systems, which appear as a series of concentric rings (lamellae). At the centre of the lamellae are channels

DISCUSSION POINT

As people get older, the amount of collagen and mineral salts in the matrix of their compact bone decreases. What effect do you think this has?

called Haversian canals, which contain blood vessels, lymphatic vessels and nerves. These connect with the periosteum (the tough membrane surrounding bones), and with the marrow (where red and white blood cells are produced). Within the lamellae there are small spaces called lacunae, where bone cells (osteocytes) are found. These secrete the bone matrix, and are linked by a series of fine channels.

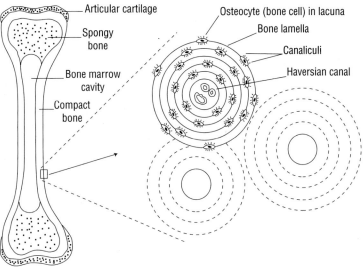
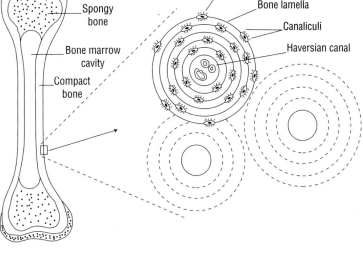

Nervous tissue

Nervous tissue is made up of nerve cells called neurons. The most important property of neurons is excitability. They:

■ are sensitive to stimuli, producing nerve impulses

■ transmit nerve impulses to other neurons or effectors (parts of the body which do things, or 'effect' action).

In doing so, they act as the body's rapid communication system.

Sensory neurons react to stimuli from the internal and external environment. Receptor organs – which control vision, hearing, smell and taste are connected directly to the brain by short nerve tracts. Other sensory information is carried to the central nervous system (brain and spinal cord) from receptor nerve endings in the joints, skin, muscles, tendons and internal organs.

The central nervous system (CNS) processes the information it receives from sensory neurons. If action is necessary, motor neurons conduct impulses from the CNS to effector organs, triggering a response such as contraction of a muscle, or secretion in a gland.

Like other cells, neurons have a cell body containing a nucleus and cytoplasm. However, they also have dendrites and an axon, fibres that project from the cell body and give it its unique shape and excitability.

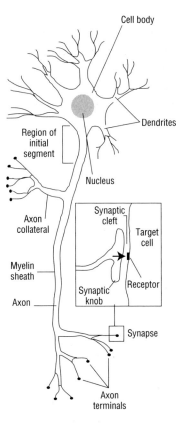

A motor neurone

ACTIVITY

Excitability depends on potassium ions inside the neuron and sodium ions outside it. Find out more about:

- how these ions enable neurons to receive and transmit impulses
- how excitability enables neurons to communicate.

Dendrites are fine branching fibres that receive impulses from other neurons and conduct them to the cell body. The **axon** is a long, single nerve fibre that conducts impulses away from the cell body. It is branched at the end, with small swellings called **boutons**, which form the junctions with other neurons. Often, the axon is covered by a **myelin sheath**, a casing of fatty materials, which insulates the fibre and increases the speed at which impulses are conducted. In human beings, most cell bodies are in the brain or spinal cord, and axons may be over a metre long in order to reach an organ.

DISCUSSION POINT

Having explored the four main tissue types, discuss how their features relate to their function. How is muscular tissue designed for movement rather than communication? Why is epithelial tissue protective rather than supportive?

3.1.3 Interpreting micrographs to identify tissue types

A **micrograph** is a photograph of a sample viewed through a light microscope. An **electron micrograph** is a photograph of a sample viewed through an electron microscope.

Scientists examine cells and tissues using a microscope. To prepare a section of tissue for viewing under a light microscope, a piece of dead tissue is preserved in a fixing fluid and dehydrated with ethanol. It is then cleaned with an organic solvent and embedded in molten wax. When the wax hardens, a thin section of the tissue is cut and attached to a microscope slide. The wax is removed, and the tissue is stained to accentuate contrasts and make it easier to see tissue and cell structures.

ACTIVITY

Ask the biology department at your school or college if they have any examples of micrographs you could look at. If possible, also borrow slides of prepared sections you can look at under a microscope.

Micrographs of epithelial tissue

DISCUSSION POINT

In a group, look at these two micrographs and identify which is simple squamous epithelial tissue, and which is stratified squamous epithelial tissue. In each case, identify key features of the tissue.

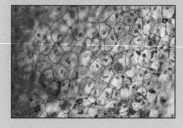 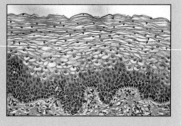

Micrographs of connective tissue

DISCUSSION POINT

In a group identify which of the micrographs on the right is of blood, and which is of compact bone. Once you have decided which is which, find the following features:

- erythrocytes
- leucocytes
- plasma
- a Haversian system
- a Haversian canal
- lamellae
- lacunae.

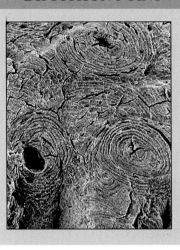

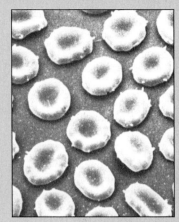

Micrograph of muscular tissue

ACTIVITY

This micrograph shows a sample of striated muscular tissue. Draw a diagram of the tissue based on the micrograph, identifying key features, and write a paragraph explaining how these key features relate to the tissue's function.

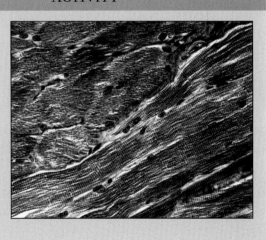

To stay alive the human body needs to deal with the environment – we need to breathe, eat, drink, get rid of waste products and to sense where we are and what's going on. The body's systems all interrelate to make these happen.

The nervous system is the dominant system of the body, providing an elaborate communication system. Working in relation to the endocrine system, the nervous system directs and integrates all of the body's activities.

The structural parts of the nervous system are the brain, spinal cord, nerves, ganglia, receptors and effectors. The brain and spinal cord comprise the central nervous system; the other parts form the peripheral nervous system.

Three main types of response are controlled by the nervous system:
- reflexes
- conscious response
- autonomic response.

Reflexes

A reflex is a quick automatic response to a particular stimulus – blinking, coughing, sneezing. Impulses from a sense organ (for example, the pain receptor in a finger as in the diagram) are carried along the sensory neurone to a dorsal root of the nerve cord. They move along a relay neurone, out of the nerve cord, along a motor neurone to the muscle. The muscle then responds to the stimulus. The example shows a pin pricking a finger and the muscles pulling the finger from the pin quickly and automatically. Such nerve connections are an example of a reflex arc.

Diagram of the main divisions of the nervous system

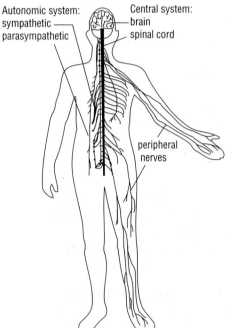

Autonomic system: sympathetic parasympathetic

Central system: brain spinal cord

peripheral nerves

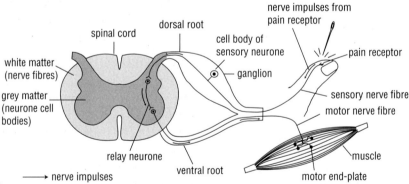

spinal cord • dorsal root • nerve impulses from pain receptor • white matter (nerve fibres) • cell body of sensory neurone • pain receptor • grey matter (neurone cell bodies) • ganglion • sensory nerve fibre • motor nerve fibre • relay neurone • ventral root • muscle • motor end-plate

⟶ nerve impulses

ACTIVITY

Find out what happens when drugs such as aspirin suppress a region of the brain which normally receives impulses from pain nerve endings. Write a brief summary of your findings.

Conscious response

This kind of response may begin with the sense organs or originate in the cerebrum of the brain.

Sense organs

These are connected to the brain or spinal cord by nerve fibres. When a sense organ is stimulated it sends electrical impulses along the nerve fibre that supplies it to the spinal cord and on to the brain.

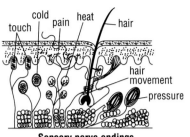

Sensory nerve endings (receptors) in the skin

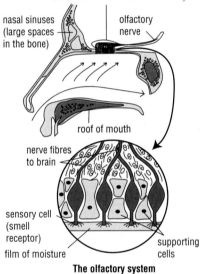

The olfactory system

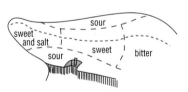

The position of taste receptors on the tongue

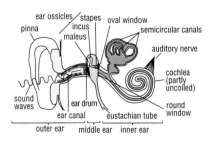

The sense organs include:

- touch receptors – these are sensitive to light pressure and help us to distinguish one texture from another
- pressure receptors – these are under the dermis and respond to heavy pressure
- pain receptors – branched nerve endings in the epidermis and other parts of the body
- temperature receptors – these help us to respond to hot and cold
- nerve receptors at the hair roots – movements of hair
- smell receptors – olfactory organs in the roof of the nasal passages
- taste receptors – the four types of taste bud (salt, sweet, sour, bitter) concentrated in different areas of the tongue
- sound mechanisms – the ear follicles which change sound waves into nerve impulses
- balance mechanisms – the semi-circular canals of the inner ear
- image receptor mechanisms – the rods and cones which form images on the retina of the eye.

The brain

Some theories say that because of the increasingly high level of effectiveness and specialisation of the sensory organs of the head of animals (eyes, ears, nose), more and more fibres entered the front part of the spinal cord. So in vertebrate animals, this region became very highly developed to form the brain. The more complex the lifestyle of the animal, the greater this brain development.

Conscious responses are thought to be the outcome of activity in the cortex of the brain. But human beings can suppress a huge amount of sensory data that comes into the cerebral hemispheres and single out the aspects they want to concentrate on.

An example of a conscious response involving your sense organs and the brain is the command to move your arm. The stages of this process are:
- you receive the command through your ear
- the message, translated into nerve impulses, travels through the auditory nerve to the brain
- the brain processes the information
- the brain then sends a motor impulse to the muscles of your arm.

A map of half of the cerebrum

Sensory areas receive impulses from sense organs. Motor areas control voluntary muscles. Association areas are connected with thought, memory, and emotion.

Speech occurs on one hemisphere only. All other areas occur on both hemispheres.

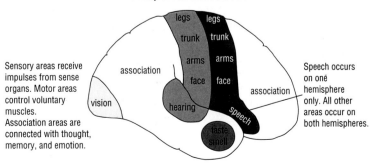

DISCUSSION POINT

List the sorts of information you are likely to be filtering out from your attention during activities such as reading your GNVQ book, meeting a friend for a chat, writing an exam or participating in a competitive sporting event.

ACTIVITY

Find out what happens to sensory information relayed to the cortex of the brain during sleep. Write an explanation of the process, describing what may occur on waking.

Autonomic response

Part of the nervous system coordinates internal, mainly involuntary, body activities such as:

- digestion
- blood pressure
- vasoconstriction
- the heartbeat
- peristaltic contractions in the alimentary canal.

ACTIVITY

Find out the main effects of the autonomic nervous system. Draw up a chart with three columns. On the left side list:

- stomach
- sweat glands
- eye iris
- pancreas
- genitals
- saliva glands
- heart
- bronchi
- urinary bladder
- gut sphincter.

At the top of the middle column put the heading 'sympathetic effect'.

In the right-hand column put the heading 'parasympathetic effect.'

Define the sympathetic and parasympathetic systems. Then describe in the appropriate column of your chart how each system affects each item listed on the left.

3.1.5 Endocrine system

The endocrine system is mainly concerned with:

- growth
- maturation
- metabolic processes
- reproduction.

It comprises a collection of glands situated around the body. A gland is an organ that extracts substances from the blood and produces one or more new chemical substances, known as secretions. An endocrine gland doesn't have ducts (unlike exocrine glands such as the salivary, gastric, mammary and sweat glands). The secretions made by endocrine glands are called hormones, and they pass directly into the blood and act on specialised tissues throughout the body.

The endocrine glands are:

- the pituitary gland
- the thyroid gland
- the four parathyroid glands
- the islets of Langerhans
- the two adrenal glands
- the two testes in males and the two ovaries in females.

Pituitary gland

The pituitary gland is sometimes known as the master gland or conductor of the endocrine orchestra because it has such a widespread effect throughout the body.

Thyroid gland

The thyroid gland secretes thyroxine, which regulates metabolism and secrets calcitoni, which regulates serum calcium levels and bone mineralisation.

Parathyroid glands

The parathyroid glands secrete parathormone, which regulates the levels of calcium in the blood.

Islets of Langerhans

These are tiny islands of specialised cells scattered throughout the pancreas. Alpha cells secrete glucagon and the beta cells secrete insulin. In a healthy person the interplay of these hormones regulate the blood glucose levels.

Adrenal glands

The adrenal gland of the cortex secretes corticosteroid hormones, which have a range of functions including:

- water balance
- anti-inflammatory properties
- influence on some of the sexual characteristics.

The medulla secretes adrenaline and noradrenaline, which are associated with any increase in emotion. They prepare the body for flight in response to fear, and fight in response to anger.

The testes

The testes glands secrete testosterone which is responsible for initiating and maintaining the male secondary sexual characteristics.

The ovaries

Ovaries secrete oestrogens, which give rise to female sexual characteristics. They are involved in the menstrual cycle. Ovaries also secrete progesterone, which plays a part in the menstrual cycle and is essential for pregnancy.

3.1.6 **Respiratory system**

A constant exchange of oxygen and carbon dioxide between the living organism and its environment is essential for survival. Respiration is the process that performs this function. The exchange takes place between the total organism and the environment and between the tissue cells and the blood. The former involves pulmonary (lung) ventilation and the diffusion of gases through the alveolar membrane of the lungs. The exchange between the cells and the blood (sometimes called internal or tissue respiration) requires transportation of the gases oxygen and carbon dioxide by the blood and diffusion of these gases between the capillaries and tissue cells.

Pulmonary ventilation or breathing consists of the movement of air in and out of the lungs (inspiration and expiration).

The respiratory system consists of the upper and lower respiratory tracts, respiratory muscles and the thorax.

The upper respiratory tract consists of the nose, mouth and pharynx. The highly vascular and ciliated mucous membrane lining the nose serves to warm, filter and moisten inhaled air. This then passes through the pharynx into the lower respiratory tract.

The lower respiratory tract consists of the larynx, trachea, bronchi and lungs.

Each major body system has several important roles. The respiratory system not only performs the vital function of external and internal respiration, but is also involved in:

Inspiration is the process in which air is drawn through the upper respiratory tract into the lungs. The contraction of the diaphragm and external intercostal muscles creates a situation in which air is drawn deep into the alveoli. The relaxation of these muscles reverses this process, and is called **expiration**.

- the production of speech and sound
- regulating the pH of body fluids through adjusting the amount of carbon dioxide eliminated
- helping to regulate the elimination of water and heat.

When the air reaches the alveoli diffusion takes place. Diffusion enables the process of internal respiration, in which oxygen is transported into individual cells. Gases move rapidly from areas of higher to lower pressure. Oxygen moves across the thin, elastic, semi-permeable membrane of the alveoli into the capillaries as a result of this pressure differential, and carbon dioxide moves in the opposite direction for the same reason.

Cell metabolism

Internal, or tissue respiration, is a vital component of cell metabolism. Every individual cell requires a supply of oxygen and the removal of carbon dioxide, a by-product of metabolism.

Homeostasis

Homeostasis (the maintenance of a constant internal environment) is explained in section 3.2. The respiratory system has an important role to play in homeostasis.

Our rhythmical breathing movements are usually done unconsciously. Adults inhale and exhale between twelve and twenty times a minute. It is thought that the brain initiates breathing rhythm; but the rate can be influenced by reflex action, the chemical composition of the blood and by conscious control.

ACTIVITY

Compare your breathing rate and depth when you are relaxed and when doing intense physical activity (or immediately after). Write up your findings. Explain why your breathing rate changes during intense activity. Summarise the effect on your active muscles: how respiration affects energy.

3.1.7 Cardiovascular system

The cardiovascular system comprises the heart, arteries, veins, capillaries and blood. The cardiovascular system distributes food, oxygen, amino acids, plasma proteins, electrolytes, hormones, enzymes, antibodies and anticoagulants) to all parts of the body. The movement of the blood in the vessels everywhere in the body continuously changes the fluid surrounding the cells so that:

- fresh supplies of oxygen and food are brought in
- toxins don't build up.

It takes about 45 seconds for a red cell to circulate once around the body.

The heart lies behind the sternum, occupying a large part of the mediastinum in the thoracic cavity. It is divided into a right and left side by the septum. The right atrium receives deoxygenated blood from the venae cavae and the coronary sinus, and forces it into the right ventricle via the tricuspid valve. From the right ventricle the blood is forced through the pulmonic semilunar valve into the pulmonary artery to be transported to the lungs for oxygenation. This freshly oxygenated blood returns to the left atrium via the four pulmonary

ACTIVITY

Investigate how carbon dioxide is transported from the tissues into the lungs.

Then, using diagrams if appropriate, explain the connection between circulation, respiration and the effects on the body's energy.

veins. It is forced through the mitral valve into the left ventricle, from which it is forced through the aortic semilunar valve into the aorta to be distributed around the body.

Oxygen dissolves in the blood in the lungs. Active tissues produce carbon dioxide and use oxygen. When the blood reaches these tissues, the raised acidity level caused by the carbon dioxide produced by the working tissues, and the low oxygen concentration, causes oxyhaemoglobin (haemoglobin combined with oxygen) to be broken down and oxygen is released to the tissues.

3.1.8 Digestive system

ACTIVITY

Explain what happens if the amount of food a person eats exceeds their needs. Describe what happens to glucose, fats and amino acids which are excess to needs.

Then explain the effects of these systems on the energy levels of a marathon runner:
■ digestive system
■ respiratory system
■ circulatory system.

Also think about how the other body systems affect the runner's energy level, for example:
■ the nervous system and sense organs
■ the endocrine system.

Food is of little value unless its nutrients enter the blood stream and are distributed to living tissues. Digestion and absorption take place in the alimentary canal. Food moves through the alimentary canal by:
■ ingestion – bringing food in through the mouth
■ swallowing – taking roughly six seconds for fairly solid food to reach the stomach
■ peristalsis – the contracting and relaxing of the circular muscles in the walls of the alimentary canal (which propels the food through the system)
■ egestion – expulsion of the undigested remains of food from the alimentary canal.

Digestion (and absorption) occurs in all the main parts of the alimentary canal: mouth, stomach, duodenum ileum and colon.

The products of digestion pass across the wall of the alimentary canal and are carried around the body in the blood. Most living cells can absorb and metabolise glucose, fats and amino acids:
■ Glucose is oxidised to carbon dioxide and water. This reaction produces ATP energy molecules, which are used for the chemical processes in the cell. For example, in muscle cells it produces contractions and it aids the production of electrical changes in nerve cell transmission.
■ Fats are also oxidised by cells to produce the ATP energy molecules needed for cell functions. Fats provide much more energy molecules than glucose.
■ Amino acids make proteins when absorbed by cells.

3.1.9 Renal system

The renal system comprises:

- two kidneys
- two ureters
- one bladder
- one urethra.

Functions of the kidneys

These crucial organs

- produce the filtrate – urine, from the blood
- help to regulate the body's water balance
- assist in the adjustment of the electrolyte content of the plasma
- assist in the adjustment of the acidity and alkalinity of the blood, so that only a slight alkalinity is maintained
- eliminate urea, urates, creatinine and uric acid from protein metabolism
- excrete the end products from drugs and toxins
- help in the maintenance of normal blood pressure.

The two kidneys lie on the posterior abdominal wall, one on either side of the spine. They are bean-shaped, surrounded by fat (for protection) and enclosed within a fibrous capsule. The outer layer of the kidney is a granular cortex, and within this is the striped medulla. At the centre of each kidney is a space called the pelvis.

Kidneys are composed of millions of nephrons. One hundred litres of blood are filtered in the nephrons each day, but only one and a half litres of urine are excreted daily. Much of the fluid is reabsorbed along the tubules, so that in a healthy person the urine only contains those substances that the body wants to get rid of.

Secretion of urine

This is controlled by the antidiuretic hormone (ADH) and aldosterone. Urine passes from the pelvis of the kidney into the ureter, where it collects in the distensible bladder. A sensory stimulus from the bladder causes the internal and external sphincters to relax, while the bladder muscle contracts to void urine via the urethra. This is a reflex act but is also usually under conscious control except in babies and young children.

Key questions

1 What is the role of the nervous system in relation to the body's activities?

2 Describe the three main types of response controlled by the nervous system.

3 From where do conscious responses originate, and how are they transmitted to the sensory organs?

4 The endocrine system has many functions. Select one of the glands that form part of this system and explain what it does.

5 Briefly describe the process of respiration.

6 Describe the process by which oxyhaemoglobin releases oxygen into the tissues.

7 Name the parts of the alimentary canal where digestion takes place.

8 Briefly describe the process by which food crosses the gut wall and enters the bloodstream.

9 List the functions of the kidneys.

10 In which part of the kidney does reabsorption of fluid take place?

11 Name the hormones that control the secretion of urine.

Homeostasis

66 When a patient is admitted with hypothermia, it is important we recognise the knock-on effect on other systems. For example, the blood pressure falls as a result of vaso-constriction, in an attempt to conserve an adequate supply of oxygen to the brain. So it is essential to monitor and record all the vital signs until homeostasis is re-established. 99

nurse on medical ward

66 New and inexperienced parents are sometimes over-cautious about their newborn's temperature and are tempted to overheat them. In an older child the negative feedback loop would give rise to obvious signs, such as flushed skin, sweating and thirst. A newborn baby is unable to complain, and is more vulnerable because the system of homeostasis may not be well established in the early months. If the parents are not observant the baby's temperature can rise to a dangerous level. 99

health visitor

66 The effects of cocaine on the body are a good example of what can happen when homeostatic mechanisms fail to work. Cocaine stimulates the central nervous system, and the result is an increased heart rate, respiratory rate and higher body temperature. The homeostatic mechanisms that control these are ineffective because of the way cocaine affects the central nervous system. The negative feedback loops are overridden. In extreme cases the failure to re-establish homeostasis in the affected systems can lead to a stroke, convulsions, respiratory failure, cardiac failure and ultimately death. 99

drugs counsellor

66 When an athlete exercises intensively their breathing rate increases, and so does the heart rate. Deeper breathing helps to increase the level of oxygen and decrease the level of carbon dioxide. The body's attempt to maintain a constant equilibrium means that training has to take into account the mechanism whereby feedback affects the body's ability to continue with aerobic exercise. 99

sports coach

Homeostasis is the process the body uses to maintain a stable environment. To understand it you will need to be aware of the principle of negative feedback in regulating the body's environment. You will need to understand how body systems control the homeostatic mechanisms for blood glucose level, body temperature, heart rate, respiratory rate and hydration, and you will also need to know about the role of ADH (antidiuretic hormone).

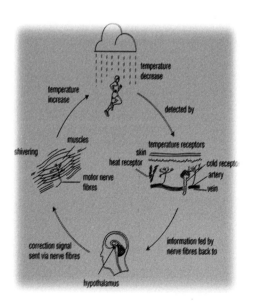

3.2.1 Homeostasis: the principle of negative feedback

The negative feedback loop

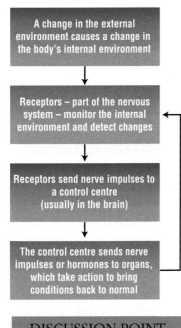

A change in the external environment causes a change in the body's internal environment

↓

Receptors – part of the nervous system – monitor the internal environment and detect changes

↓

Receptors send nerve impulses to a control centre (usually in the brain)

↓

The control centre sends nerve impulses or hormones to organs, which take action to bring conditions back to normal

DISCUSSION POINT

Why do you think this is called a negative feedback loop?

Homeostatic mechanisms are the processes by which the body maintains homeostasis – a stable internal environment in which cells can function. It is not an absolute constancy, but is a dynamic balance that varies within narrow limits.

Enzymes control all chemical processes which take place within cells. The chemical processes are very sensitive to the conditions in which they work, and a slight fall in temperature or rise in acidity can slow down or stop a vital chemical reaction. To prevent this from happening, homeostatic mechanisms ensure that the composition of tissue fluid around cells remains stable despite changes to the external environment.

The nervous system and hormones control homeostasis. A wide range of homeostatic mechanisms takes place in the body. Most follow the same pattern, known as the negative feedback loop.

Many homeostatic mechanisms take place in the body, including processes that concern the control of:
- blood glucose level
- body temperature
- heart rate
- respiratory rate
- hydration.

3.2.2 Homeostatic mechanisms

Blood glucose level
Blood sugar is the amount of glucose in the blood. This is usually about 1 mg of glucose per 1 cm^3 of blood.

Cells need a constant supply of glucose to generate the energy they need to function. (Brain cells rely entirely on glucose for energy, and can be permanently damaged by a low blood sugar level.) Because of this, the body uses homeostatic mechanisms to ensure there is a steady amount of glucose in the blood – a constant blood sugar level.

The digestive system breaks down carbohydrates eaten during a meal to produce glucose, which passes into the bloodstream. The pancreas (which is near to the stomach) detects that the blood sugar level has risen, and releases a hormone called insulin.

Insulin:

- enables glucose to pass into body cells more easily by increasing the permeability of the cell membrane to glucose
- activates the enzymes inside the cells which make use of glucose
- converts glucose into glycogen, where it is stored for use in the future (this takes place in the liver).

If the pancreas detects that the blood sugar level is falling, it produces less insulin and fewer glucose reactions take place. The amount of glucose in the blood then increases, until levels are back to normal.

If the blood sugar level falls very low, the pancreas stops secreting insulin and produces another hormone called glucagon. This converts the sugar stores of glycogen held in the liver into glucose, which enters the bloodstream until the blood sugar level has stabilised.

During exercise or in response to stress, the adrenal glands produce another hormone – adrenaline – which helps to regulate blood sugar levels. Like glucagon, this converts glycogen stores into glucose, enabling the cells to generate more energy.

Body temperature

Human beings are homeotherms – like other mammals and birds. We maintain a constant body temperature (about 37 °C) whatever the temperature of the outside environment. Unlike animals such as reptiles, human beings can generate their own heat and don't have to rely on the sun from day to day.

The hypothalamus at the base of the brain acts as the body's thermoregulatory centre. It:

- checks the temperature of blood as it passes through the brain
- receives nerve impulses from receptors in the skin and around internal organs about changes in the temperature of the environment outside the body.

If blood temperature is rising, the interior hypothalamus sends nerve impulses to organs of the body which control mechanisms to prevent overheating. If blood temperature is falling, the posterior hypothalamus sends nerve impulses to organs of the body which control mechanisms to conserve heat. Action is taken to bring the body temperature back to normal.

This is the negative feedback loop for controlling body temperature. What action does the body take in each case?

If temperature is rising:

- blood vessels in the skin get wider (vasodilation) and more blood is directed to the skin, making it red and warm (the heat is then lost from the skin's surface by conduction, convection and radiation, causing cooling)

ACTIVITY

Draw a diagram to show the negative feedback loop for maintaining blood sugar levels.

Find out about diabetes mellitus. What part of the loop doesn't work efficiently in patients with diabetes mellitus that began in childhood? How is it treated? How does this form of the disease compare with that associated with ageing?

DISCUSSION POINT

What factors may cause body temperature to rise and fall?

ACTIVITY

Try to detect the cold sensitive receptors in the skin by running the point of a pencil slowly across the back of the hand.

- sweat glands make more sweat, which is evaporated from the skin's surface using heat from the blood
- hairs on the skin lie flat, allowing air currents to pass across and cool the skin
- panting causes more heat to be lost as air is breathed out
- behaviour changes – clothes are removed and cold drinks taken.

If temperature is falling:
- blood vessels in the skin become narrower (vasoconstriction) and less blood is directed to the skin
- sweat glands stop producing sweat
- muscles beneath the skin contract, creating goose bumps and raising hair on the skin – this acts as an insulator, trapping warm air
- the body starts to shiver due to the contraction of skeletal muscles – this creates heat
- behaviour changes – clothes are put on and hot drinks taken.

ACTIVITY

Carry out some experiments to demonstrate the changes that take place in the body when temperature rises and falls. How can you observe these changes physically? Explain why each of these changes occurs.

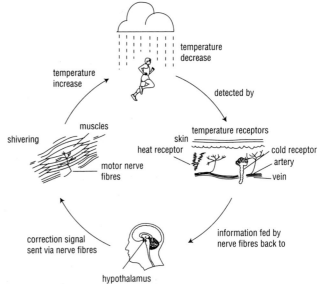

Heart rate

Throughout the day there are slight variations in the volume and viscosity of the blood. There are also changes in the heart rate in response to altered levels of activity and changes in the emotional state.

Complex homeostatic controls are needed to control the heart rate. The negative feedback loop for heart rate starts in the cardiac centre, which is situated in the medulla oblongata.

When the heart rate increases, for example during exercise, the blood pressure becomes elevated, and the levels of the metabolites carbon dioxide and lactic acid in the blood are raised, with a corresponding decrease in oxygen tension. This causes vasoconstriction and increased resistance. A decrease in the pH also causes vasoconstriction.

The cardiac centre controls the heart rate by sending impulses from specialised pressure-sensitive nerves, known as pressoreceptors, which are activated by an increase in blood pressure, and chemical-sensitive nerves, known as chemoreceptors, which are activated by elevated levels of metabolites such as carbon dioxide and lactic acid. These parasympathetic impulses from the cardiac centre travel via the vagus nerve to the sino-atrial node, the atrio-ventricular node, and the atrial muscles in the heart, and the effect is to slow the heart rate down.

Conversely sympathetic impulses originating in the cardiac centre have the effect of increasing the heart rate.

In addition to this homeostatic mechanism, chemoreceptors in the aortic arch and the carotid arteries are sensitive to the levels of carbon dioxide and oxygen levels in the blood, and pressoreceptors which are sensitive to changes in the blood pressure, send nerve impulses to the cardiac centre. This system is known as the cardiac reflex, and impulses originate from outside the central nervous system, particularly in response to emotions.

Respiratory rate

Respiration – or breathing – is the process by which the body draws in oxygen from the atmosphere to the lungs, and pushes out carbon dioxide as a waste product. This consists of a cycle of inspirations (breathing in) and expirations (breathing out) which are controlled by homeostasis.

Skeletal muscles between the ribs and in the diaphragm bring about breathing. The movement of these muscles is triggered by nerve impulses from a respiratory centre in the brain. This centre consists of three distinct areas:

- the medullary rhythmicity area – this controls the rhythm of breathing, producing nerve impulses which either cause inspiration and inhibit expiration, or vice versa
- the apneustic area – this can produce nerve impulses which stimulate the medullary rhythmicity area to change the depth of breathing
- the pneumotaxic area – this can produce nerve impulses which stimulate the medullary rhythmicity area to change the breathing rate.

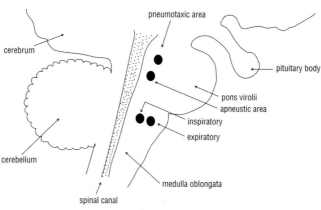

<table>
<tr><td colspan="2">

DISCUSSION POINT

The homeostatic mechanisms explained in this section are interrelated. Give as many situations as you can think of in which homeostasis is active when a cyclist competes in a long-distance race. Consider temperature, blood sugar, water, respiratory rate and heart rate control.
</td></tr>
</table>

If the blood's water content is low:

- nerve impulses stimulate the pituitary gland to release more ADH to the kidneys
- the collecting ducts become more permeable to water
- more water is reabsorbed from the kidney nephrons (urinary tubules) into the blood
- the level of water in the blood increases
- concentrated urine is produced, and urinary flow decreases.

If the blood's water content is high:

- osmoreceptors are not stimulated, and the pituitary gland releases less ADH to the kidneys
- the collecting ducts become less permeable to water
- less water is reabsorbed from the kidney nephrons (urinary tubules) into the blood
- the level of water in the blood decreases
- diluted urine is produced, and urinary flow increases.

The respiratory centre is sensitive to a range of signals from the body which show that breathing rate needs to change. For example, during exercise a rise in blood carbon dioxide causes an increase in the concentration of hydrogen ions in the blood, which is sensed by the respiratory centre. In addition, chemoreceptors (chemical receptors) in the aortic arch and the carotid arteries are sensitive to the levels of carbon dioxide and oxygen in the blood, and send nerve impulses to the respiratory centre. Breathing occurs at an increased rate and becomes deeper, in order to expel carbon dioxide from the body and take in more oxygen.

As well as being controlled by homeostasis, variations in breathing can be controlled at will. For example, an individual may choose to breathe at a different rate, or to hold their breath.

Hydration

As well as needing glucose, cells depend on a constant, regular supply of water. To ensure that they receive this, the human body relies on a homeostatic mechanism involving the kidneys.

The negative feedback loop for water regulation begins with special receptors in the hypothalamus, called osmoreceptors. Rather than directly detecting the amount of water in the blood, these detect the osmotic potential of the blood. For example:

- if the blood is more concentrated than normal, it contains less water and more sodium chloride (salt)
- if the blood is less concentrated than normal, it contains more water and less sodium chloride.

In response to changes in osmotic potential, the osmoreceptors send nerve impulses to the pituitary gland, which secretes antidiuretic hormone, ADH (also known as vasopressin).

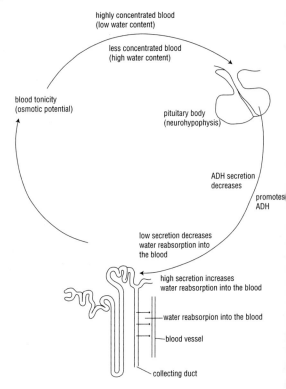

3.2.3 Effects of ageing on homeostasis

The main homeostatic mechanism affected by ageing is control of body temperature.

Maintenance of body temperature

During most of people's lives, their body temperature is efficiently controlled by homeostasis. However, newborn babies and older people often struggle to maintain a consistent body temperature:

- A baby's brain may not be mature enough to react to changes in temperature. They also lose heat quickly because they have a large surface area in proportion to their body volume and are often bald. (Hair helps to insulate the body.)
- An older person's cells may be unable to react efficiently enough.

As a result, babies and older people are particularly at risk from hypothermia. Sally, a care assistant who works with older people, explains:

66 *I'm always on the lookout for signs of hypothermia in the winter. Clients who live alone, away from their families, are particularly susceptible – they're often too proud to ask for help, and try to pretend everything's fine. Some of my older clients are confused, and don't keep their homes warm enough or eat and drink properly. Others simply can't afford to. I take steps at the first sign of a client having a low temperature – older people are less able than we are to reverse the effects of hypothermia.* 99

3.2.4 Normal body ranges which are regulated by homeostasis

The previous pages explain that homeostasis regulates:

- blood glucose level
- body temperature
- heart rate
- respiratory rate
- the level of water in the body.

Homeostasis maintains all of these at a 'normal', or average level. If levels deviate a long way from this norm, becoming very high or very low, they become 'abnormal' or 'pathological'.

Normal levels usually fall within a range rather than being a precise figure. Values not only vary between people, but also change in the same person depending on exercise, when they last ate, and level of excitement.

Normal body temperature is around 37 °C. This is the temperature at which the body's enzymes work most efficiently.

ACTIVITY

Find out more about:

■ the causes of pyrexia and hypothermia

■ the signs and symptoms of pyrexia and hypothermia

■ how to care for patients with pyrexia and hypothermia.

Produce a leaflet for families explaining normal ranges for body temperature; what might cause abnormalities; how to recognise high or low body temperature; and how to care for individuals with pyrexia and hypothermia.

Body temperature

Normal body temperature can vary slightly for several reasons:

■ the temperature in the rectum is usually slightly higher than in the mouth, which is slightly higher than the armpit

■ a child's temperature is usually higher than an adult's

■ temperature increases at ovulation during the menstrual cycle.

Causes of an abnormally raised temperature may include:

■ infection by bacteria or viruses

■ damage to the thermoregulatory centre in the hypothalamus (for example, following a head injury or heat stroke)

■ damage to body tissues (for example, caused by tumour growth, burns or scalds).

As the body temperature rises, the enzymes start to speed up. A patient with a high temperature is said to have pyrexia (or hyperthermia), and may show the following signs and symptoms:

■ rapid respiration

■ headache

■ hot, flushed skin

■ feeling cold and shivery

■ dry mouth

■ fast pulse

■ aching limbs

■ sweat

■ delirium

■ loss of consciousness

■ convulsions.

It is considered a medical emergency if the body's temperature rises to 41 °C, when enzymes start to be destroyed by the heat and stop working. If body temperature rises above 44.4 °C to 45.5 °C, it causes death.

Conversely, if body temperature falls to below 35 °C, the person is said to be suffering from hypothermia. Older people are especially at risk from hypothermia, in particular if they are confused, have difficulty with mobility, or have limited money for heating and food. Someone with hypothermia may show the following signs and symptoms:

■ slow respiration

■ slow pulse

■ shivering

■ cold, pale, mottled skin

■ mental slowness, loss of consciousness

■ numbness of hands and feet.

It is considered a medical emergency if the body's temperature falls to 34.4 °C.

ACTIVITY

Find out about:

- hyperglycaemia
- hypoglycaemia.

Write a paragraph explaining how each involves a variation from normal blood sugar levels.

Blood sugar

The normal level of glucose in the blood – blood sugar level – is about 1 mg of glucose per 1 cm^3 of blood.

Water

This can be monitored by urinary output. On average:

- men produce between 30 and 50 ml of urine an hour
- women produce between 25 and 45 ml an hour.

If an individual is producing abnormally small amounts of urine, this may mean that there is not enough water in the body fluids or they are retaining fluid. If they are producing abnormally large amounts of urine, this may mean they have taken in a lot of fluid (for example, it is the natural response to drinking heavily).

ACTIVITY

Carry out research to find out the signs and symptoms of too much water in the body, and too little water in the body. When might each situation occur? Investigate the effects of drinking alcohol on the normal control mechanism. Write a brief report.

ACTIVITY

Devise a series of experiments to establish 'normal' respiratory rates, and to investigate what causes deviations from the norm. (You may find it helpful to look at section 3.3.)

Respiratory rate

During quiet breathing, inspiration (an intake of breath) lasts about two seconds, and expiration (breathing out) usually lasts about three seconds. An adult's normal resting respiratory rate is between 13 and 17 breaths per minute. During exercise, this may increase to as many as 80 breaths per minute.

Respiratory rate also varies with age, for example, babies take between 30 and 40 breaths per minute.

3.2.5 **Heart rate**

ACTIVITY

Talk to a nurse or doctor about how they monitor one of the aspects described in this section. Ask them to explain:

- normal body ranges for the aspect you choose
- how they detect variations from the norm
- what causes variations
- what the possible implications are of variation from the norm
- how they treat variations.

At rest a healthy adult's heart rate will be between 60 and 80 beats per minute. This rate can increase with exercise or emotions by a factor of three. As with the respiratory rate, heart rate also varies with age – a baby's resting heart rate per minute is about 110–130, and this slowly declines until maturity is reached.

ACTIVITY

Maximum heart rate (Max HR) and maximum volume of oxygen (VO_2) are directly related. Athletes use these measurements in order to fine-tune their training. Ask a member of the gym staff about how these measurements are established for individual athletes, and how this information is used for training.

Key questions

1 What is homeostasis?

2 What is a negative feedback loop?

3 Give five physical changes which take place when the body temperature is falling.

4 What is the role of insulin in homeostasis?

5 Describe what happens if the blood's water content is low.

6 Why does respiratory rate increase during exercise?

7 What are dangerously high and low body temperatures?

8 What is the normal blood sugar level?

9 What is the normal heart rate in a healthy adult?

10 How does ageing affect regulation of body temperature?

66 Our instruments have to be regularly calibrated to ensure accuracy when taking measurements. We have to be totally confident that the measurements are accurate, as the consequences of errors when working in such a critical environment can be life threatening. Staff training in using equipment correctly, monitoring and recording results is also part of the ward procedure to minimise the possibility of mistakes. 99

nurse manager in intensive care unit

66 Even a routine task such as taking someone's temperature has risks. If the person is agitated or confused on admission, it may not be appropriate to take a sublingual temperature. So we have to use common sense and discretion in deciding how and when to carry out the procedure. 99

care assistant in residential home for older people

66 It can be a frightening experience for a sick child to come into hospital. Staff need to be sensitive and engage the child's trust before attempting to take routine measurements of vital signs. If a child is anxious the pulse rate will be raised and the measurement won't be an accurate reflection of their resting heart rate. 99

children's nurse

Physiological measurements of individuals in care settings

Monitoring bodily functions enables us to understand what is happening inside the body. Routine monitoring of clients receiving health or social care services can help identify any dysfunction of homeostatic systems. In this section you will learn about the various functions that can be monitored, the equipment that is used, factors that can afffect the readings, the expected range for the measurements you take and possible causes of any deviations from the range.

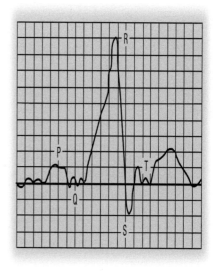

3.3.1 Monitoring the cardiorespiratory system

How efficiently the cardiorespiratory system is functioning gives an important indication of an individual's overall health. This can be monitored using a range of techniques which are simple, quick and non-invasive (they don't involve introducing anything into the body). They include measuring:

- pulse rate
- temperature
- blood pressure
- breathing rate
- lung volumes.

Pulse rate

Pulse is the rhythmical throbbing of the arteries as blood flows through them. Contraction of the heart's ventricles forces blood into the main arteries, creating a wave of pressure. This wave – the pulse – can be felt wherever an artery is near to the surface of the body and crossing a bone or other firm tissue. An individual's pulse rate shows how often their heart is beating.

Pulse rate is usually measured in the wrist, where the radial artery crosses the bones. However, it can also be felt at:

- the carotid artery, on either side of the neck
- the brachial artery, on the inner arm
- the temporal artery, on either side of the forehead.

As well as measuring pulse rate to find out how fast the heart is beating, feeling the pulse can give other indications of an individual's state of health. While counting the number of beats, doctors and nurses also check whether:

- the pulse's rhythm is regular
- the pulse feels strong or weak
- the artery feels soft or hard (hardness).

DISCUSSION POINT

Why do you think medical staff usually measure pulse rate at the wrist, rather than another part of the body? When might it be difficult to feel a pulse at the wrist?

Monitoring pulse rate

1 Press two fingertips lightly against the wrist, just below the thumb. Make sure you don't press too hard, and don't use your thumb because this has its own pulse.

2 Feel the pulse where the radial artery crosses the wrist.

3 Using a clock or watch with a second hand, count the number of beats in a minute.

For a resting adult, pulse rate is usually between 60 and 80 beats per minute.

For a baby, pulse rate is usually about 130 beats per minute.

For a young child, pulse rate is usually about 100 beats per minute.

ACTIVITY

Find out:

- possible causes of an irregular pulse
- possible causes of a weak pulse
- possible causes of an artery which feels hard.

Remember to think about these points when you monitor pulse rate yourself.

Causes of variations

A pulse rate which is faster than normal can be caused by:

- exercise
- fear
- fright or excitement
- fever
- illness.

Working in pairs, measure your own and your partner's pulse rate when you have been resting, after gentle exercise (such as walking), and after vigorous exercise (such as running). After exercise, keep measuring the pulse rate every two minutes until it has returned to normal. Make sure that the exercise you choose is safe for both of you.

Record your results in a chart, and then draw graphs showing pulse rates against time. Explain why the pulse rate took time to return to normal after vigorous exercise.

A slow pulse rate can be caused by fainting and some heart disorders. However, it can also be a sign of fitness, showing that the circulatory system is functioning efficiently.

Blood pressure

Blood pressure is the pressure which blood exerts on the walls of the arteries as it flows through them. Maintaining normal blood pressure is essential, so that the blood can supply body tissues with oxygen and nutrients.

Blood pressure is measured using a piece of equipment called a sphygmomanometer. This consists of an inflatable cloth cuff connected to a pressure gauge. The pressure gauge may be:

- a vertical tube up which a column of mercury is pushed by the rising pressure (this is called a manometer)
- a cylinder with a dial attached (this is called an aneroid).

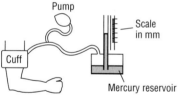

The raised pressure inflates the cuff and simultaneously pushes the mercury up the manometer.

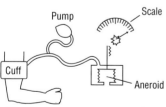

The raised pressure compressses the aneroid and moves the needle on the scale.

Measuring blood pressure

Safety point: only measure blood pressure if someone trained is with you.

1 Wrap the inflatable cuff around the upper arm, above the elbow (so that the reading is taken at a point level with the heart).

2 Place the stethoscope bell over the brachial artery at the elbow, just below the cuff.

3 Make sure that the arm is straight and relaxed with the elbow resting on a surface.

4 Inflate the cuff with air until the pulse disappears – which should be about 110–120 (millimetres of mercury). This should flatten the artery and stop blood flowing through it, and no pulse should be heard through the stethoscope. Don't leave the pressure this high for more than a few seconds, as there is no blood supply to the arm.

5 Gradually release the pressure in the cuff, listening carefully through the stethoscope.

6 When you hear blood rushing through the artery, with a loud knocking sound at every beat, write down the measurement on the pressure gauge. This is the systolic blood pressure (the pressure in the blood vessel as the heart contracts).

7 Carry on releasing the cuff pressure until you can't hear any more sound, and write down the measurement on the pressure gauge. This is the diastolic blood pressure (the pressure between heartbeats).

8 Blood pressure is written as a fraction. Write the systolic pressure over the diastolic pressure to give the full blood pressure reading.

In a healthy adult, blood pressure is usually about 120/80 mmHg.

ACTIVITY

Working in the same pair as when you measured pulse rates, and with a trained person present, use a sphygmomanometer to read your partner's blood pressure when they have been resting, and after exercise.

Design a chart or table to record your results.

ACTIVITY

Abnormally low blood pressure is called hypotension, and occurs as a result of shock, including:

- haemorrhagic (hypovolaemic) shock
- cardiogenic shock
- anaphylactic shock
- eurogenic shock
- septicaemic shock.

Find out more about these types of shock. What causes them?

ACTIVITY

Patients in hospital have their pulse rate, blood pressure and breathing (respiratory) rate taken regularly. During a visit to your local hospital or contact with nursing staff, ask for a copy of a chart they use to record this information. If it is unclear, ask them how they fill it in.

Then make a copy of the chart, and transfer the results of your own monitoring onto the chart.

Blood pressure varies with every heart beat, and can be drawn like a wave showing the peaks and troughs of pressure.

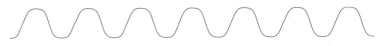

Blood pressure wave

Abnormally high blood pressure is called hypertension. It can be caused by many factors, including:

- anxiety
- pregnancy
- lack of exercise
- excess weight
- too much salt in the diet
- smoking.

However, in 95% of cases no clear cause can be identified.

It can also be a sign of renal disease, some tumours, and atherosclerosis (hardening and narrowing of the arteries). High blood pressure is dangerous because it often doesn't cause any symptoms, but the heart and major arteries are damaged by years of working at too high pressure. This can lead to heart attacks and strokes (cardiovascular accidents), so it is important to treat high blood pressure even if there are no symptoms. This is why doctors and nurses always check patients' blood pressure during routine clinical examinations.

Breathing rate

Breathing is the process by which the body draws in oxygen from the atmosphere to the lungs, and pushes out carbon dioxide as a waste product. This consists of a cycle of inspirations (breathing in) and expirations (breathing out). Breathing rate is the number of breaths taken in a minute.

Breathing is usually controlled by homeostasis, from the respiratory centre in the brain. However, it can also be controlled consciously.

Monitoring breathing rate

Using a clock or watch with a second hand, count the number of breaths taken in a minute. This can be hard to see. Look for signs such as raising chest, shoulders and abdomen, and listen to breathing noises.

- In adults, the usual breathing rate is between 13 and 17 breaths per minute.
- After strenuous exercise, this may rise to 70 to 80 breaths per minute.
- Babies breathe faster than adults, taking about 40 breaths per minute.

ACTIVITY

Working with the same pairs as before, measure your partner's breathing rate when they are relaxed and resting, after gentle exercise, and after vigorous exercise. After exercise, measure their breathing rate every two minutes until it returns to the baseline value. Remember that breathing rate can be controlled, and try to ensure that your results are as authentic as possible.

Design a chart to record your results, and then draw a graph showing breathing rates against time.

Measuring peak flow

1 Take a deep breath, then blow into the mouthpiece as quickly as possible.

2 Repeat this twice, and take the highest reading obtained.

3 Repeat the process over a period of time, as peak expiratory flow varies at different times of the day.

4 Find the average result.

In a healthy adult, peak expiratory flow is usually between 400 and 600 dm^3 of air per minute.

Lung volumes

During breathing, the volume of the lungs changes – increasing as air is drawn in, and decreasing as it is pushed out. This changing lung volume can give a good indication of the health of the lungs, showing whether there is any obstruction to the respiratory pathway.

Measurements taken to test lung function include:
- peak flow – the maximum rate at which air flows out of the lungs
- tidal volume – the volume of air breathed in and out in a normal breath
- vital capacity – the maximum amount of air which can be breathed in and out.

Peak flow

Peak expiratory flow estimation – measurement of the speed at which air flows out of the lungs – is carried out using a peak flow meter. This is a simple piece of equipment consisting of a calibrated meter attached to a mouthpiece.

People with asthma often have a low peak expiratory flow, as narrowing of the trachea and bronchi prevents air flowing out as quickly as usual. Some asthmatics use a peak flow meter to monitor their peak expiratory flow every day, and drugs are adjusted accordingly. If a patient uses a broncho-dilator inhaler (a drug which widens the air passages) it is useful to measure the peak flow before and after using the inhaler.

Peak expiratory flow also varies with:
- age – rising from childhood to adulthood, then falling after middle age
- sex – men tend to have a higher peak flow than women
- size – larger people have a higher peak flow than smaller people.

ACTIVITY

The graph below shows normal peak expiratory flow rates for women of different ages and heights.

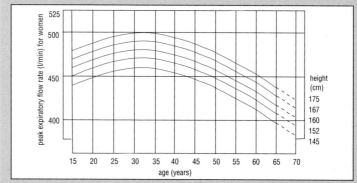

Investigate peak expiratory flow rates in your GNVQ group, relating your findings to height and sex. Ask your tutors to take part in the experiment, so that your sample includes people of different ages. Does anyone in your group have asthma?

Following the format of the graph above, produce a visual presentation of your findings.

Measuring tidal volume and vital capacity

1. Breathe into the spirometer mouthpiece normally.

2. A drum containing a mixture of gases inside the spirometer inflates and deflates with the breaths. This moves a piston, which causes a recording pen to move on a chart, tracing the pattern of breaths. This trace shows the tidal volume.

3. Breathe out and in as deeply as possible.

4. The spirometer trace shows the vital capacity.

In a healthy adult, tidal volume is about 0.4 dm^3.

In a healthy adult, vital capacity is usually between 3 and 5 dm^3.

ACTIVITY

If possible, use a spirometer to measure your own tidal volume and vital capacity. You should only use a spirometer if there is a trained person present.

Keep a copy of your spirometer trace in your portfolio, labelling your tidal volume, vital capacity, inspiratory reserve volume, expiratory reserve volume and residual volume. Alongside the trace, give each measurement in figures and explain what it means.

Tidal volume and vital capacity

Breathing is described as tidal because air flows in and out of the lungs. The volume of air taken in and then let out during one normal breathing cycle is called the tidal volume. The maximum volume of air that can be taken in and let out, by breathing as deeply as possible, is called the vital capacity.

Tidal volume and vital capacity are measured with an instrument called a spirometer.

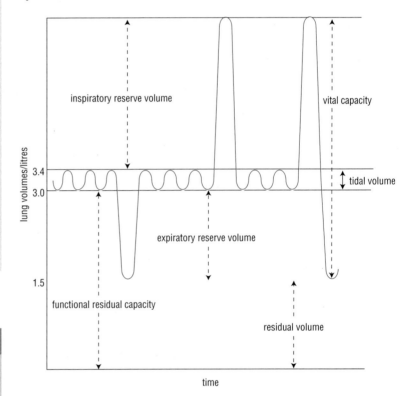

A typical spirometer trace

Using a spirometer can also provide other information about lung volumes, as the spirometer trace above shows:

■ inspiratory reserve volume – the extra air which can be drawn into lungs by breathing deeply

■ expiratory reserve volume – the extra air which can be forced out of lungs after a normal breath

■ residual volume – the amount of air left in the lungs after expiration. This is usually between 1 and 2.5 dm^3.

3.3.2 **Additional routine measurement**

Body temperature

Body temperature is explained on pages 151–152. It is usual to measure and record body temperature of a patient in hospital at least once a day. In adults the temperature is usually taken by inserting a thermometer under the tongue for a period. Increasingly, electronic ones are being used because they offer a more accurate and speedier reading. For reasons of safety in the case of a young child it would be usual to place the thermometer in the armpit, and adjust the measurement by adding one degree to the result. In a baby the temperature is recorded by carefully inserting a thermometer into the rectum, and adjusting the result by subtracting one degree from the result. It is important that a trained member of staff supervises you when taking a rectal temperature. Measurements of temperature are recorded on the same chart that is used for pulse, respiration and blood pressure.

ACTIVITY

Write a paragraph explaining why a young child or older person is more susceptible to hypothermia (a low body temperature).

Key questions

1 What measurements are taken to monitor the cardiovascular system?

2 What does the pulse rate measure?

3 Name three situations in which the pulse rate may be elevated.

4 What is the normal range for a child's heart rate?

5 How long does it usually take to measure the body's temperature?

6 Why is it potentially unsafe to take an oral recording of the temperature in a child?

7 Briefly describe the signs and symptoms of hypothermia.

8 Describe the terms systolic and diastolic in relation to blood pressure.

9 What is the upper level of a normal blood pressure in an adult?

10 When measuring blood pressure, why is it important that the patient is relaxed and rested?

11 What does breathing rate measure?

12 What is measured using a peak flow meter?

13 Why do people with asthma often have a low peak expiratory flow rate?

14 Give three reasons for variations between individuals' peak expiratory flow rates.

15 A spirometer is used to measure tidal volume and tidal capacity. What do these terms describe?

SECTION **3.4**

Safe practice, accuracy of results and accurate analysis of results

You must be aware of potential health and safety risks that apply when carrying out monitoring activities and using equipment in the workplace. You also need to know how to reduce these risks.

❝ Following safety procedures is an integral part of being a professional, for the safety of practitioners and patients. Taking short cuts can lead to mistakes – they can, and sometimes, do have tragic consequences. ❞

local authority health and safety inspector

❝ With the new electronic blood pressure monitors it is possible to get bizarre results simply because the patient moved or talked during the procedure. ❞

primary healthcare nurse

❝ Being conscientious about recording results neatly and clearly assists with accurate analysis. Also a clear understanding of plotting points on a chart or graph is essential so that other members of staff can quickly see the patient's status. ❞

care assistant in a nursing home

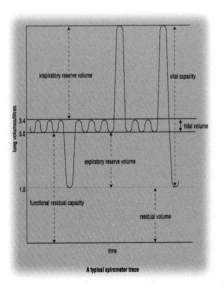

A typical spirometer trace

3.4.1 Guidelines and regulations

It is essential when using equipment to measure a patient's physiological status that you understand good practice about potential health and safety risks.

Nursing

A Code of Professional Conduct is issued by the United Kingdom Central Council for Nursing, Midwifery and Health Visiting (UKCC). This states:

66 *Each registered nurse, midwife and health visitor shall act, at all times, in such a manner as to justify public trust and confidence, to uphold and enhance the good standing and reputation of the profession, to serve the interests of society, and above all to safeguard the interests of individual patients and clients.* 99

In the case of a pre-registration student, a qualified member of staff is responsible for ensuring that the student is competent to perform the task, and is adequately supervised.

The UKCC considers record keeping a fundamental part of nursing, midwifery and health visiting practice. It issues Guidelines for records and record keeping. The UKCC states that: 'record keeping is process and it is not an optional extra to be fitted in if circumstances allow.' It suggests that its newly issued Guidelines for records and record keeping are read in conjunction with the Code of professional conduct and the Guidelines for professional practice. All these publications are available free of charge by writing to the Distribution Department, UKCC, 23 Portland Place, London W1N 4JT.

Social work

The Central Council for Education and Training in Social Work (CCETSW) issues guidelines for safe practice for social workers. It may be contacted at Derbyshire House, St Chads Street, London WC1H 8AD.

For all professionals

The basis of British health and safety law is the Health and Safety at Work, etc., Act 1974. The Management of Health and Safety at Work Regulations 1992 (the Management Regulations) make even more explicit what employers have to do to manage health and safety at work. The main responsibility on employers is to carry out a risk assessment and record the significant findings of the risk assessment. The Health and Safety Executive (HSE) leaflet *5 Steps to Risk Assessment* gives details of what a risk assessment involves, and this varies according to the nature of the workplace. Leaflets are available free from HSE Books, PO Box 1999, Sudbury, Suffolk CO10 6FS.

The Workplace (Health, Safety and Welfare) Regulations 1992 clarify and consolidate existing law, and establish a consistent set of standards for most workplaces, schools, colleges and universities. A copy of these regulations should be available for you to read in your workplace. It is advisable to familiarise yourself with the relevant section for your setting.

The Reporting of Injuries, Diseases and Dangerous Occurrences Regulations 1995 (RIDDOR) came into effect on 1 April 1996. They require employers to keep records of any potentially dangerous occurrence in the workplace and certain incidents must be reported to the HSE. These regulations may not directly involve you, but it is wise to familiarise yourself with them.

As a student, the requirements of your Local Education Authority (LEA), the Department for Education and Employment (DfEE) and the Association for Science Education must be strictly observed during any of the procedures explained in this section.

3.4.2 **Safe practice**

ACTIVITY

Contact a healthcare practitioner. Find out the protocol for using a thermometer in their setting. Ask about the risks of failing to follow the protocol.

The thermometer

Inserting a glass thermometer into a patient's mouth may not always be advisable. In the case of a patient who is confused or unconscious, and in babies and young children it is advisable to take the temperature using the axilla or the rectum. Always make sure that a trained member of staff supervises you.

Hygiene is also paramount when using a thermometer and you should follow the procedure laid down for cleaning thermometers. Cross-infection is an increasing hazard in care situations. Never be tempted to take short cuts. You must follow the established protocol for your workplace.

The sphygmomanometer

You should practise recording blood pressure under the supervision of a trained colleague until you become proficient in this technique.

A common mistake with learners is to keep the cuff inflated too long. This means occluding the blood supply to the arm, which is both painful and potentially dangerous. Always tell the patient that the procedure may cause a sensation of discomfort when the cuff is inflated, but that in no circumstances should it be painful. Release the pressure immediately if the patient complains of pain.

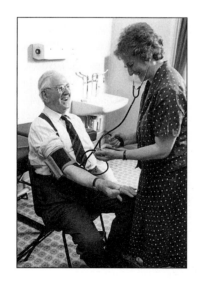

A column of mercury is contained within the glass manometer. Take care when handling the sphygmomanometer since it is possible to break the glass if you are careless, particularly when closing the container. In the event of a spillage of mercury, ensure that it is disposed of safely according to health and safety regulations. Report the incident to a trained member of staff.

(Keep up to date with European legal requirements; for example, phasing out the use of mercury in health monitoring equipment is under consideration.)

Peak flow meter and spirometer

When using the peak flow meter and spirometer, the disposable mouthpiece must be changed between patients. It should be safely disposed of after use in the appropriate bin bag.

It is also advisable to ensure that the patient is seated comfortably because the procedure may cause the patient to feel dizzy. It is even possible that they may faint, especially if they have impaired lung functions.

The peak flow meter should be regularly cleaned according to the manufacturer's instructions, since it is a potential source of cross-infection.

3.4.3 Accuracy of results

You need to know the possible sources of error in the practical monitoring systems and how to estimate and reduce the risk of error. Errors occur because of:

■ the monitoring process
■ the limitations of the monitoring equipment.

To reduce the possibility of errors influencing the results, you need to consider both these possibilities. Be vigilant about using the correct procedure. Check that equipment has been correctly calibrated. If you are concerned about the accuracy of the results when using a specific measuring instrument:

■ use a second instrument as a control
■ check the results with a trained practitioner.

Thermometer

- Ensure that the thermometer is intact and has been cleaned according to established protocols.
- If you are using a glass mercury thermometer, check that the column of mercury is at zero before use.
- Check that the patient has not recently had a hot or cold drink or food.
- Use a watch with a second hand to check that the thermometer is in place for the correct time.

If in doubt about the result, repeat and check the result with a trained member of staff.

DISCUSSION POINT

What might be the risks to patients of failing to take and record their temperature accurately? Consider a variety of situations, for example:

- routine temperature monitoring of a newly born baby
- monitoring of the temperature of a young person in hospital with a chest infection
- routine temperature monitoring of an older person in a nursing home.

DISCUSSION POINT

Discuss each other's views about the potential for inaccurate reading of a patient's blood pressure.

Sphygmomanometer

- Ensure that the equipment is in good working order.
- Check that the patient is comfortable and relaxed.
- Ask the patient to keep quiet and still during the procedure.
- Check that the cuff is the right size and ask the patient to keep their arm straight.

If in doubt about the result, repeat the procedure and inform a trained member of staff.

ACTIVITY

Investigate the risks of trainees recording inaccurate results. What training do new practitioners require before they can be judged competent at taking a patient's blood pressure?

ACTIVITY

Find out if there is any margin for error in the measurement of blood pressure, or whether the measurement must be strictly accurate. Justify your findings.

Peak flow meter and spirometer

- Check that the equipment is in good working order.
- Zero the equipment before use.
- Ensure that the patient is relaxed and rested before taking measurements.
- Check that the patient has not recently taken any medication (e.g. a broncho-dilator) that may affect the result.

If in doubt about the result, repeat the procedure and inform a trained member of staff.

3.4.4 Accurate analysis of results

To be effective in monitoring patients, you need to be able to:

- plot graphs, for example to record blood glucose levels, temperature, breathing rates, changes in heart rate
- use fractions and decimals to record physiological values
- determine and interpret rates of change from linear and non-linear graphs, for example changes in breathing rate and oxygen consumption from spirometer traces
- use formulae, for example to express electrolyte concentrations.

Purpose of monitoring

By monitoring and then analysing the cardiorespiratory system, medical staff are able to draw valid conclusions about an individual's physiological status. This analysis may be:

- statistical – involves looking at the measurements as a set of figures to analyse an individual's status (for example, comparing the measurements with normal values)
- transformed – involves using formulae and graphical techniques to interpret measurements (for example, drawing a graph to analyse a patient's blood pressure over time)
- for clinical relevance – involves identifying physical dysfunction by monitoring the cardiorespiratory system (for example, identifying respiratory problems by measuring lung volumes).

171

JANET HARVEY

Janet Harvey is 55 years old. She is 1.6 m (5' 3") tall and weighs 85 kg (13 st 5 lb). Janet has always smoked cigarettes and even now, although she has cut down, she still smokes ten cigarettes a day. Two years ago Janet suddenly developed a severe pain like a vice in the centre of her chest and down her left arm. In hospital, they told her she had had a heart attack. Ever since, Janet has experienced a similar, but milder, pain if she hurries or gets upset. It is particularly bad if she tries to walk up a hill. She is very upset about her condition as she has had to give up her job in a bank, and finds it difficult to do housework or go to the shops.

Janet is suffering from angina after having a myocardial infarction. Angina is a pain caused by the heart muscle not having enough oxygen. Janet has had hypertension for many years and this, along with the smoking, is a major risk factor.

Janet is seen regularly by her general practitioner because she says her angina is getting worse and she is getting breathless.

DISCUSSION POINT

What advice do you think the doctor might give Janet?

DISCUSSION POINT

How do these measurements differ from the normal values?

JANET'S CARDIORESPIRATORY MEASUREMENTS

The doctor examines Janet.

- Her pulse rate is 110 and her heartbeat is irregular.
- Her blood pressure is 190/110.
- Her respiratory rate is 25 breaths per minute.
- Her peak flow is 300 dm^3 per minute.

ACTIVITY

From the results of monitoring your own cardiorespiratory system in section 3.1.1, write up an analysis of your physiological status.

THE DOCTOR'S CONCLUSIONS

The doctor completes her examination of Janet. She draws the conclusion that a disturbance of the heart rate may have made Janet's heart beat less strongly and worsened her angina.

Earlier sections focused on primary source data – data you collected yourself. However, medical staff often rely on secondary source data – data collected by other people – to provide further insight into an individual's physiological status.

This secondary source data may include:

- electrocardiogram (ECG) traces
- blood cell counts
- electrolyte concentrations in body fluids
- spirometer tracings.

ECG traces

Electrocardiograms – or ECGs – enable medical staff to monitor an individual's heart activity.

Each contraction of the heart muscle is stimulated by an electrical impulse called the cardiac impulse. This impulse starts in the sino-atrial (S-A) node of the heart, and travels across the muscle fibres of the atria, causing them to contract. It then spreads to the ventricles via the atrio-ventricular node and the Bundle of His (a conducting system of fibres), causing both ventricles to contract at the same time.

The heart's electrical activity can be monitored using an ECG recorder. Electrodes connected to a monitor are attached to a client's wrists, ankles and across their chest. These amplify the electrical activity taking place in the heart, so that it can be displayed on screen or as a trace on graph paper. The speed and rhythm of waves of electrical activity recorded can help doctors to diagnose a range of heart problems. Most modern ECG machines read the traces automatically, compare them with data stored on a computer, and print out a diagnosis.

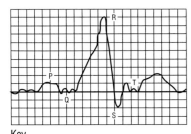

Key
P = Atria contract
QRS = Ventricles contract
T = Heart relaxes

The ECG trace on the left is normal for a healthy adult. The waves show the speed and rhythm of the electrical impulse passing through the heart:
- the P wave shows the contraction of the atria
- the Q, R and S wave shows the contraction of the ventricles
- the T wave shows the ventricles relaxing again.

This normal pattern of waves changes in individuals with heart disorders. Constant ECG monitoring of patients who have had a heart attack can alert medical staff to further problems. In some cases, for example patients with angina, an ECG is taken during exercise on a treadmill. This can reveal abnormalities not seen if the individual is resting.

JANET HARVEY'S ECG

Janet's doctor decided she needed some more information from tests which she could not do herself. She ordered:
- an ECG
- a chest X-ray
- a full blood count
- a urea and electrolytes profile.

This test confirmed that Janet's irregular heartbeat was caused by atrial fibrillation. This is important because it can be treated.

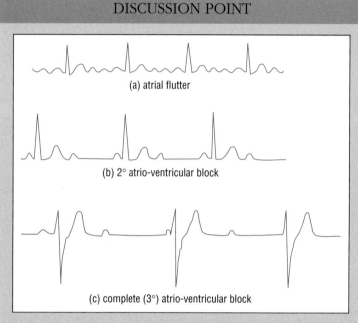

(a) atrial flutter

(b) 2° atrio-ventricular block

(c) complete (3°) atrio-ventricular block

The ECG trace above was taken from a patient with a heart disorder. Compare it with the normal ECG trace above, and discuss the differences you can see.

Blood cell counts

The study of blood and its diseases is called haematology.

A blood cell count is one of the most commonly used sources of data on an individual's physiological status. A small sample of blood is taken and sent for laboratory analysis. The blood cell count may involve looking at:

- the number of red blood cells
- the number of grams of haemoglobin per dm3
- the volume occupied by red blood cells when they have settled (packed cell volume)
- the number of white blood cells
- the number of different types of white blood cells
- the appearance and size of red and white blood cells
- the number and appearance of platelets.

Under normal conditions, blood is made up of each of these cells in particular proportions. Blood cell counts outside the normal range can provide important information about an individual's health.

Look back to the chart on page 134 to remind yourself of the structure and function of different types of blood cells. In a normal person, a blood cell count would show 5 million red blood cells in 1 mm^3 of blood – over a thousand times as many red cells as white. The different white cells would be found in the following proportions:

Normal values for haematology tests

Haemoglobin (Hb)	Men: 13.5–18.0 g per 100 ml blood
	Women: 11.5–16.5 g per 100 ml blood
Red blood cell count	Men: 4.5–6 million per ml
	Women: 3.5–5 million per ml
Packed cell volume	Men: 40–55%
	Women: 36–47%
White blood cell count	$4.0–11.0 \times 10^9$ litre

Differential white blood cell count:

Neutrophils	65%
Lymphocytes	8%
Monocytes	24%
Eosinophils	2%
Basophils	1%

Blood cell counts outside these normal ranges can indicate a wide range of illnesses and infection, including anaemias, blood disorders and leukaemias.

ACTIVITY

Look at the blood cell counts for the three patients below. Identify abnormalities and suggest what may be causing them.

	Patient 1	Patient 2	Patient 3
Erythrocytes per mm^3	3 million	5 million	4.75 million
Total white cell count	4,500	42,000	6,000
Neutrophils	65%	4%	64%
Monocytes	8%	1%	9%
Lymphocytes	24%	95%	23%
Eosinophils	2.5%	–	1.5%
Basophils	0.5%	–	1.5%

Find out how sickle-cell anaemia can be detected through a blood cell count.

Electrolyte concentrations in body fluids

The study of the composition of body fluids takes place in the clinical chemistry department of hospitals.

Electrolytes are substances that carry an electrical charge when dissolved. For example, sodium chloride (common salt) dissolves in body fluids to make positively charged sodium (Na^+) and negatively charged chloride (Cl^-).

Body fluids contain a range of electrolytes, including:

- sodium, potassium, calcium and magnesium (positively charged)
- chloride, phosphate, sulphate and nitrate (negatively charged).

These electrolytes need to be in balance for healthy functioning of the body. For example, too little potassium in the body can cause tiredness, faintness, abnormal heart rhythms, nausea, cramps and even death in extreme cases.

The table on the left shows normal values for different substances in body fluid.

Na^+	134–147 mmol/dm^3
K^+	3.4–5.0 mmol/dm^3
Urea	2.5–7.0 mmol/dm^3

ACTIVITY

Electrolyte concentration is usually monitored by testing levels in the blood. Find out what concentration of sodium and potassium you would expect to find in the blood.

What could be the causes and effects of too little sodium in the blood? How could it be treated?

What could be the causes and effects of too much potassium in the blood? How could it be treated?

ACTIVITY

Compare Janet's results with normal values. What is the abnormality?

Low blood levels of potassium can be caused by some drugs such as diuretic therapy. Find out what a diuretic is.

JANET HARVEY'S LABORATORY TESTS

Janet Harvey has the following results from the laboratory.

Hb	12.5 g/dl
White blood cell count	6.6×10^9/l
Na^+	145 mmol/l
K^+	2.9 mmol/l

Janet has been having a diuretic to treat her high blood pressure. Her doctor knows that the low serum K^+ may have caused, or worsened, her atrial fibrillation. She prescribes oral potassium supplements.

ACTIVITY

Talk to a doctor or nurse about the importance and purpose of using both primary and secondary source data to monitor an individual's physiological status.

Spirometer tracings

Spirometer tracings are often taken by one member of staff, and used by another as secondary source data to analyse an individual's physiological status.

For more information on spirometer tracings, see page 164.

Key questions

1 What is the pulse?

2 What are the normal pulse rates for a resting adult, a baby and a young child?

3 Explain how you would use a sphygmomanometer, and what you would use it for.

4 What causes high blood pressure?

5 What is the normal breathing rate for adults, and what may it rise to after exercise?

6 Explain peak flow, tidal volume and vital capacity.

7 What equipment would you use to measure lung volumes?

8 What does an ECG show?

9 What is measured during a blood cell count?

10 What might a red blood cell count of 3 million cells per 1 mm^3 of blood suggest?

11 What are electrolytes?

Assignment

Produce the results of monitoring the physiological status of individuals to show your understanding of human body systems. Include information about:

■ routine measurements of at least three human body systems

■ safe practice in taking measurements

■ the interactions between the human body systems

■ immediate structures and the systems involved in each homeostatic mechanism monitored.

Key skills

You can use the work you are doing for this part of your GNVQ to collect and develop evidence for the following key skills at level 3.

when you	you can collect evidence for
	communication
deal with people when taking body measurements	key skill C3.1a contribute to a group discussion about a complex subject
research into correct use of equipment, considering health and safety legislation and how RIDDOR applies	key skill C3.2 read and synthesise information from two extended documents about a complex subject, one of these documents should include a least one image
explain the structure, function and interrelationship of human body systems; record measurements effectively	key skill C3.3 write two different types of document about complex subjects; one piece of writing should be an extended document and include at least one image

when you	you can collect evidence for
	application of number
record measurements of at least three human body systems using appropriate equipment	key skill N3.1 plan, and interpret information from two different types of source, including a large data set
use fractions and decimals to record physiological values; determine and interpret rates of change from linear and non-linear graphs; use formulae to express electrolyte concentrations	key skill N3.2 carry out multistage calculations to do with (a) amounts and sizes (b) scales and proportion (c) handling statistics (d) rearranging and using formulae; work with a large data set on at least one occasion
plot graphs and explain the meaning of any deviations from the range	key skill N3.3 interpret results of calculations, present findings and justify methods; use at least one graph, one chart and one diagram
	improving own learning and performance
agree methods for measuring and monitoring the physiological status of individuals	key skill LP3.1 agree targets and plan how these will be met, using support from appropriate others
make and record measurements	key skill LP3.2 use the plan, seeking and using feedback and support from relevant sources to help meet the targets, and use different ways of learning to meet new demands
review methods, accuracy and handling of sources of error	key skill LP3.3 review progress in meeting targets, establishing evidence of achievements, and agree action for improving performance
	working with others
plan the collection of data in small groups, and plan to take measurements from people	key skill WO3.1 plan the activity with others, agreeing objectives, responsibilities and working arrangements
work in pairs when taking appropriate measurements; work with the subject(s) of measurements	key skill WO3.2 work towards achieving the agreed objectives seeking to establish and maintain cooperative working relationships in meeting responsibilities
review the effectiveness and accuracy of collaborative work	key skill WO3.3 review the activity with others against the agreed objective and agree ways of enhancing collaborative work
	problem-solving
recognise possible sources of error in the practical monitoring systems	key skill PS3.1 recognise, explore and describe the problems, and agree the standards for its solution
find ways of estimating and reducing these errors	key skill PS3.2 generate and compare at least two options which could be used to solve the problems, and justify the option for taking forward
apply methods for estimating and reducing errors	key skill PS3.3 plan and implement at least one option for solving the problem, and review progress towards its solution
review the identification of the errors and their correction	key skill PS3.4 agree and apply methods to check whether the problem has been solved, describe the results and review the approach taken

UNIT **4**

Factors affecting human growth and development

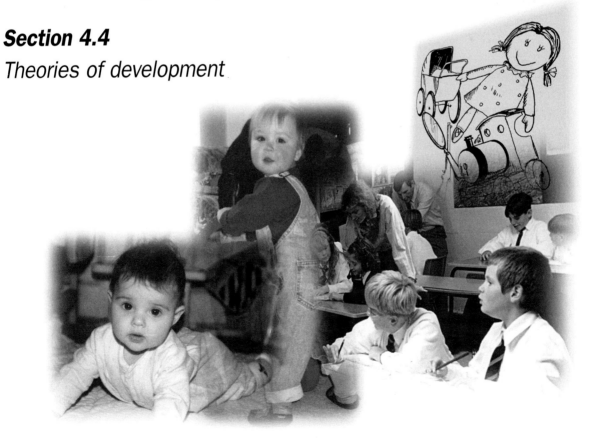

About this unit

This unit explores the concepts and theories of human growth and development. It aims to give you a basic understanding of every stage of life and this will contribute towards your knowledge base for working with people.

You will learn about:

- development from infancy to later adulthood
- skills developed through the lifespan
- the range of factors that can influence growth and development: including genetic, environmental and socioeconomic factors
- theories of development.

The unit links with and builds upon unit 3 Physical aspects of health.

66 *Teaching is a challenge – but it is rewarding to see a child suddenly grasp an idea. I teach children who have physical disabilities and learning difficulties. We have one little girl of nine years old who was overjoyed because she managed to lift a spoon to her mouth for the first time last week – we all could have cried with joy for her.* 99

teacher in a special school

66 *It can get distressing here. We had a man of 52 who lost his job as a manager of an office a year ago. He tried everything to find a new job, but felt as if he was on the scrap heap. His wife had left him, and he had become short of money and had to lose his house. He got so down. I feel the day centre has helped to bring him back from the brink but it is upsetting to see people who have got to such a state through no fault of their own.* 99

mental health nurse in a mental health day centre

66 *We have a lot of dependent elderly people here, but it is homely and happy. The nurse in charge always seems to have a smile and a good word. We have old time music and singalongs most days and a lady who organises activities. The staff know what they have to do and our manager is fair if she tells you off. She says it is better to have quality of life when you're old so we do everything to make today a good day, every day.* 99

care worker in a nursing home

Human development

It is important to consider human growth and development across the whole lifespan and be able to explain the key factors relating to human development. In this section you will find out about the maturation process, and how and why to observe and measure human development.

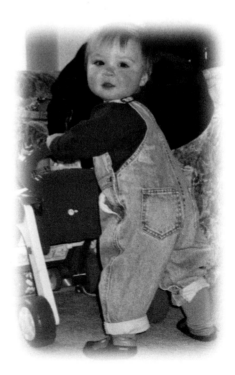

4.1.1 Periods of life

Health and social care practitioners need to understand how individuals change, develop and feel, so that they can recognise and meet their needs effectively. This includes understanding the process of maturation, from birth to late adulthood.

The periods of growth and development are:
- infancy (birth to 2 years)
- early childhood (2 to 8 years)
- puberty and adolescence (9 to 18 years)
- early adulthood (19 to 45 years)
- middle adulthood (46 to 65 years)
- later adulthood (65+ years).

If you are familiar with babies you will know that they learn how to:
- recognise key people in their lives and respond in different ways
- recognise and respond to stimuli such as sound, movement or touch
- move and hold themselves up as they grow bigger and stronger
- understand and talk as their brains develop.

Humans continue to grow and change throughout their lives through a process of development that is partly genetic and partly social and environmental.

Many people grow up to be healthy members of society, and they need relatively little professional health or social care for much of their lives. But sometimes children are born with inherited or fetal development problems. Other people may experience disease, accidents, or social problems later in their lives.

Because of improvements in living conditions and medicine, more people in the West are living longer. This affects individuals and society as a whole. There is a growing industry to support and care for older people, people with disabilities and those who are suffering from long-term illness, both in their own homes and in sheltered or residential settings.

The rate at which people develop over time varies according to:
- age
- health and disease
- nutrition
- genetic inheritance
- environment
- levels of stimulation and activity.

People develop a range of skills and abilities across their lifespan.

DISCUSSION POINT

Why do you think it is important for practitioners to be able to make judgements about stages of development in adults as well as children?

Important skills and abilities related to development include:

- gross and fine motor skills
- intellectual ability
- emotional development
- language skills
- social skills.

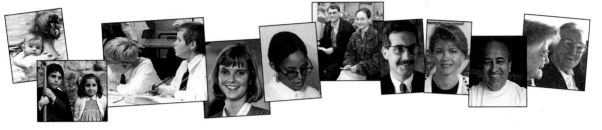

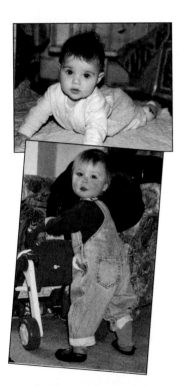

Human development is sequential: it follows a recognised order. Even after accident or disease we can see a pattern of events occurring as people change. These patterns occur in all of the areas of skill and ability.

The nervous system develops in a particular manner, which is termed 'cephalocaudal' – from head to the base of the spine and from the midline to the extremities. This explains, to some extent, the sequence of events from the time a baby develops the ability to hold up its head through to the time the child learns to walk.

Throughout an individual's lifespan change occurs continuously.

There are periods of rapid change that seem to be followed by calmer less dramatic periods. Different theorists have described these in different ways, for example:

- Bee (1992) refers to transitions and consolidations
- Reigal (1975) uses the phrase 'developmental leaps' to describe the periods of rapid change.

Infancy (birth to 2 years)

Over the last hundred years it has become apparent that the newborn baby has immense cognitive and perceptual ability, and an amazing capacity to learn. Within a few hours of birth infants can distinguish between an adult's different facial expressions and will often try to imitate them.

The first two years of life are a period of rapid growth and development. The newborn baby has yet to make sense of the world and is totally reliant on others to ensure survival. But step by step the baby begins to take control and learn to manipulate the surroundings.

DISCUSSION POINT

Try to think of other patterns and sequences that relate to the way people develop and change over their life. See if you can encompass all life stages.

183

Early childhood (2 to 8 years)

At the age of two the skills which the child has developed in previous years allow the child's experience of the world to expand. Increased mobility and language encourage increased independence and experience.

A greater diversity of people and environments influence the development of the child as he or she begins to explore the world on their own. Major transitions such as starting nursery and primary school increase the breadth and depth of the child's experience.

The childhood years are a journey from dependence to increased autonomy.

Puberty and adolescence (9 to 18 years)

Puberty (the beginning of sexual maturity) begins between the ages of nine and 14 and may continue up until the age of 20 or 21, depending on the individual. Puberty involves the maturation of the primary sexual organs:

- ovaries in females
- testicles in males.

It also involves development of the secondary sexual characteristics:

- growth of hair around genitals and armpits for both sexes
- chest and facial hair in males
- changes in the shape of breasts and hips in females
- changes in depth of voice, which is more significant in males.

Adolescence signals a time of change in biological, social and cultural aspects of life. It is a period of life that involves the transition from childhood to the adoption of the full adult role.

ACTIVITY

This life stage involves events that are often termed 'rites of passage'. These involve events such as becoming eligible to vote and a lot of other less formal events. List as many rites of passage as you can that occur in your own culture during adolescence. Then do the same for an adolescent from a different culture.

DISCUSSION POINT

In the UK, as in other Western countries, the age of puberty seems to be starting about four months lower each decade. Can you think why this might be?

The influence of the peer group is perhaps the most significant during this stage of life. The adolescent spends more and more time away from the family with groups of their own age. Physically, young people grow very rapidly particularly during a period around the time of puberty – the pre-pubescent growth spurt. The dramatic rate of growth can account for the large appetites which some teenagers have and their need for more sleep.

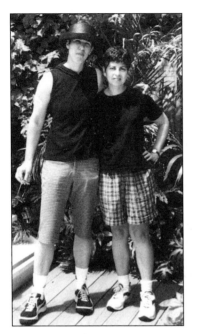

Early adulthood (19 to 45 years)

Early adulthood bestows upon the individual the rights and privileges that the adolescent has been striving for. And with these come the increased responsibilities of the adult role.

During adulthood most people form long-term relationships with a significant other person. They may set up home with them and perhaps have a family of their own. These relationships may be formalised by marriage between two adults of the opposite sex. However, same sex relationships are becoming increasingly accepted by some within our society and may serve a similar purpose.

The young adult is at the peak of physical functioning. The body develops quickly with physical activity and heals quickly following injury. Performances of many physical (and some mental, such as higher mathematics) tasks peak between the late teens and early thirties.

Middle adulthood (46–65 years)

Adults often 'slow down' as they get older. But it is possible to stay fit and healthy by eating sensibly and getting enough exercise. Loss of mental ability is compensated for by increased knowledge and experience, so that peak performance in mental spheres is more common among people in their thirties, forties or fifties than for those in their twenties. Adult life can be described in terms of stages and roles as shown in the box below.

Stages and roles in adult life

Stage	Description	Roles
1	adult is newly partnered, with no children	role of partner is added
2	first child is born	role of parent is added
3	oldest child is between two and six	role of parent has changed
4	oldest child is between six and twelve	role of parent has changed again as child enters school
5	oldest child is adolescent	role of parent changes again
6	oldest child has left home	sometimes called the 'launching centre' phase, as parents assist child to become independent
7	all children have left home	dramatic change in parental role; sometimes called the 'empty nest' or post-parental stage
8	one or both of the spouses has retired	sometimes called ageing family

DISCUSSION POINT

Age and ageing might be related to biological phenomena. But their meanings are socially and culturally determined. We take for granted terms such as adolescence and childhood. These are socially recognised descriptions of life stages and they possess certain cultural characteristics. Discuss what it means to say that the concept of age is socially or culturally determined.

ACTIVITY

What do you think about middle adulthood (46–65)? Do you agree with the ideas of Beard, above? Find out about the work of Hareven (1995). What are his views about middle adulthood?

Because of industrialisation and increasing interest in social welfare and insurance, society became interested in the limits of individual usefulness in the workplace and issues were raised about when old age insurance or pension ought to be paid.

Psychologist George Beard (*Legal Responsibility in Old Age*. Based on researches into the relationship of age to work. New York: Russels 1874) asked questions such as 'What is the average effect of old age on the mental faculties?' He tried to determine at what age the 'best work of the world' had been done and he suggests that:

- 70 per cent of creative works were achieved by the age of 45
- 80 per cent were achieved by the age of 50.

Bear in mind that things were different in Beard's time; generally people did not live much longer than the age of 64.

Beard thought that 30 to 45 was the optimal period of life. As far as we know, Beard's was the first attempt at scientific inquiry into the relationship between ageing and efficiency and it set the scene for the concept of retirement from work. (from Hareven, T.K. 'Changing Images of Ageing and the Social Construction of the Life Course' in Featherstone, M., Wernick, A. *Images of Ageing* London: Routledge 1995)

Hareven (1995) describes how life stage descriptions come into being:

66 *The discovery of a new life stage is itself a complex process. First, individuals become aware of the specific characteristics of a given stage of life as a distinct condition among certain social classes or groups. This discovery is then made public and popularised on a societal level. Professionals and reformers define and formulate the unique conditions of such a stage of life, and then it is publicised in the popular culture. Finally, if the conditions peculiar to this stage seem to be associated with a major social problem, it attracts the attention of public agencies, and it becomes institutionalised: its needs and problems are dealt with in legislation and in the establishment of institutions aimed directly to meet its needs. Such public activities, in turn, affect the experience of individuals going through such a stage.* 99

Later adulthood (65+ years)

In 1900, the average life expectancy in the UK was 49 years. Now it is usually considered to be over 70 years. The process of ageing can be considered as a gradual deterioration in function and capacity to respond to environmental stress. This process varies enormously between individuals, depending on their particular combination of genetic make-up, lifestyle choices, environment and experiences. Physical changes which occur to a greater or lesser degree in older people include:

- slowing of physical responses
- slowing of cognitive responses

- slower recovery times
- greater susceptibility to illness – particularly the diseases associated with ageing.

Although it is true that there is an increase of disease with age, and that some physiological function slows and is reduced, there are also a lot of myths and stereotypes that surround ageing. For example, younger people often refer to their elders as 'senile', either in a joking or insulting manner. The word senile means old, but it is often associated with loss of intellect. It is inaccurate to infer that older people have less intellectual ability than younger people. Studies consistently show that intelligence does not deteriorate with age, although recall may take longer.

DISCUSSION POINT

Consider this statement on intelligence and ageing. Discuss how this is relevant to the way care workers deal with older people.

ACTIVITY

There are several theories suggesting why humans age. One is the biological clock theory, summarised briefly below. Find out more about this, or another theory on ageing, and explain it. If appropriate, include a series of diagrams in your explanation.

Is there a biological clock?

The rhythms of the body's daily activities are regular and cyclical, revolving around a 24-hour day and night. There are also longer-term rhythms, such as monthly cycles. Research with animals shows that these rhythms persist even when the obvious sources of stimulation – food, other animals – are not present. These rhythms show themselves in patterns of electrical and chemical activity in nerve cells and ribonucleic acid (RNA) content. Is the slowing down of age a sign of a clock ticking slowly over the entire course of a person's life?

4.1.2 **Measuring and observing human growth and development**

The first years of life are a period of rapid physical development. Babies and small children are weighed, measured and checked for sensory development at child health clinics to ensure that they are progressing 'normally'. The information is recorded on a centile chart.

Measuring growth – centile charts

Centile charts are a means of assessing growth patterns. Centile charts used in the UK show growth within a 'normal' range, which covers 97% of the population of the UK. The exact average (mean) is 50%. The chart indicates the range within which children's weight and height are expected to fall, by a shaded curve. The range considered normal is quite wide although most people will be more or less consistent in their centile position throughout their childhood. However, it would cause concern if a child's weight declined from the eightieth to the fortieth centile, even though both are within the normal range, because it might indicate deterioration in health. Rates of growth need to be monitored for each individual, not just against the normal range.

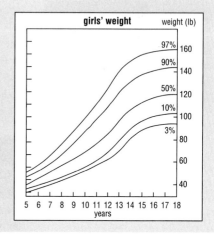

Normal development

Most babies and young children will:

■ lift their head by three months

■ sit unsupported by six to eight months

■ start trying to crawl around six months

■ be crawling by nine months

■ pull themselves upright holding onto furniture by ten to twelve months

■ walk unaided by ten to sixteen months

■ learn to kick or throw a ball by eighteen months to two years

■ learn to pedal a tricycle by two to three years.

Health and social care professionals frequently use information like this (above) to assist in assessing the needs of individuals. Different developmental stages are often referred to as 'norms'. The psychologist A. E. Gesell has written extensively about developmental norms, collecting information from many other theorists and practitioners.

There are many ways to collect information about development. Frequently longitudinal or cross-sectional studies are carried out.

Cross-sectional studies	Studies in which different groups of individuals of different ages are all studied at the same time.	This is a relatively quick method of study that can give us a lot of information. It can often tell us a lot about differences at different times of life but it does not tell us about sequences.
Longitudinal studies	Studies in which the same subjects are observed over a period of time.	This is more time consuming but gives us information about sequence.

Many different methods are used to collect information relating to development. We use the information to establish norms and averages. However, we must be aware of the limitations of such information and that each person's development is influenced by their own unique circumstance. It is very difficult to identify and describe what is normal with accuracy.

DISCUSSION POINT

There are significant problems in conducting good scientific research into development because of:

■ the range of variables involved

■ the length of time it takes to study one element of development in an individual

■ the lack of variable control.

Physical development is the easiest aspect to study. Suggest ways in which you might determine the normal physical growth rate of children. What factors might affect the growth rate?

Key questions

1   What are the six periods of life? Put down the ages of each.

2   What six factors determine the rate at which individuals develop over time?

3   What key skills and abilities are related to human development?

4   What does the term 'cephalocaudal' mean?

5   Describe 'rights of passage'. At what life stage are these often a feature?

6   The life expectancy of individuals is now beyond what age?

7   What information will a centile chart provide?

8   If a child's height or weight measurement changed from the eightieth centile to the fortieth centile, what would this indicate?

9   At what stage in life is peer group influence thought to be most significant?

189

SECTION **4.2**

Development of skills and abilities

People develop a range of skills and abilities throughout life. These can be broadly grouped into the following four developmental areas: physical, intellectual, emotional and social. Within each area we can focus on particular skills and abilities. However, the areas, skills and abilities are all interlinked.

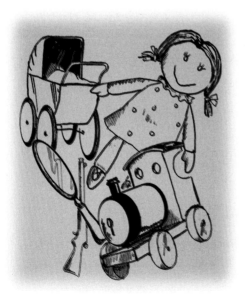

> **66** Some people have particular needs because of cultural or religious reasons. They come to light during personal care assessments and are taken into account like any other needs. **99**
>
> *occupational therapy services manager*

> **66** Karen used to babble happily as a baby. We did not realise she was deaf at first. She has special help. Her teachers are helping her to learn to communicate and she is able to make us understand most things. **99**
>
> *mother of a profoundly deaf child*

4.2.1 **Physical development: gross and fine motor skills**

Gross motor skills are skills involving posture and the large movements related to locomotion – e.g. sitting, crawling, standing, walking.

Fine motor skills are skills involving hand to eye coordination, and precise manipulation – e.g. grasping, picking up objects, writing.

The development of motor skills is an area of physical development that is carefully monitored by health professionals during early years of life. It is also an area that can be affected by disease. Professionals such as physiotherapists and occupational therapists are frequently involved in helping individuals to regain their gross and fine motor skill ability.

ACTIVITY

Find out about the role of these therapists and the principles that underpin the treatment when they are helping a person regain motor skill ability after disease or accident.

The development of these skills usually occurs in the early years of life. By the age of about six all the fundamental skills are in place but continue to be refined and perfected into adult life as we develop abilities as hobbies or skills:

■ swimming
■ embroidery
■ football
■ snowboarding
■ use of a keyboard.

As adults we are able to learn a host of new motor skills, for example, driving a car. There are thousands of examples. The necessary movements and coordination that allows us to develop these new skills have been learnt in childhood.

Month	Motor	Social	Hearing and speech	Eye and hand	Month
1	Head erect for few seconds	Quieted when picked up	Startled by sounds	Follows light with eyes	1
2	Head up when prone (chin clear)	Smiles	Listens to ball or rattle	Follows ring up, down and sideways	2
3	Kicks well	Follows person with eyes	Searches for sound with eyes	Glances from one object to another	3
4	Lifts head and chest prone	Returns examiner's smile	Laughs	Clasps and retains cube	4
5	Holds head erect with no lag	Frolics when played with	Turns head to sound	Pulls paper away from face	5
6	Rises onto wrists	Turns head to person talking	Babbles or coos to voice or music	Takes cube from table	6
7	Rolls from front to back	Drinks from a cup	Makes four different sounds	Looks for fallen object	7
8	Tries to crawl vigorously	Looks at mirror image	Shouts for attention	Passes toy from hand to hand	8
9	Turns around on floor	Helps to hold cup for drinking	Saya 'Mama' or 'Dada'	Manipulates two objects at once	9
10	Stands when held up	Smiles at mirror image	Listens to watch	Clicks two bricks together	10
11	Pulls up to stand	Finger feeds	Two words with meaning	Pincer grip	11
12	Walks or side-steps around pen	Plays	Three words with meaning	'Holds' pencil meaningfully	12

The *Concise Oxford English Dictionary* defines **intellect** as '*the faculty of reasoning, knowing and thinking as opposed to feeling*'.

Cognition refers to the way people make sense of the world through what they know and learn about it. **Cognitive development** is the development of skills that make this possible.

Intellect is extremely difficult to define. During the centuries many theorists have tried to define and describe its development.

Many aspects of intelligence are taken for granted until a problem arises. We expect to be able to interpret situations and scenes, plan activities and draw on the memory of events and information we have experienced before.

A fundamental idea relating to intelligence is that of *schema*. Schemas can be described as mental representations, which include plans of action and factual knowledge.

> A **schema** is a mental framework or structure that encompasses memories, ideas, concepts and programmes for action which are relevant to a particular topic.

Schemas are a central concept within the work of developmental psychologist Jean Piaget (see page 231). Piaget suggested that at birth an individual has a very small range of sensory and motor schemas such as looking, tasting, reaching, which develop to allow us to categorise and compare, eventually leading to complex analysis and reasoning. He proposed that an individual progresses from those simple to complex schemas through three basic processes:

- assimilation
- accommodation
- equilibration.

Assimilation is the process of taking in new information or experience. For example, a child assimilates new objects into their sucking 'schema' as they try sucking on fingers, toys or maybe soap.

Accommodation will then occur as the child realises that some objects are more suckable than others! Accommodation is the modification of the existing schema to fit the new experience.

As individuals absorb and adapt the new information and experience, Piaget suggested that they required a periodic sorting out or restructuring of all the information. He called this process equilibration – a striving to get things in balance and make overall sense.

This model of intellectual development led Piaget to describe particular stages in cognitive development, which are discussed later in this section.

It was once thought that intellectual abilities reached a peak between the ages of 20 and 30 and then began to decline. More recent studies suggest that this depends how you measure and define intellectual ability:

- Where intelligence involves the acquisition of knowledge and skills from daily living there may be improvement well into late adulthood.

Language is an organised system of symbols used to communicate in speech, writing and signs. Language in all humans develops through the same stages, irrespective of culture.

■ Where the intelligence relies on speed of thought and mental agility, we may see a decline with age as this ability is more closely related to changes in the central nervous system.

Language development

Babies can usually make noises from birth. A baby's development of language starts with cooing and babbling noises that are not affected by the language its parents or carers speak, whether people talk to it or whether the child is deaf. These noises are sometimes called 'pre-language'.

The pattern of communication is apparent in very young babies. A carer can talk and smile to the baby and it will soon realise that if it responds with facial expression and noise the carer will respond with more smiles and talk. This turn taking is part of the pattern of our everyday communication.

Between the ages of ten and twelve months, babies start to say their first recognisable words, and by 18 months they understand more than they can say. Parents help in the development of speech by:
■ chatting to their babies, and to each other
■ rehearsing phrases
■ repeating them
■ completing sentences.

Phases of language development

As with many other areas of development there appears to be a developmental process that follows common steps:

1   Pre-linguistic phase – the period before the child speaks his or her first words. During this stage babies can discriminate between many speech sounds and intonation patterns. Cooing and then babbling occurs. Cooing is repetitive vowel sounds, that often run up and down in pitch and tone; babbling is a combination of consonant and vowel sounds. When babies are babbling it sounds as if they are playing with the sounds. Bates (1987) refers to this as 'learning the tune before the words'.

2   Receptive language and the use of gestures – at around the age of eight to nine months infants begin to use gestures that have clear meaning. This can be seen with games like 'peekaboo', waving bye-bye and the way in which infants reach out and grasp to demonstrate that they want something. Studies demonstrate that the child's understanding of language between the ages of nine and eighteen months increases from understanding of around 17 words to 50 words. Their understanding of words appears to be greater than their ability to express them.

3   Expressive language – the term used to describe the child's ability in speaking and communicating orally. This includes aspects of language style and the development of grammar.

To acquire language effectively, children need three types of competence:

- linguistic competence – such as adding on 's' to words to form a plural
- cognitive competence – the desire and ability to convey meaning or understand someone else's meaning
- communicative competence – relating to other people and a whole social environment.

Some elements of language competence are built in, such as the ability to distinguish between subject and object. Others are learnt, through listening and trying out and through a developing awareness of self and others.

People may lose the ability to speak or understand language because of illness, which can be most distressing for them and their carers. There are different ways of establishing and maintaining communication including:

- sign language
- technology
- touch.

66 *I am the only person who can understand my mother. She had a stroke last year and has not been able to speak since. But she can understand what I am saying if I speak clearly and don't use too many words. She makes me know what she wants by pointing to a large card we have made with different pictures – a cup for a drink, or flowers when she wants to go into the garden. It is difficult but we manage.* **99**

daughter caring for her mother at home

ACTIVITY

Identify the techniques Kay is using to encourage Adam, aged three, to develop language. Adam has just spotted a lorry passing in the street:

Adam (pointing): 'Kay see lorry?'

Kay (moving down to his level): 'Did you see a lorry, Adam?'

Adam (continuing to point): 'Lorry, lorry.'

Kay: 'Have you got a lorry like that Adam?'

Adam: 'Adam lorry.'

Kay: 'Do you play with your lorry, Adam?'

(Lorry drives away.)

Adam (pointing) 'Lorry gone, lorry gone.'

Kay 'Yes, the lorry has gone now.'

Adults sometimes use similar techniques to help each other in a conversation. See if you can spot them when you talk to your friends.

4.2.3 Emotional development

Emotion enables us to feel rather than just think and reason. The psychologist John Bowlby has helped us to understand the behaviour of children and adults through his attachment theory.

Bowlby paid particular attention to the bond between parent and child when he was asked to study children who had been orphaned after the Second World War. He argued that babies are born with an innate tendency to create strong bonds with their care givers to ensure survival. He suggested that there was a need for one central care giver in the early years of life and that attachment was essential for healthy psychological development in the same way that vitamins and minerals are essential for healthy physical development.

Earlier theorists suggested that attachment is related to the satisfaction of basic needs such as hunger, thirst and the reinforcement of social signals and pleasant experiences. These theories are termed 'behaviourist'. They led to rigid and distant approaches to care which revolved around well-regulated schedules to meet physical needs.

Bowlby's studies had an impact on the way we practise health and social care today, recognising the importance of a prime care giver. Practices such as a named nurse, key worker and the move towards adoption and fostering rather than residential child care are examples of the way care has evolved since Bowlby's work.

Attachment behaviour continues throughout people's lives. The formation of a bond is described as falling in love, maintaining a bond as loving someone, and losing a partner as grieving over someone.

Many parents can identify five emotions in their one-month-old babies:

- interest
- surprise
- joy
- anger
- fear.

Experimental evidence shows that very young babies respond to the shape of a particular face and quickly learn to distinguish their mother's face. A baby is able to recognise and bond with its mother soon after birth. A very young baby will turn its head to follow the sound of its mother's voice.

The state of mind of the mother can affect the state of mind of the baby. If a mother is upset, the baby will sense her distress.

❝ *When I am really tired and upset I give the baby to my partner or my mother. Because they are feeling calm this seems to settle the baby.* ❞

mother of three-week-old baby

ACTIVITY

A study performed by a psychologist called H. F. Harlow in 1959 using young rhesus monkeys supported Bowlby's theories. Look up this study in a psychology book under 'attachment'. Consider how the results would have to be different to support the behaviourist approach.

DISCUSSION POINT

How do parents recognise these emotions? Do you think other people (i.e. those who are not the parents) might be able to identify them too?

Role of interaction

Throughout life, people interact with others in various ways. The first and most important bond is with carers, but gradually friends also become important and influential. Researchers who interviewed children about their best friends identified three stages of friendship:

- age five to seven – no real feelings of liking or disliking, no understanding of another's feelings (egocentric); friendships easily started and finished; based on proximity and sharing things
- age eight to eleven – mutual interests, responding to other's needs, tendency to form cliques
- age twelve and over – deeper, more enduring friendships, sharing thoughts, feelings and secrets; friends give comfort and support, and act as confidants and therapists.

Positive close relationships enhance self-esteem and social skills. Friendships can offer close relationships in place of a family and are increasingly important with age. Negative close relationships, whether with friends or family, can have the opposite effect.

❝ *Although I loved my father, he was always saying that we were rubbish. I could never do anything right. I was convinced that I was stupid. But when Mum remarried, my new Dad was very different. He had time for us and he even helped me with my schoolwork. He showed me that I was really all right. I'm going to do my exams next year and have been put up a group at school.* ❞

15-year-old girl

❝ *James always wears his emotions on his sleeves! You can always tell when he is upset, angry or bored. He doesn't have to say anything.* ❞

James's colleague

Babies and young children usually show their emotions without restraint. The tantrums that are so common in children around the age of two are often due to an inability to cope with strong emotions such as anger and the forceful feelings they release. On the other hand, babies quickly learn the pleasure of amusement and become adept at evoking pleasure-giving responses for their carers.

As life progresses, social codes of behaviour begin to mould how people express emotions. Boys may still be taught that it is 'babyish' to cry. Girls may still be encouraged not to show anger. Children who cry a lot may be labelled 'crybabies', and this belittles their behaviour. People can be trained, encouraged or shamed into showing or concealing their feelings and emotions.

Different cultures have different ways of showing their emotions. Grief, for instance, is displayed in a variety of ways, according to the norm or tradition of the cultural group.

> ### DISCUSSION POINT
>
> Choose a cultural group that is different from your own and find out its traditional ways of expressing grief and happiness.
>
> How might people from other cultures understand this behaviour? Why is it important that people should demonstrate their grief in a way that is comfortable to them?

Social skills

Norms define appropriate behaviour and attitudes for particular social situations and social roles.

Beliefs are a set of ideas (religious, political, racial) which individuals, groups or societies accept and regard as centrally important. They may depend upon faith rather than rationality.

Values are ideas or ideals that individuals, groups or whole societies consider to be of supreme importance. They can be described as a moral code or a set of priorities. Values often underpin the norms of a society and give them their particular characteristics.

ACTIVITY

Identify the norms, beliefs and values of a group that you belong to. Identify a group different from your own and do the same, listing and explaining the norms, beliefs and values.

Socialisation is learning the norms or rules of behaviour and acquiring (or rejecting) the belief systems of a family and society in general.

Social skill development involves the internalisation of the norms, values and beliefs that allow an individual to function in their culture. However, groups of people living in the same society frequently hold different values and beliefs.

The process by which an individual takes on the norms, values and beliefs of a society is called socialisation. Socialisation happens to everybody, through the primary influences of parents and family and the secondary influences of education, work and contact with other people.

Health and social care practitioners need to be aware of the different norms, values and beliefs of the groups they work with. It enables practitioners to:

- respect individuals
- understand and meet their needs
- consider how society has influenced their development.

66 *When I meet some forms of social behaviour which can seriously affect health I can't help but be upset. Alcohol is the one I get most upset about. It's the failure of people to realise that their habits are harmful to themselves and to those they live with.* 99

doctor in charge of health screening, private hospital

66 *We are hoping to influence people's choices about their lifestyles and give them information about how they could make positive changes. So we have to make sure that information is accessible and attractive to the right audience by thinking about how people see themselves in society. For example, we have found from research that many women don't take exercise because they don't see themselves as the 'sporty type'. But by no means all types of exercise have to involve sport – so we now know that many women need more information about how they can exercise without being 'sporty'.* 99

physical activity manager

The process of socialisation

As people grow up and grow older, many inherited and environmental factors combine to make them into unique individuals. Environmental factors include the culture, values, ideas and attitudes of:

- parents and other family members
- teachers
- friends and others in their peer group
- employers and people they meet at work
- religious institutions
- the mass media – mainly newspapers, TV and radio.

The process of socialisation continues throughout life. Sociologists describe two main stages of socialisation:

- primary – the process of children growing up to become adults
- secondary – the process of adults interacting with the culture of a particular society at a particular time.

❝ *In our family Father makes the decisions. I don't always agree but it is his right.* ❞

mother in a Pakistani family

Family

Primary socialisation takes place within the family. Family, friends and neighbours are all strong influences. Young children learn firstly from their prime carer, usually the mother, and then from other members of the family. Family systems vary greatly, so there is really no standard experience. In a multicultural society, practitioners need to be aware of the variety of experiences and sensitive to the way these may affect people's behaviour.

As well as family members, other factors related to the family affect people's lifestyles and the process of socialisation. They include where the family lives, the economic status of parents or adult carers, and the number and type of siblings (brothers and sisters).

DISCUSSION POINT

You may know the term 'streetwise'. What does it means to you? Does family influence play a role in whether someone is streetwise? Or are other processes of socialisation more influential?

DISCUSSION POINT

Do any of these Family Policy Studies Centre statistics surprise you? Can you spot areas that could become trends? Do you think the rise in the number of children living in poverty is likely to increase or decline over the next generation? Support your views.

Useful statistics

The facts of life in Britain

- There are 16.3 million families.
- Almost 38% of babies are born outside marriage, compared with 7.2% in 1964.
- The number of children living in poverty rose from 1.4 million to 4.4 million between 1968 and 1998.
- The number of children living in a one-parent family has nearly trebled in 25 years, from 1 million to 2.8 million.
- More than 40% of all marriages are remarriages, compared with 20% in 1971.
- 150,000 children live in families of divorced couples, nearly double the 1971 figure.
- The average age of mothers giving birth is 29, compared with 26 in the 1970s.
- Nearly 25% of women born in 1973 are expected to be still childless at age 45.
- 80% of dependent children still live in a family with two parents.
- More than 80% of fathers still live with their children.
- The birth rate is 1.73 per woman.
- Except among those aged 50 to 59, nearly 75% of people are members of families including three living generations.

Source: Family Policy Studies Centre (2000)

Vital statistics *(thousands)*	1984	1994	1995	1996	1997
Live births	729.6	750.7	732	733.4	725.8
Deaths	644.9	627.6	641.7	638.9	632.5
Migrant inflow	201.1	253.2	245.5	272.0	285.0
Migrant outflow	163.9	190.8	191.6	216.0	225.0
Net migration	37.2	62.4	53.9	56.0	60.0
Marriages	395.8	331.2	322.3	317.5	N/A
of which:					
Remarriages (one or both parties)	136.8	130.3	130.2	132.2	N/A
Divorces (England and Wales)	144.5	158.2	155.5	168.9	N/A
Average household size (GB)	2.59	2.44	2.4	N/A	N/A
Percentage of one-person households	10	11	12	N/A	N/A
Life expectation at birth *(years)*					
Males	71.5	73.9	N/A	N/A	N/A
Females	77.4	79.2	N/A	N/A	N/A
Infant mortality (deaths per thousand live births)	9.6	6.2	6.2	6.1	N/A
Legal abortions in England and Wales (thousands)	147.9	161.5	154.3	166.4	167.8
Deaths *(thousands)* **due to:**					
Cancer	155.9	158.6	157.9	156.3	154.1
Heart disease	214.7	188.6	187.3	181.9	174.7
Respiratory disease	65.9	90.9	101.6	99.2	103.1
Road accidents	6.0	3.9	3.7	3.7	3.8
All other accidents	9.2	8.2	8.3	8.7	8.8
All causes	644.9	627.6	645.5	636.0	629.7

ACTIVITY

Select one topic and its statistics from the 'vital statistics' above. Specify and comment upon current social or health policy in the area you selected e.g. migration, marriage, abortion, disease.

DISCUSSION POINT

Using the statistics on the right, compare and comment on the relationship between the number of marriages and the number of divorces in 1985 and 1997. Do you think a trend is emerging as shown by the statistics from 1985 to 1997?

Year	Total marriages	First for both parties	First for one party only	Remarriage for both parties	Divorce
1985	346389	221927	67531	56931	160300
1986	347924	220372	68976	58576	153903
1987	351761	226308	69092	56361	151007
1988	348492	219791	69419	59282	152633
1989	346697	218904	69185	58608	150872
1990	331150	209043	67013	55094	153386
1991	306756	192238	63159	51359	158745
1992	311564	191732	66296	53536	160385
1993	299197	181956	64551	52690	165018
1994	291069	174200	64009	52860	158175
1995	283012	166418	63975	52619	155499
1996	278975	160680	64653	53642	157107
1997	272536	156907	62911	52718	146689

Source: Office of National Statistics

People in households by family type					
	1961	1971	1981	1991	1998
Couples					
Dependant children	38	35	31	25	23
Non-dependent children	10	8	8	8	7
No children	26	27	26	28	28
Lone parents					
Dependant children	2	3	5	6	7
Non-dependent children	4	4	4	4	3
Multi-family households	3	1	1	1	1
One-person households	11	18	22	27	28
Two or more unrelated adults	5	4	5	3	3
All families (millions)	13.7	14.5	14.8	15.7	16.3
All households (millions)	16.3	18.6	20.2	22.4	23.6

Percentages (exept where stated)

Source: Family Policy Studies Centre (2000)

DISCUSSION POINT

Some people have a different attitude to lone parents who are in that position through divorce or voluntary separation, to those who are one parent through the death of a partner. What attitudes have you encountered in these cases? What do the differences in people's attitudes say about the modern family as a social construct?

Some people choose to be lone parents or to live with rather than marry the other parent of their children. Others may be alone due to marriage breakdown, divorce, separation or the death of one of the partners. Remarriage and step-parenting are becoming more common.

There are alternatives to the traditional family. Communes such as the kibbutzim in Israel have existed for a long time. A **kibbutz** is a community of families and individuals which cooperates in work and in raising children.

Cohabitation is the name given to the state in which a couple live together in a sexual relationship without being married. This is increasingly common in the UK and many other countries: figures from 1994 suggest that 10% of men and women aged between 18 and 49 were cohabiting. Many cohabiting couples who choose to have children no longer feel compelled to marry. In 1995, 34% of babies born in England and Wales were to unmarried women.

Families in which the parents are gay or lesbian are also increasing, although many people still do not accept this concept. Some gay or lesbian couples have entered into 'marriages' and are bringing up the biological children of one of the partners.

DISCUSSION POINT

Will the family survive as a social construct? What do you think families might be like in the UK 50 years from now?

Peer groups are people who have a similar status in some way, for example, in age or profession. The word 'peer' means 'equal'.

Peer group

In today's society, more mothers work and many more children attend nurseries and day care. This provides opportunities to come into contact with their peers from an early age. Some group friendships last a long time, sometimes even a lifetime.

DISCUSSION POINT

What peer groups are you part of? How do these different groups influence your behaviour?

Peer group relationships tend to be more democratic than those between parents and children. They also open out important opportunities for new knowledge and experimentation. With their peers, young people:

- develop their own tastes and fashions, e.g. in clothes and music
- experiment with ways of challenging the values of their primary socialisation, such as families
- gain knowledge and experience of lifestyles different from their own.

Work

In most cultures, work is one of the most important settings for socialisation. It is only within industrial societies that people 'go out to work'. In less industrialised societies, work is near or within the home or on the land associated with the home.

DISCUSSION POINT

Some people say of health or social care work: 'I could never do that type of work.' How might their socialisation make them not want to work in health or social care? How does your socialisation contribute to your interest in this type of work?

People's jobs affect their behaviour in many ways. Some people such as hospital workers or police officers work irregular hours. Many jobs have developed their own language and norms, as one staff nurse on an accident and emergency ward describes:

66 The humour shared between hospital staff would be socially unacceptable at the dinner table of non-medical people. But it allows us to face traumatic and difficult situations with a sense of proportion. 99

Education

Education plays an important role as a socialising influence. Every child in the UK must receive formal education until the age of 16. The great majority of children go to school but a few are educated at home. Schools are formal institutions with their own rules and codes of behaviour. All children attending state schools now follow a national curriculum so that there is a degree of uniformity to the knowledge and skills to which each child is introduced.

Education can be seen as a way of helping to equalise individuals in society, and this was the rationale for the comprehensive system introduced in Britain in the 1960s. There is an opposite argument that says that education in its present form ensures that inequalities in our society will continue. Bernstein's description of linguistic codes shows that children who have acquired an 'elaborated' code find it easier to cope with formal academic education. There is a tendency for children with a 'restricted' code to come from a lower socioeconomic background than those with an elaborated code.

Socialisation in schools also takes place in more subtle ways. Sociologists describe a concept called 'the hidden curriculum', first described by Ivan Illich in 1971. He found that a lot of what is learnt in school has nothing to do with the formal content of the classes, but is about things like discipline and regimentation.

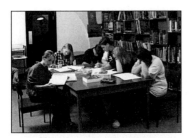

DISCUSSION POINT

What have you learnt at school, apart from the subjects you studied? What will you really take away from your years of schooling into future life?

What are schools for?

Ivan Illich, a critic of traditional educational approaches, argued that schools have four main purposes. They:

- provide custodial care – keeping pupils off the streets and in a controlled (safe?) environment
- help to distribute people between occupational roles – academic ability, skills developed and certificates awarded guide and restrict young people in terms of their future occupation
- teach dominant values – including moral and political values
- allow children and young people to acquire socially approved skills and knowledge – how to behave in a socially acceptable way, work as a team, listen and communicate.

DISCUSSION POINT

Formal education might reduce the influence that the family and peer groups have on the socialisation process. What do you think about this?

Religious institutions

Several values are common to many religions. Most religions use sets of symbols and are linked to rituals or ceremonies that are carried out by groups of believers. Some religions believe in a god or gods, others in a divine force. Many think with reverence about an important figure.

Religion is 'the belief in, worship of, or obedience to a supernatural power or powers considered divine or to have control over human destiny' (Collins English Dictionary).

Three influential monotheistic (belief in one god) religions in the world today are Judaism, Christianity and Islam. The oldest of the world's major religions is Hinduism, which is a polytheistic religion (with a belief in many gods). Other religions such as Buddhism and Taoism relate to natural harmony, which is believed to unite all creatures and facets of the universe.

The strength of belief influences the behaviour of the believer. If the parents in a family are active believers, their children will be brought up in a religious environment. When people come to a religion later in life the effect may be different. In contemporary UK society, many people do not take an active part in religion. The decline in the influence of religion is known as 'secularisation'.

The media

The modern world is dependent on communications. The mass media – newspapers, magazines, cinema, radio, television and the Internet – are all influential channels that have a powerful effect on the information audiences receive and the way in which it is interpreted.

The media help to shape people's cultural identity. For example, many TV soaps confirm how we live or make us behave in a different way because we like or have learnt from the way the characters behave. Often these programmes highlight important issues of the day. Examples include dealing with a friend suffering from HIV/AIDS, the breakdown of a marriage and how it affects children in the family.

Some media messages may concern anyone working in health and social care. For example, the media have been blamed for portraying an image of models as 'waifs': girls seeing these images strive to match them and may enter the spiral of strict dieting that may lead to anorexia nervosa.

The media are a method of control as well as a channel of information. An important aspect of secondary socialisation is learning to ask these questions:
- Who is passing on this information?
- Why are they doing it this way?

Social constructs

Personal constructs are how people develop a personal concept of themselves, others or things that is not necessarily shared by other people. Social constructs reflect a shared view held by society as a whole.

Social constructs are not fixed. They are open to re-evaluation and review in the light of new information and changes in the way people think. But with social constructs, just as with personal constructs, it is possible to have stereotypical ideas about people or roles.

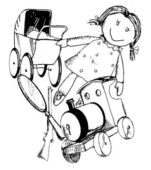

Some of the most powerful and influential social constructs are made about:

- people's roles – especially in relation to their sex and their family role
- power – the relative power of individuals to one another and the power of social structures, such as the idea of the free market
- deviance – behaviour that is not normal or socially acceptable, including criminal behaviour
- health and illness.

Gender

Gender socialisation starts as soon as a child is born. Even parents who believe they treat children equally probably act differently with boys and girls. These differences are reinforced by many other cultural influences. On the whole, society has different expectations of boys and girls.

66 *We still comment when a girl is admitted to the ward with a football injury – we are surprised.* 99

orthopaedic ward sister

Feminists say that the role of women in relation to men is a result of socioeconomic factors and can be changed. In the last 25 years, they have challenged many of the gender constructs affecting women, especially in their demands for equal pay, equal opportunities at work and abortion on demand. Since the 1960s, women have become more active in the workplace. During the last 20 years there has been an increase in the numbers of :

- women in management
- female doctors
- men in secretarial work
- men caring for children at home.

> ### DISCUSSION POINT
>
> Do you think it is acceptable for a man to be a midwife? Do you and others around you have a gender construct of this role?

But as you saw in unit 1, research shows that women still face gender barriers and stereotypes at work. They are lower paid, more likely to be in part-time, low-paid or repetitive low-skill work and still face a 'glass ceiling' – an invisible barrier to progression in a career. At home, they still undertake the bulk of household tasks.

Development of personality

> ### DISCUSSION POINT
>
> Are the patterns of behaviour that you see in yourself and other people there from birth, or were they learnt?

> **Personality** is a unique combination of each individual's bodily and mental characteristics, formed by experience and shown in their attitudes, interests, abilities and behaviour.

Personality develops during childhood and adolescence and can continue to change throughout life. Social psychologists explain the development of personality in different ways. Some believe that inherited factors play the most significant role; others argue that environmental factors are the key. It is difficult to be sure either way because there are so many variables and some

What are the variables that usually make it difficult to reach conclusions about the relative importance of inherited and environmental factors on the development of personality?

Dimensions of personality

■ neuroticism – describes people who have a tendency to worry, are temperamental, self-pitying, self-conscious, emotional and vulnerable

■ extroversion – describes affectionate, talkative people who are likely to be active, fun-loving, passionate, and who join in

■ openness to experience – this is characteristic of people who are imaginative, creative, original, curious, liberal and willing to explore inner feelings

■ agreeableness – people who are soft-hearted, trusting, generous, acquiescent, lenient and good-natured

■ conscientiousness – people who are hard-working, well-organised, punctual, ambitious and persevering.

of them are impossible to control. Some elements of personality can be researched using identical twins who have not been brought up together. Other work focuses on children who have been deprived of stimulation because of illness or lack of contact with other people.

The psychologist Hans Eysenck, working in the 1940s and 1950s, believed that personality is biologically based and lodges within the cortex of the brain. He proposed that personality could be looked at in terms of three ranges of behaviour:

■ neuroticism versus stability
■ extroversion versus introversion
■ psychoticism versus intelligence.

Eysenck suggested that introverts are more easily conditioned, more conforming, have a lower sensory threshold and therefore feel pain more acutely. Extroverts seek greater excitement and dangerous pastimes. Contemporary researchers have identified several aspects of personality that they say remain constant over periods of time and in a variety of situations. They are shown in the box on the left.

DISCUSSION POINT

How are descriptions like these of people's personality types relevant to care? Find two or three specific examples showing how they influence health and social care today. You could find evidence in newspaper or journal articles, or by asking people you know who work in the care sector. Write up your examples in the form of case studies.

Alternative theories that discuss influences relating to the development of personality are found in sections 4.3 and 4.4.

Key questions

1 What is the difference between fine and gross motor skills?

2 List at least five fine and five gross motor skills.

3 How does Bowlby's theory of attachment differ from that of the behaviourists?

4 What is the difference between receptive and expressive language?

5 How does secondary socialisation affect primary socialisation?

6 In what ways do work and religious institutions contribute to socialisation?

7 What are social constructs?

8 Why do social constructs change over a period of time?

SECTION **4.3**

Factors affecting development

Many factors influence the way we develop. Some have positive effects and others negative effects. In this section you will explore genetic, socioeconomic, and local and global environmental factors, and how they are interrelated.

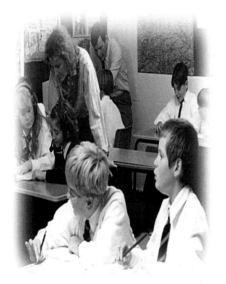

66 *It's odd how the two sisters are so different: same parents, same school, same house – but they are like chalk and cheese!* 99

primary school teacher

66 *Parents can put a lot of pressure on young people to perform well. Parents are often trying to persuade their children to gain what they see as a better life, but the students may not know why they are doing it. 'Who am I doing this for?' is the sort of question we often hear. If they are studying all the time it can create conflict with their need to be with their peer group, which is important when you're young. There are conflicting loyalties – they worry about who they should align themselves with.* 99

counsellor at a young people's counselling and information centre

66 *Many of the people I see live in poor, damp surroundings. It is hard for them to improve things without help from outside agencies. I am sure that many of their children's health problems are caused by the damp conditions.* 99

health visitor

4.3.1 Inherited and environmental influences

The nucleus of each human cell contains 23 pairs of chromosomes, half of each pair from the female and half from the male parent. Each pair of chromosomes contains many pairs of genes, which carry information about specific features of the offspring, one from each parent. Genes are either:

- dominant – the gene that has dominance over its opposite gene
- recessive – the gene which is inhibited by the dominant gene.

The genetic information in each cell of a human being influences the development and activity of the cell and the whole organism. It is widely accepted that genes control a lot of physical characteristics that are part of development. Increasingly many geneticists argue that inherited factors influence all areas of development.

It is also widely accepted that environment and experience influence the extent to which genetic potential is reached and maintained. A simple example of this is our understanding of the abnormal growth and development of cells which cause some forms of cancer. Some types of skin cancer are caused by ultraviolet radiation in sunlight. The rays alter the DNA (deoxyribonucleic acid) in the cells of the skin, changing the way they develop. In this example the environment influences the cells' development.

We also know that diet affects growth and development.

People inherit physical characteristics from their parents, such as hair and skin colour. Do they also inherit personality? There are two ways of studying the effects of genes on personality and behaviour. The first is to look at how genes specify the functions of the nervous system. This is done by finding out the pathways that link chromosomes to behaviour. The second is to look at the effects on behaviour of genetic changes, through selective breeding or mutations.

There is evidence that mutation in a single gene can have effects on behaviour. For example, babies who carry abnormal genes that make them unable to metabolise the amino acid phenylalanine have relatively low intelligence (which can be partly offset through diet). A study of one Dutch family with a history of violence discovered an inherited defect in the gene that makes monoathine oxidase (a chemical involved in metabolising adrenaline). The genetic defect on its own does not make members of the family more violent, but it does make them less able to deal with the social pressures that lead to violence.

Some diseases are linked to the sex chromosome: they appear only in one sex but are carried by the other biological parent to their offspring. Examples include colour blindness and haemophilia. Other diseases can be linked to specific combination traits in the parents, for example cystic fibrosis.

Evidence that behaviours and personality traits can have a genetic link, as well as physical characteristics, comes from comparing identical twins who are

ACTIVITY

As a child you may have been told to eat lots of certain foods because they affect a certain area of development. Many people were told that eating fish helped the brain develop, for example. Research the suggested links between diet and intelligence. Do you think that the theories can be either proved or discounted? Are we what we eat? What are your views?

The genetic make-up of an individual is called its **genotype**. The characteristic being studied – such as colour blindness, height or personality – is called the **phenotype**.

DISCUSSION POINT

Geneticists can now identify genes that carry susceptibility to many diseases, such as heart disease, certain forms of cancer, sickle cell anaemia and Huntington's chorea. It may be possible to eradicate genetically orientated disease. What practical problems might there be in doing this? What ethical problems are there?

brought up separately and identical twins brought up together. Both sets of twins have similar scores on intelligence tests. Aspects of their personality such as introvert or extrovert behaviours are also influenced by genetic factors.

In most of these cases, it is impossible to locate a single gene that is responsible for the similarities. They are probably a result of a combination of genes (known as 'polygenes'). As with the Dutch family, it is the interaction between individuals and their environment and its effect on the whole genotype that makes genetically inherited characteristics significant.

ACTIVITY

A central issue within many debates surrounding human development is the 'nature–nurture' controversy. Philosophers such as Descartes, Plato and more recently Locke, all had views relating to this issue. Find out about the arguments for the nature and nurture sides of the debate from a book on psychology. Try to work out how current thinking differs from that of the ancient philosophers.

How do inherited and environmental factors affect people's physical, linguistic, cognitive and emotional development?

Physical development

The likeness of physical features in families clearly demonstrates that genes play a significant role in passing on certain characteristics from one generation to another. There is now clear evidence that some malignant diseases such as breast cancer and heart disease are also carried in genes.

This discovery has increased the amount of screening done during pregnancy. It has also started to revolutionise the counselling services required to support people who are planning to have children. Potential parents need to know whether they are likely to pass on a genetically carried disease. The changing of gene patterns will allow children who previously would have died or been disabled to be born healthy.

The lifestyle of a child's biological parents and/or their carers also affects physical growth. For example, smoking during pregnancy is known to produce smaller babies and smoking around children is known to exacerbate certain conditions such as asthma.

Linguistic development

All children are born with the ability to learn language – grammar, vocabulary, sounds. Which language or languages and dialects they actually learn depends on the community that they grow up in. The first influence is the immediate family, and then as their social groups expand, other influences come into play. People continue to learn and develop language throughout their lives, as they move between different social groups or learn new things.

DISCUSSION POINT

Socially excluded children may suffer from poor language development. Why do you think this may happen?

Four main views about language development are summarised in the chart below.

Theory	Name of theory	Person who developed theory
Language is learnt through practice or reinforcement and imitation. In families where parents talk more to the children, the children develop a wider-ranging vocabulary.	learning theory	Skinner (1957)
People are born with the ability to formulate and understand language. The brain is pre-programmed with the rules of grammar. Language is specific to a species, but almost all children learn language at the same age and in the same sequence.	nativist theory	Chomsky (1959)
Language depends on cognitive development, controlled by the development of the nervous system. Language develops as children interact with their environment. The child prompts the development.	cognitive theory	Piaget (1952)
Language is a means of social interaction. Children develop language for social reasons of their own, not just because they need it to survive in their environment.	social theory	Bruner (1983)

Cognitive development

Piaget (see page 231) believed strongly that cognitive development was due to an interaction between the environment, learning and genetic influences.

ACTIVITY

Arrange to visit two schools or nurseries, one of which should be for children with learning difficulties. Observe for half an hour how the children are playing and interacting with others. Describe what you see and compare the two. Produce a table or chart showing:

■ how their behaviours matched the expected developmental norms for children of that age

■ the main differences between the two groups.

DISCUSSION POINT

Look at some case studies of children who have suffered from emotional deprivation and privation. Can you see a difference between the two types of suffering and their effects?

Emotional development

Family life, and in particular parental influences, affects the emotional state of children. Bowlby (see page 220) thought that maternal deprivation would result in an inability to establish relationships in later life, with a possible risk of antisocial behaviour. Other psychologists differentiate between two states where emotional needs are not met:

■ deprivation, which has short-term effects

■ privation, the effects of which are long-term.

209

4.3.2 **Environmental influences**

How do the way a child is brought up, the type and method of education, expectations of society and other influences affect their development?

Probably the best-known theorist to link development with environment was Abraham Maslow (1908–1970). He thought that individuals are born with a basic drive to fulfil their own potential and to achieve what he called 'self-actualisation'. Maslow was particularly interested in the developments of needs, which he divided into:

- physiological needs – food, warmth, shelter
- safety – physical and psychological
- love and belonging
- esteem
- self-actualisation.

Maslow argued that physiological needs must be met first, then safety needs and so on. Each stage was a foundation for the next and a weakness in fulfilment of a lower stage would have a negative impact on the stage above.

The theories of Freud and Erikson are discussed in section 4.4.

Socioeconomic factors

Socioeconomic factors include:

- housing
- employment status
- education
- relative wealth (income)
- environment
- nutrition
- access to health services
- social class
- age profile.

These have a continual effect on the development of the individual throughout their life, and the factors are closely linked. For example, employment or unemployment may determine an individual's income; this in turn may affect the quality and location of their housing.

Housing

Improved, affordable housing was one of the main aims of Beveridge's welfare state (see section 5.1). Many studies have indicated the link between poor housing conditions and premature death or chronic illness. Families living in poor-quality housing often experience cramped, damp conditions with fewer resources. The result can be a stressful environment with increased incidence of illness. Although individual development will occur, the pace of development is often impeded in childhood and the onset of late adulthood is hastened.

DISCUSSION POINT

Look at Maslow's hierarchy of needs. What might be the result on someone's self-esteem if their need for love and belonging were not fulfilled?

Being homeless also affects a person's health. A person is classified as homeless if they are without a home and have no legal right to housing, or if threats of violence prevent them from exercising this right. If the homelessness is intentional, the local authority has no legal duty to rehouse the person.

There is a direct link between life expectancy and poverty. Individuals living in poverty are less likely to experience a lifestyle that helps to delay the degenerative changes linked to ageing – so they may age more quickly than those who have access to health-giving resources.

Employment status

At any one time only a minority of the adult population are in paid employment. The young, older people, a high proportion of women, those living off unearned income and unemployed people are all outside the adult workforce. But many of these people work just as hard as those in paid employment.

66 *I had to give up my job. Now I have both my parents living with us. My mother has arthritis and can't get around much. My father used to look after her, but now he has Alzheimer's disease.* **99**

42-year-old woman

In our society, as in most, having a job is important for wellbeing. It provides:

- money – without the income from work, anxieties about coping with day-to-day life tend to multiply, as do problems of housing, nutrition and other health-related factors
- activity level – employment often provides the opportunity to gain and exercise skills and capacities; it also offers a structured environment in which people's energies may be absorbed
- variety – a job provides access to contexts that contrast with domestic surroundings even when the tasks involved are relatively dull
- structure – for people in regular employment the day is usually organised around the rhythm of work; those who are out of work may get bored or apathetic
- social contacts – friendships and opportunities to participate in shared activities with others
- personal identity – employment is usually valued for the sense of stable social identity it offers, and self-esteem is often bound up with the economic contribution people make to the household.

ACTIVITY

Various demographic characteristics can be linked to employment rates. Look at recent statistics for the area of your local authority in one of these:

- disability
- chronic ill health
- suicide
- a specific disease, e.g. stomach ulcers.

Then find out the percentage unemployment figure in the same area. Can you link the statistics to the employment/unemployment rate? Explain your findings in a brief report.

DISCUSSION POINT

The purpose of employment is varied; it is not just about providing income. Identify the areas of development that are influenced by an individual's employment. How might the employment of a parent influence the development of their children?

Education

Education – learning – occurs throughout an individual's life. Formal education involves learning from instruction, from exposure to information and other resources, and from training. Examples of formal education include:

- instruction in the knowledge and skills needed to manage a diet, for instance for individuals suffering from diabetes
- the national curriculum, which is designed to help students acquire skills and abilities during the years of compulsory schooling.

In countries where the level of literacy is low, there may be a direct link between education, health or wellbeing, rates of development and the way people cope with the change in their lives, including:

- contraception and birth control
- basic health precautions
- access to public health and social services
- access to job opportunities.

In a country like the UK where the level of education is fairly high, the link between education and health may not be so direct. But it is still there, mixed in with other socioeconomic factors. People with better education tend to have better jobs, live in better housing and have healthier lifestyles than those with a poor education.

There is a lot of discussion about whether increased education can speed up the rate of cognitive development and intelligence. In 1999, the Prime Minister, Tony Blair, announced the launch of the Head Start programme in the UK. This programme of preschool educational provision is targeted at areas of poor educational achievement and high levels of unemployment and illness.

Piaget's theories suggest that children advance their knowledge and ability largely as a result of biologically related cognitive changes. He thought that children should be offered new stimuli but only when they were ready for them: '*each time one prematurely teaches a child something he could have discovered himself, that child is kept from inventing it and consequently from understanding it completely*' (Piaget, 1970).

Vygotsky (1896–1934) took a different view, suggesting that cognitive development requires guidance from those with greater knowledge. He felt that development would be inhibited and slowed if this was not available. An investigation by L. Freund supports Vygostky's views. She set up an experiment which involved testing preschool children's ability to identify and place doll's-house furniture appropriately. This established baseline ability. She then divided the children into two groups, leaving one group to play on their own while the other received guidance and instruction by playing with their mothers. Finally she tested the improvements of each group in the doll's-house furniture sorting activity. She found the group that had guidance showed dramatic improvement, whereas the other group showed little change. Section 4.4 contains further information on Vygotsky's work.

From one point of view, education can be seen as a great equaliser – through education, everyone will have an equal chance in life. Another view is that the quality of people's educational opportunities are largely determined by their social status. Children from middle-class backgrounds go to better schools, do better in exams and have a higher chance of going on to further and higher education than children from working-class backgrounds. In this way, the education system reinforces the social and class structure of the country.

Education doesn't stop at the age of 16, 18 or 21. It can also be seen as a lifelong opportunity for personal development. For example, women who did not achieve their educational aims in their youth may return to formal education when their children are old enough. The number of women returners entering college courses at all levels is increasing.

> The term **wealth** covers economic resources including property, vehicles, investments and pension rights.

Relative wealth and income

In all societies there are inequalities of both wealth and income, although its extent will vary both geographically and over time. For example, there are wider differences in income between the average and the top 5 per cent in Britain than in Japan and those differences in Britain were greater in 1997 than they were in 1979.

Both wealth and its opposite, poverty, are relative terms defined by reference to the living standards of the majority in any given society. Subsistence poverty is when there is a lack of basic resources needed to maintain health and effective bodily functioning.

ACTIVITY

Find out about the government White Paper, Saving Lives: Our healthier nation 1999. It sets out targets to reduce deaths from cancer, coronary heart disease and stroke, accidents and suicide by the year 2010. Investigate the emphasis the White Paper places on the role of poverty and social exclusion in relation to individual development and wellbeing. How does the Government hope to tackle these problems?

Environment

Environmental factors which can affect health include:
- geographical location
- pollution levels
- air quality
- proximity to specific hazardous areas.

There is a link between people's level of income and the impact of the environment upon health. For example, car accidents account for almost half of all child injury deaths. Cheap cars without modern safety features increase chances of traffic death, so inequalities of income are directly related to the likelihood of being killed or injured in car accidents.

At home, people can to some extent control the environment. For example, they can decide whether they want the windows open or shut, but may not be able to have the heating on as much as they would like, because of cost. Services to the home, or substances such as food brought into the home, are often subjected to quality control through legislation concerning the quality and safety of food and electrical appliances.

Relevant ONS publications include:

- *Occupational Health* – gives a picture of changing patterns of health in different occupations and provides figures for sickness absence from work
- *Communicable Diseases* – gives information on infectious diseases, analysed by age, sex and health authority regions.

The work environment is controlled through legislation and regulations including:

- The Health and Safety at Work Act (HASAWA)
- Control of Substances Hazardous to Health (COSHH)
- The Reporting of Injuries, Diseases and Dangerous Occurrences Regulations (RIDDOR)
- Manual Operations and Handling Regulations
- The Lifting Operations and Lifting Equipment Regulations
- The Provision and Use of Work Equipment Regulations.

In the community, records are kept of notifiable diseases so that:

- there is a current picture of the number and types of infection in the community
- prevention measures can be quickly implemented
- adequate provision of hospital and community services can be maintained
- appropriate research can be carried out.

ACTIVITY

Vehicle emissions raise the levels of pollution in our towns and cities. Identify the main pollutants. List ways of managing the situation to reduce pollution. Explain how your ideas might help the health and social wellbeing of an affected community.

If you are interested, explore the work and research into new developments to reduce vehicle emissions.

Nutrition

The importance of balanced nutrition has become more apparent in the last century. The most obvious effect is on the individual's physical development but there is gathering evidence to suggest that nutrition influences cognitive function and behaviour.

66 *An increasing number of parents inquire about the types of snacks we provide for their children. Many want reassurance that we do not give them food with a lot of additives or sugar as they believe it affects their child's behaviour.* 99

manager of day nursery

ACTIVITY

The occurrence of poor nutrition in individuals today allows us to study how development is affected. Find out more about two conditions: anorexia nervosa and obesity. Identify how they can alter development.

Studies show that rates of development change as diets improve. Increased height and weight occur particularly in European populations. European populations are taller and heavier than they were in the Sixteenth Century.

Different rates of development are not only noticeable over time but in different populations of the world. This suggests that the environment and perhaps the diet of each population influences development.

Nutrition during pregnancy and early life is particularly important. The link between increased levels of folic acid intake in pregnant women combined with the reduction of babies born with spina bifida is one example of how nutrition can affect health and development.

Studies of infants who experience malnutrition in the first two to three years of life and whose mothers suffer malnutrition during pregnancy, show that the infants grow more slowly and that there may be permanent effects on the development of the brain and nervous system. During the last three to five months of pregnancy and the first three years after birth, there is rapid growth of the extensions of the nerve cells (dendrites) and the covering of nerve cells (myelin). The effects of the malnutrition appear to be permanent even if good nutrition is established after this time.

Access to health services

Different groups of people access health care with greater or lesser frequency. Sometimes this is because of the state of their health or their life-stage.

How we respond to sickness and ill health is influenced by a number of factors, such as age, sex, social class and ethnicity. Similar factors influence the way in which we access health care and preventative services such as screening.

It was noted in the Black Report (1980) that social classes 1V and V were less likely to visit their doctors in the early stage of illness or make use of preventative services when compared to the higher social classes.

ACTIVITY
Find out about the classification of social classes as used in the Black Report 1980. You could visit a reference library and ask for details of the report. Or contact your local authority or the Office of National Statistics to find out the meanings of IV and V. Find out the other classifications as well.

In some areas of Great Britain minority ethnic groups tend to have a lower uptake of services. Cameron (1989) suggests that this may be due to the service provider making assumptions about the amount of care provided by the extended family.

Another example of how racial stereotypes may influence the provision of services is the disproportionately high referral of Afro-Caribbean people to psychiatric services (Littlewood and Lipsedge, 1986).

You will find further material on access to care in section 5.6.

DISCUSSION POINT

Malnutrition may be just one consequence of poverty. What other factors related to poverty could account for the slow growth and other negative effects on the nervous system?

ACTIVITY

Find information about the client groups that cost the National Health Service the most.

Visit a health centre and make a record of the age profile of the people waiting to see the doctor (obtain permission first).

DISCUSSION POINT

Women of all social classes consult their doctors more than men. Why do you think this is? Is it possible that this will change as the role of men and women in the family change?

Social class

Class refers to the distinctions between individuals and different groups in society, such as occupational groups or social classes.

In Britain, which class people belong to stems from economic factors affecting the material circumstances of their lives and the circumstances of their birth. Although there is some social mobility – movement of people from one class to another – family and cultural background still create powerful social and cultural barriers to mobility. The White Paper, Saving Lives, identifies differences in the health of various social classes. For example, research has found that poor housing increases the chance of death and injury by fire.

Age profile

An accurately forecasted age profile of a population is important for planning. In the case of health and social care services, which are particularly expensive, this profile is essential. Health authorities are responsible for planning to meet the health needs of the population and local authorities are responsible for planning to meet social care needs.

The age profile may make the balance of needs different. For example, in Britain people are surviving to a greater age. This has implications for:

■ the types of service required, such as community nursing, residential care homes, nursing homes

■ the amount of services.

Demography is the statistical study of populations in terms of their size, structure and composition, and changes in these over time.

Other socioeconomic factors: life events

Divorce

Divorce is becoming increasingly common in our society. In 1994, there was more than one divorce for every two marriages. The divorce rate was 13.4 per 1,000 marriages compared to 5.9 per 1,000 in 1974. Changes in legislation have made it easier to dissolve unhappy marriages: 'no-fault' divorce laws were first introduced in 1971 and revised in 1996. It is a widely held belief that a good divorce is less harmful than the discord caused by family rows; however, see the Cockett and Tripp research on the next page.

Divorce statistics present only part of the picture: legal separations and couples living apart are not included in the figures. However, studies show that children from reordered families (where separation, divorce or remarriage has occurred) are more likely to have health problems, require help at school, have a higher level of conduct disorders, have problems with psychological adjustment and suffer from low self-esteem.

Cockett and Tripp (1994) found that children from reordered families experienced more problems (shaded column) than children from intact families:

Self-image		Social life		School work		Behaviour		Health	
Re-ordered family	Intact family	Re-ordered family	Intact family	Re-ordered family	Intact family	Re-ordered family	Intact family	Re-ordered family	Intact family
60%	28%	38%	12%	37%	13%	30%	5%	25%	10%

Relevant ONS (Office for National Statistics) publications include *Marriage and Divorce Statistics*, which has figures for the regions in England and Wales and details of the grounds for divorce. You can find out more from the ONS web site: *http://www.ons.gov.uk*.

ACTIVITY

What are the major events or stages in life? List ten or twelve. Then get together with three or four other people and look at each other's lists. How many can you add to your list from theirs?

What influence do you think each event has on development?

Accurate information is required so that the needs of these groups can be identified and plans made to support them.

Transition and change

People experience similar broad changes in their lives. For example, most people experience loss (of parents, family or friends). Many of these events are expected, but they may still cause stress. Some are unexpected, like the onset of an illness or the death of a close friend. Divorce is a life change that is thought to influence development. Many of these events partly influence an individual's development.

Many changes are part of the normal developmental pattern and the transition from one life-stage to the next. People's ability to cope with these changes, whether they are expected or unexpected, varies and depends on many factors, including their:

■ age and maturity
■ past experiences
■ personality
■ degree of support
■ level of knowledge and understanding of the situation.

A lot of research has been carried out into the positive and negative effects of change. In 1967, a scale was published indicating the impact of life events. It was based on research involving 5,000 people and aimed to identify what life events preceded illness. The events were then ranked.

217

Stress chart

The higher the stress score, the greater the risk to your health.

Rank	Life event	Stress
1	Death of spouse	100
2	Divorce	73
3	Marital separation	65
4	Jail term	63
5	Death of a close family member	63
6	Personal injury or illness	53
7	Marriage	50
8	Dismissed at work	47
9	Marital reconciliation	45
10	Retirement	45
11	Change in health of a family member	44
12	Pregnancy	40
13	Sex difficulties	39
14	Gain of a new family member	39
15	Business readjustment	39
16	Change in financial state	38
17	Death of a close friend	37
18	Change to a different line of work	36
19	Change in number of arguments with spouse	35
20	Large mortgage repayments	31
21	Foreclosure of mortgage or loan	30
22	Change in responsibilities at work	29
23	Son or daughter leaving home	29
24	Trouble with in-laws	29
25	Outstanding personal achievement	28
26	Wife begins or stops work	26
27	Begin or end school	26
28	Change in living conditions	25
29	Revision of personal habits	24
30	Trouble with boss	23
31	Change in work hours or conditions	20
32	Change in residence	20
33	Change in schools	20
34	Change in recreation	19
35	Change in church activities	19
36	Change in social activities	18
37	Small mortgage repayments	17
38	Change in sleeping habits	16
39	Change in number of family get-togethers	15
40	Change in eating habits	15
41	Vacation	13
42	Christmas	12
43	Minor violations of the law	11

Expected transitions

Change can always be stressful, but when it happens at an appropriate time it is not so frightening.

66 *When mothers go into labour with a full-term baby they are ready for the baby to be born. Although they are sometimes concerned that the process might be painful they are not usually frightened, just apprehensive. If on the other hand it is a premature labour, they may be frightened for the new baby and for themselves.* 99

midwife

Events such as weddings, 21st or 50th birthday parties and funerals help people to cope with the transition from one stage of life to another by formalising it as a social ritual. More generally, life changes can be expected and planned for. Psychoanalyst Erik Erikson suggested that people's personalities develop throughout their lives in eight stages (see page 228).

Changes in childhood can be traumatic, and people working with young children need to be sensitive to the signs. The head of a childcare centre explains:

66 *With transitions like the birth of a brother or sister, or for example if mum or dad is ill, how they react depends on the character of the child. But it will nearly always show in some way or another. Small children may regress – a little one who is dry may start to wet again. Sometimes it comes out in imaginative play.* 99

Good, effective support can make a difference to their later development:

66 *Staff may observe children showing that they feel stressed. In these situations the carer must adjust accordingly and provide the extra support and reassurance needed. Children need to be made to feel special and that they have rights. If they come through difficult situations with the right support, they learn how to empathise as they get older.* 99

Adolescence is a time when people change in many ways, physically and socially, and establish a sense of identity outside of the family. Parents and families must also come to terms with these changes.

The physical age of 40 years may be seen by some people as a 'mid-life crisis'. Hormonal changes for women may cause stress. Children may be growing into adolescence or adulthood at this time and facing emotional difficulties themselves. Some people see this time as a positive stage when they have accepted themselves and feel content with their lives.

Old age can be a time when the changes are greatest since childhood, and the sense of loss can be great:

66 *When people move in they are often giving up the home of a lifetime. All they can bring with them is some personal belongings and small items of*

> **DISCUSSION POINT**
>
> Discuss the mid-life stage in terms of Maslow's hierarchy of needs (page 210).

furniture. It's a major bereavement for them and they need a lot of emotional support and care at this time. It is common for a new resident to be rude, unhappy or totally withdrawn. Staff here recognise that we have to spend a lot of time building up trust and reassuring new residents. **99**

manager of a residential care home for older people

Some life events involve individuals in loss, for example when a child leaves home. Even when the experience is mainly happy it can also involve loss, such as when first-time parents experience joy in their baby but also sadness at the loss of freedom. There is a common pattern of behaviour in situations where loss is experienced. Often the depth of the loss is marked by the length of time it takes to go through the pattern.

Psychologist John Bowlby distinguished five phases of grief and mourning:

- initial shock, denial, concentration on the lost person
- anger
- appeals for help
- despair, withdrawal, disorganisation
- resolution, reorganisation and new focus.

Mr Graham was admitted to psychiatric care because he was suffering from increasing bouts of uncontrollable anger. As a result of his behaviour he had lost his job, and his son refused to see him any more because he found his father's anger too difficult to handle. On admission to the ward, Mr Graham took out his anger on female staff and broke several windows.

After several weeks of therapy it was discovered that Mr Graham's wife had been killed in a road accident ten years previously. Mr Graham had not accepted this and never talked about it with anyone. He still laid the table for her at meal times and bought birthday and Christmas presents for her.

After treatment Mr Graham made a full recovery and was reunited with his son. The diagnosis was delayed grief syndrome.

Symptoms of grieving

- loss of appetite
- anxiety
- withdrawal
- depression
- guilt
- sleep disturbance
- panic attacks
- crying
- lack of concentration
- difficulty in sleeping or excess sleepiness
- poor memory

DISCUSSION POINT

Why do you think Mr Graham's condition might have arisen? Identify the stages in his grief pattern with reference to Bowlby's five phases.

Grieving ends when the person reconstructs their sense of self, and comes to terms with the situation and accepts it, though they may always feel sad about it. Some common symptoms of grieving and adjusting are shown in the box on the left.

Positive changes such as promotion at work, moving house and pregnancy can also be stressful and require coping strategies.

Unexpected transition

Examples of this might include:

- being a victim of crime
- becoming disabled
- serious illness
- breakdown of significant relationships
- death of a friend or relative.

Other stressful events which are becoming more common – though they are often unexpected – are redundancy and divorce.

Divorce is one of the most common unexpected life events. One in three marriages ends in divorce, mostly within the first seven years. Reactions vary according to what the marriage was like, and whether there are children involved.

Studies have shown that people who are unemployed experience more psychological difficulties and poorer health than when they were in work. For may people, work is part of their overall identity. The loss of status, social contacts and sense of purpose can lead to a loss of self-esteem. For some people this can lead to an increased chance of depression, alcoholism or even suicide. Attempted suicides are eight times more common among unemployed people. They are most likely to occur during the first month of unemployment.

DISCUSSION POINT

Studies in the United States found that more than 80% of children attending psychiatric clinics came from reordered homes. Do you think that this could be related to the grief mechanism in some way? Should other factors be considered too? If so, what might they be?

4.3.3 **Local and global environmental factors**

ACTIVITY

Find out about the BSE crisis in Britain. Describe the difficulties scientists have in determining whether BSE has been transmitted to humans from cattle.

Governments and pressure groups are increasingly concerned about the effect that human beings have on the environment and how local and global practices can cause long-term harm to the health and development of populations and individuals.

A recent example is the concern about bovine spongiform encephalitis (BSE). There is evidence to suggest that this disease can be transmitted from one species to another in the food chain. The human form of this disease causes dramatic damage to the nervous system that can result in young adults dying prematurely.

Pollution

The expression '*as mad as a hatter*' probably arose from the damaging effect of mercury on the nervous system. In the Nineteenth Century, mercury was used extensively in the hat-making process. The damage mercury caused to the nervous system affected the behaviour of the hat makers and they were considered to be mad. Although mercury poisoning is no longer a significant problem to human beings, many other chemicals that get into the air, water and food can cause problems.

Damage to the environment is frequently caused by agricultural and industrial practices, although legislation exists in European countries to ensure that the damage is minimised.

Nitrates used as fertilisers can get washed into rivers and lakes and consequently into water supplies. Small levels of nitrate in drinking water can damage the haemoglobin of children.

There has been concern that use of oral contraception raises oestrogen levels in rivers. It is thought that this has resulted in infertility and feminisation of fish populations. Some scientists think there may be a link between the rise in oestrogens in the water and in our food, to reduced sperm counts in many human males.

ACTIVITY

In 1986 an explosion at a nuclear reactor in Chernobyl caused high levels of radiation in surrounding areas. This lead to widespread damage to plant life and the death of some people.

The threat of high levels of radiation are not disputed. Why do governments tend to promote the use of nuclear power?

Radioactivity in a variety of forms is in our surroundings all the time. This is known as background radiation. Levels of radiation are carefully controlled but it is known that higher levels of radiation may cause changes to the genetic information carried by cells. If this occurs to human sperm and ova it can be transmitted to children and cause deformities. High levels of radiation are also known to cause some forms of leukaemia. Nuclear power stations are used throughout the world to produce electricity. If accidents occur and radioactive material escapes, damage and death can occur to all forms of life.

ACTIVITY

Mobile phones may damage the functioning of the brain. Find out about the effect that radio waves from mobile phones and radio transmitters are thought to have, and how we can protect ourselves as individuals and whole societies against the damage.

Key questions

1 How has improved antenatal and post-natal care influenced the development of individuals over recent years?

2 Give an example of how environmental factors can alter the genetic material in cells.

3 What is the meaning of the term 'genotype'?

4 Briefly describe the nature/nurture debate.

5 What needs did Maslow identify as necessary for individuals to reach their potential?

6 Give two examples of how lifestyle can influence development.

7 How do Skinner, Chomsky, Piaget and Bruner differ in their explanation of the influences on language development?

8 Describe some effects that socioeconomic factors can have on development.

9 How does education help people to take control of their lives?

10 What effects are thought to be related to high levels of nitrates and oestrogen in the food chains and water supply?

11 What other local or global environmental influences can affect human development?

SECTION **4.4**

Theories of development

There are many theories of development and many views about influences on human development are held by psychologists. Each theory places a different emphasis on the extent to which various factors influence development, and on the importance of stages of development. In this section you will consider the strengths and weaknesses of the theories and how they relate to modern thinking.

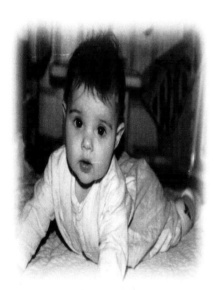

66 *We grow and change in more of a spiral way than in a straight line. We go backwards as well as forwards. Perhaps we can only go forwards if we go backwards and regress into childlike feelings first. Growth is working with the rhythms, not proceeding from some depressing reality to a perfect harmonious self in the future.* 99

Chaplin 1988 Counsellor

66 *Nature has equipped babies with all the necessary equipment to make sense of their environment. As long as you ensure that your baby experiences the rich environments around her, she will learn from it!* 99

a grandmother encouraging her daughter to take her baby out into different settings

4.4.1 Arnold Gesell

Arnold Gesell (1880–1961) was one of the early developmental psychologists. He is said to exemplify the 'nativist' school of thought. He believed that development was genetically determined and the associated abilities and characteristics merely unfolded with age. His work focused mainly on development during childhood as he considered development to be complete when an individual reached adulthood.

Genetic maturation was the term Gesell used to describe 'genetically programmed sequential patterns of change'. Psychologists such as Gesell did not believe theories which suggest that development is an interaction of the biological processes and the environment.

Gesell's studies suggested that development happens regardless of practice or training. You do not have to practise the changes occurring during puberty; you learn to walk regardless of teaching. This is the nature side of the nature versus nurture debate.

In 1929 Gesell and Thompson reported a study on twin girls in which they were both given training for motor skills, one for a longer period than the other. They reported that there was no difference in the age at which either child had learnt motor skills. However, in 1983 Fowler looked again at the evidence and reported that there were differences. The child who had received the training for longer was more dexterous and generally better at motor skills. The differences persisted into the teenage years.

This emphasis on innate qualities was typical of the era, perhaps related to the view that the status and ability of individuals were determined by God.

DISCUSSION POINT

In today's society some people think we should be free to use genetics to select characteristics of our children, an idea sometimes referred to as 'designer babies'. How does this relate to ideas of theorists such as Gesell? Can we predict the development of future adults by manipulating their genes? Should we?

4.4.2 Sigmund Freud

Freud (1856–1939) worked in medicine. He practised as a psychotherapist and much of his work originates from self-analysis, and analysis of case studies, including the dreams, of his patients.

Freud was the founder of psychoanalysis. He suggested that unconscious processes govern behaviour. The most basic is an instinctual sexual drive he called 'libido', which he thought was present at birth and was the motivating force behind virtually all our behaviour. Freud also introduced the concept of defence mechanisms – automatic, unconscious strategies for reducing anxiety. Examples include:

- repression
- denial
- projection.

Freud suggested that the human mind was like an iceberg, four-fifths of which is below the surface:

- The surface is the part we are aware of – the conscious level.
- The pre-conscious level is the area where the waves lap at the iceberg and we drift in and out of awareness.
- But the most important part, that motivates our behaviour and emotions, is not visible. Freud called this the 'unconscious'. If the unconscious is disturbed it gives rise to inappropriate behaviour.

He proposed that unresolved conflicts in the unconscious mind gave rise to difficulties in later life.

Freud explored the unconscious mind by a method known as free association, which encourages individuals to talk about anything that comes into their minds, however shocking or ridiculous it may be. He also analysed dreams and slips of the tongue. The slips of the tongue are often referred to as 'Freudian slips', and he suggested these were the true expression of unconscious thought.

Personality development

Freud developed a theory to explain personality development that is known as psychoanalytic or psychodynamic theory. He thought that the personality consisted of three main elements:

Id	Ego	Super ego
The id consists of basic instincts present at birth. The id strives for instant gratification of need. It includes sex drive (libido) and aggression.	The ego is realistic and acts as an interface between the mind and reality.	The super ego has a sense of duty, responsibility and conscience.

According to Freud, both the id and the superego are unrealistic and demanding. They are always in conflict battling to influence the ego. The ego developed the practical compromise between the other two demanding aspects. Freud described the ego as maintaining 'dynamic equilibrium'. The ego develops as the child grows.

> ### DISCUSSION POINT
>
> What do you think Freud might suggest that the following phrase means?
>
> *That was a beautiful homemade fake.*

A lot of Freud's work focused on resolving the id/superego conflict and strengthening the ego.

Freud's work suggests that early experiences determine adult personality. He identified stages within the first five years of life, which he thought determined the sexual orientation of adult life. Sexual energy – libido – was the most important factor in the developments he discussed.

Oral stage	A child's libido is focused on the mouth and it derives pleasure and satisfaction from oral activity.
	Freud suggested that if children were not weaned correctly, they would not move on to the next stage and they would become 'orally fixated'. As adults they would have excessive interest in oral activity. If a child derived too much pleasure from sucking they may become too trusting and gullible. If the child derived too much pleasure from biting and chewing this could lead to verbal aggression and sarcasm.
Anal stage	After weaning, the child's libido becomes focused on the anus and they derive pleasure from defecating. Problems could arise at this stage if parents were too harsh during toilet training, leading to anal retention – holding on to faeces. As adults these children would hold on to their possessions in an obsessive manner.
	If parents were too lenient the child could become anal-expulsive, leading to adults who are unrealistically generous and giving.
Phallic stage	During this stage the libido is focused on the genitals. In boys this led to an unconscious longing to possess their mothers, putting them in competition with their fathers. As the father is larger and more powerful, the boy infant develops a fear for the way the father may deal with the competition – an unconscious castration threat anxiety. To deal with this anxiety the boy tries to become an ally of the father, taking on his masculine behaviour. In this way the boy hopes the father will see him as an ally, thus reducing the threat.
	Girl infants become aware that they do not have a penis and experience penis envy. This is resolved by a desire to have a baby which acts as a penis substitute.
	The girl experiences similar conflict with her mother as the boy has with the father. The origin of the conflict is the unconscious belief that she has been castrated and this is the mother's fault. Like the boy infant she resolves this by emphasising her femininity.
	In the male, the conflict is called the Oedipal conflict; in the female, the Electra conflict.
Latency stage	As a result of resolution of the conflict the libido has no specific focus but is spread throughout the body. This period lasts until puberty.
Genital stage	At puberty once again the libido becomes focused on the genitals and satisfaction is sought by relationships with the opposite sex.

Freud believed that the successful transition through the stages led to the development of the child's sexual identity.

Freud's theories were greatly influenced by the society in which he lived and his theories have been widely criticised. One major criticism is the lack of material evidence. His samples were limited and did not reflect the populations he was studying. Some psychologists regard his work as little more than elaborate stories while others feel they provide useful insights into the developing mind.

DISCUSSION POINT

What effect do you think Freud's theories may have had on childcare practices?

What did Freud believe was the result of unresolved conflicts?

4.4.3 Erik Erikson

Another major influence on psychoanalytical theories about the development of personality was Erik Erikson (1902–1994). He shares most of Freud's basic assumptions, but argues that identity is not fully developed until adult life. Personality is seen to develop throughout life, in a similar, sequential way to physical development. Erikson identified eight stages, shown in the chart below, during which the personality developed in different ways. The first four stages relate to the infant and child, the remaining four to adolescence onwards.

Stages	Personality development
oral sensory	basic trust versus basic mistrust
muscular–anal	autonomy versus shame and doubt
locomotor–genital	initiative versus guilt
latent sexuality	industry versus inferiority
puberty and adolescence	identity versus role confusion
young adulthood	intimacy versus isolation
adulthood	generativity versus stagnation
maturity	ego integrity versus despair

DISCUSSION POINT

Compare Erikson's description of the stages of personality development with the chart on page 185 showing how roles change through life. How do the two charts relate to each other? Why do you think Erikson devotes four stages to the early years of life?

4.4.4 B. F. Skinner

The work of Skinner (1904–1990) was an extension of the behaviourists such as Pavlov and Watson. Pavlov discovered that dogs would salivate as soon as their food was brought into the room. The salivation was an automatic response to the stimulus of food; the dogs did not have to learn to salivate at the sight of food. Pavlov discovered that if the dogs were repeatedly given a new stimulus, the ringing of a bell, just before bringing the food into the room, with continual repetition the dogs would salivate on the ringing of the bell. This was called a 'conditioned response'.

The principle behind this type of learning is called 'classical conditioning'.

Skinner extended Pavlov's work. He argued that all behaviour is caused, shaped and maintained by its consequence. Skinner believed that if a response resulted in a positive consequence, such as a reward, this would strengthen the response and increase the likelihood of it being repeated and maintained. The term he used to describe this is 'positive reinforcement'.

The opposite of this, 'negative reinforcement', occurs when an unpleasant consequence is avoided and this also helps to strengthen and maintain particular behaviour.

ACTIVITY

List ten or fifteen behaviours you have maintained because of reinforcement. Decide whether positive or negative reinforcement has been the most influential for at least five of the behaviours you have identified.

4.4.5 **Alfred Bandura**

A different way to explain learnt behaviour was put forward by Alfred Bandura (born 1925) during the 1960s and 1970s. Bandura believed that learning in humans was more complex than how it had been described by Skinner and other behaviourists. He developed what has become an important part of social learning theory.

Social learning

Bandura suggested that learning occurs through observation of the behaviour of others. The person who is observed is called the 'model' and so this type of learning is often called 'modelling'.

Bandura did not dispute the ideas of Skinner but proposed that the role of reinforcement was different. Skinner felt that reinforcement, whether positive or negative, gave the learner information that allowed them to predict the consequence of imitating the behaviour in different settings. Bandura suggested that reinforcement served as a motivational force to learn. If the learner values the consequence of the behaviour they are more likely to repeat this behaviour. This can be illustrated by the experiment he carried out using a BoBo doll.

BOBO DOLL EXPERIMENT

Three groups of nursery children were chosen to watch a short film with three different endings. Each child would see an adult model attacking an inflatable doll (the BoBo doll). He hit it with a mallet, threw it on the floor, sat on it, punched it, kicked it across the room and threw balls at it. At the same time he shouted aggressively at the doll.

■ The first group of children saw the model being given sweets at the end of the film for such a good performance.

■ The second group of children saw the model being told off and smacked for his bad behaviour.

■ The third group of children did not see any reward or punishment.

The children were than given the opportunity to play with the BoBo doll and their behaviour was recorded. The results showed that the groups that had seen the behaviour rewarded or where there was no consequence for the behaviour, were more likely to be aggressive towards the doll. The group that saw the behaviour punished were less likely to be aggressive towards the doll.

DISCUSSION POINT

How realistic was Bandura's experiment? Do you think it contributes to current arguments about the effect of television on people's behaviour?

4.4.6 Vygotsky

ACTIVITY

Examples of this type of interaction are: a child being helped by a relative to develop their cookery skills from making simple chocolate crispie cakes to producing and icing the family Christmas cake, and an employee asking advice from their employer on how to gain promotion.

Can you identify times when your development in a certain area could have been a lot slower or might not have occurred at all without the interaction with others?

If we reflect on how we have developed over our lifetime, we may identify many times when others have assisted our learning. Our interaction with others often allows us to progress and deal with increasingly more complex ideas, situations and problems. The interactions may involve being given explanations, demonstrations, encouragement to take a problem a step further. We often seek advice from others. Sometimes we want knowledge and explanation; or we may want others to sanction or reward our actions.

Vygotsky (1896–1934) suggested that social interactions provide a scaffolding that encourages development of the individual.

The intellect, according to Vygotsky, consists of basic mental functions and innate capabilities such as attention and sensation. Cultural influences, transmitted by people with greater knowledge and language skills, develop these basic capabilities into more complex higher skills.

An important part of Vygotsky's work focused on what he termed the 'zone of proximal development (ZPD)'. Vygotsky described the ZPD as the difference between what a child can achieve on his or her own and what he or she can achieve with help and guidance from others. Without social interaction the child will only achieve sufficient knowledge and skill to survive; the understanding of wider principles, and abstract and complex concepts, will not occur.

The ZPD is an area of potential development that can be stimulated by social interactions. This is in conflict to Piaget's ideas which suggest that an individual needs to be of a certain stage of organic maturation before certain types and stages of learning can occur.

Vygotsky also explored the relationship between language and thought. He suggested that as children develop, they develop language for two different purposes:
- language for thought
- social language for interaction with others.

He recognised that both children and adults use language to direct thoughts and plan actions.

Some ideas of Vygotsky are shown below.

Pre-intellectual language	Language developed by hearing it from others; it is not associated with thought.
Pre-linguistic thought	The infant gathers experiences and memories and structures them to create meaning.
Social linguistic stage	Around the age of two pre-intellectual language and pre-linguistic thought come together. Thought becomes verbal and speech rational.
Egocentric speech	Often apparent in young children. The child verbalises their thoughts but they are not directed at a listener.
Inner speech and social speech	Inner speech is the language we use to think with. It is often different from social speech, which we use to convey our thoughts to others and interact with them. Inner speech is often abbreviated and telegraphic.

ACTIVITY

Much of the language we use requires little cognitive activity (thinking). This is described as 'affiliative' rather than 'cognitive'. Write down or tape a short conversation between two people. Try to identify which aspects are cognitive and which are affiliative.

Vygotsky's work was carried out in the 1920s but was suppressed by the Stalin government in Russia. His ideas became available in the West during the 1960s. This perspective, which emphasises social interactions, is currently popular and has significant influence on work in early education, health and social care.

4.4.7 Jean Piaget

Some theories of developmental psychologist Jean Piaget (1896–1980) were discussed on page 192. Piaget carried out influential studies, and although they are frequently criticised, he provided the foundation for much current thinking.

Piaget's findings on cognitive development in children, from experiments in the 1950s, are still considered fundamental by some psychologists, though they are challenged by others. Piaget investigated:

- spatial awareness
- object permanence
- conservation
- hypothetical constructs
- abstract thinking.

Spatial awareness is important because many things people do require them to locate objects using their senses: seeing, hearing, touching and awareness of the movements and positions of their own bodies (kinaesthesis). Some children have considerable problems in knowing where they are in space and this may prevent them from understanding which is the left and right side of their body, or the geography of a building. It may also prevent them being able to dress easily or judge distances and directions. The box below shows the normal development of sensorimotor coordination in children.

Age	Normal development
one month	follows objects with eyes and head
two to three months	predicts future position of moving objects; takes interest in close objects, including their arms
three months	directed arm movements, looks between grasped objects and hand
three to four months	watches how two hands work together
five months	controls actions of both hands/arms, reaches rapidly and grasps objects

Conservation experiment with beakers of liquid

Part 1 of experiment

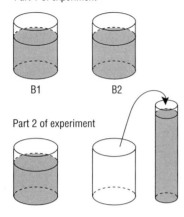

B1   B2

Part 2 of experiment

Conservation experiment with plasticine

Part 1 of experiment

plasticine 1   plasticine 2

Part 2 of experiment

plasticine 1   plasticine 2

By the age of eight months, children demonstrate curiosity about objects such as toys, but only if they can see them. If the toy is hidden, they lose interest. At about the age of twelve months babies start to understand that if the toy rolls out of sight it still exists behind whatever is obscuring it. This is what babies are exploring when they throw toys away from them for others to pick up and give back – they are learning that the toy still exists. Piaget called this 'object permanence'.

The ability to understand concepts of number, mass or volume seems built into humans, like the ability to acquire language. At around the age of six or seven, children learn to distinguish between different sizes, shapes and patterns that contain the same number, volume or mass of substance. This principle of conservation is needed for understanding maths and is important for the development of logical thinking.

Watching children play can be delightful: they have such vivid imaginations: a corner of the garden becomes their house, the stones are tables and the sticks are spoons. Scenes like these demonstrate that young children have the ability to think in the abstract and develop hypothetical constructs through cognitive techniques of assimilation and accommodation. As adolescents and adults this ability is used to build 'what if' scenarios, which enable ideas to be thought through and tested before implementation.

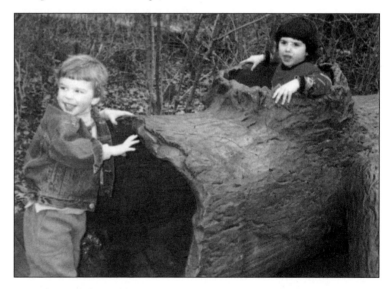

Assimilation is when perceptions are modified by what people already know. Accommodation is when existing structures of knowledge are modified by perceptions.

Piaget's work on egocentricity demonstrates how young children are only able to see things from their own point of view.

ACTIVITY

Research Piaget's theory of egocentricity. Set out the key points as a set of notes and describe one of his experiments.

Piaget's original experiments were carried out in 1952, Borke's in 1975. It may be that the two sets of children had experienced different cultural environments, such as a greater experience of more sophisticated television programmes that present various perspectives. What do you think?

Modern research does not always agree with Piaget. Borke set three-year-olds and four-year-olds a perspective task using the character Grover from the children's television programme Sesame Street. He asked them to describe what Grover could see as he drove along in a fire engine. He found that children could decentre (put themselves in the place of Grover) to a greater extent than Piaget had suggested was the norm.

The table below shows how activities and relationships can ease the transition from one stage of development to another.

Age	Transition	Activity	Important Relationships
1	Trust versus mistrust	Consistent, stable care	Mother
2–3	Autonomy versus shame	Independence from parents	Parents
4–5	Initiative versus guilt	Exploration of environment	Basic family
6–11	Industry versus inferiority	Acquisition of knowledge	Family, neighbours, teachers
12–19	Identity versus role confusion	Seeking coherent personality and vocation	Peers, in-groups, out-groups
20–39	Intimacy versus isolation	Deep and lasting relationships	Friends, lovers
40–64	Generativity versus stagnation	Being creative and productive for society	Spouse, children
65+	Integrity versus despair	Review and evaluate life	Spouse, children, grandchildren

Key questions

1 According to Erikson, what are the eight stages of the development of personality?

2 What do recent genetic discoveries add to our understanding of the development of personality?

3 What is Gesell's theory of controlled development?

4 How did Freud describe the roles of the id, ego and superego?

5 How did Freud think children develop gender identity?

6 What are the meanings of 'positive' and 'negative reinforcement'? How did Skinner think they influenced learning?

7 What can we learn from Bandura's experiment with the BoBo doll?

8 What did Vygotsky mean by the zone of proximal development?

9 What did Piaget think were the main stages of cognitive development?

10 How did Piaget and Vygotsky differ in their views on how children learn?

Assignment

Carry out a study of the human development of two individuals at different life stages (the youngest must be at least eight years old and the other at least 19 years old). You need to show you understand the way that individuals have developed and why this has been the case. Your study must include:

- the growth and development of the two individuals at different stages of their development
- how two major skill areas developed in each individual
- factors that affect human growth and development
- theories of development and learning.

Key skills

You can use the work you are doing for this part of your GNVQ to collect and develop evidence for the following key skills at level 3.

when you	you can collect evidence for
	communication
use an older person for one of the studies and family members as the case studies	key skill C3.1a contribute to a group discussion about a complex subject
investigate the theories of stages of development	key skill C3.2 read and synthesise information from two extended documents about a complex subject; one of these documents should include a least one image
describe theories of development and relate them to individuals; trace the development of different individuals at different life stages	key skill C3.3 write two different types of document about complex subjects; one piece of writing should be an extended document and include at least one image
	application of number
record appropriate routine measurements to monitor the human growth and development of two individuals	key skill N3.1 plan, and interpret information from two different types of source, including a large data set
interpret and present measurements monitoring human growth and development	key skill N3.3 interpret results of calculations, present findings and justify methods; use at least one graph, one chart and one diagram
	improving own learning and performance
set targets for learning and revision when preparing for external assessment	key skill LP3.1 agree targets and plan how these will be met, using support from appropriate others
prepare and revise for external assessment	key skill LP3.2 use the plan, seeking and using feedback and support from relevant sources to help meet the targets, and use different ways of learning to meet new demands
review performance and agree methods for improvements in the future	key skill LP3.3 review progress in meeting targets, establishing evidence of achievements, and agree action for improving performance

UNIT 5

Health, social care and early years

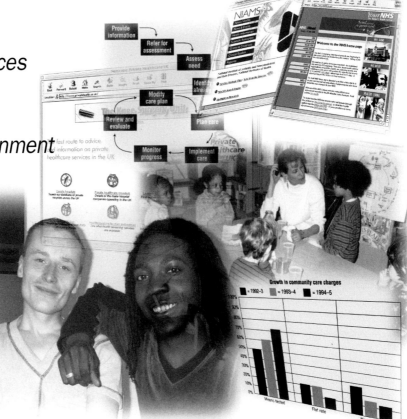

About this unit

It is important for practitioners working in health or social care and early years services to understand how their services have developed and how they are structured and funded. This unit covers:

- the origins and development of health, social care and early years services
- national and local provision of services
- access to services
- the funding of services
- how services are organised
- informal carers.

Although most people look first to their family doctor or local pharmacist for advice on health matters, dentists, optometrists or ophthalmic practitioners also provide essential care to meet everyday needs.

> 66 *Community health services staff offer a range of services for people wherever they are, in their homes, schools, clinics and even in streets. These services include health visiting, school nursing, chiropody, occupational, speech and language therapy. Services such as district nursing and psychiatric nursing and physiotherapy can enable people with short-term or long-term disabilities to be cared for in their own homes. Other specialist staff, such as midwives, provide care across hospital and community settings.* 99
>
> Health Services White Paper (December 1997)

> 66 *Children are cared for in many ways and almost all children receive a mix of informal care from parents and relatives in their homes and more formal care in other settings. . . Parental care is complemented by a range of other services, such as parent and toddler groups, family centres, one o'clock clubs and toy libraries focused on meeting the needs of children with their carers. . . Childminders, nurseries and out-of-school clubs focus on meeting the needs of children while their parents work.* 99
>
> Meeting the Childcare Challenge (November 1998)

> 66 *Community care means providing the right level of intervention and support to enable people to achieve maximum independence and control over their own lives.* 99
>
> Caring for People, Department of Health White Paper (1989)

Origins and development of services

The whole of your life, and that of your parents, has been spent under the welfare state – a comprehensive package of health and social care 'from the cradle to the grave' that developed throughout the Twentieth Century. The greatest development came during and after the Second World War. The last 20 years have brought major changes and an increasing challenge to the assumption that the state can and should cover all eventualities at no direct cost to the user. This pace of change still continues into the new century.

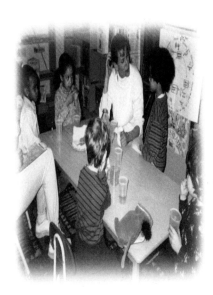

5.1.1 **Development of services**

Social policy refers to the whole range of ways in which government affects the lives of individuals. It includes, but is not restricted to, welfare policies.

The way in which health, social care and early years services have been developed is through the social policies of different national governments and their interpretation of the attitudes, opinions, needs and wishes of their populations.

Since 1945, government social welfare policy has gone through several broad phases of philosophical approach:

- the welfare state – a full provision of health and welfare services
- market economy – the provision of health, social care and early years services through commissioning contracts
- mixed economy – the provision of health and social care services through a mixture of statutory, voluntary and private organisations
- integrated care – a closer joint working between health and social services.

As you will read in this section, the election of a Labour Government in 1997 has brought about a rethink of social policy in many areas – not least health, social care and early years. Keep yourself up to date on these changes by reading newspapers and journals, and by using the Internet, and following up specific references.

Start with the Government's web site (*http://www.open.gov.uk*) which will give you access to the web sites of all government departments and agencies.

Welfare state

Although the roots of the welfare state lay much earlier with a free child health service and public housing, its form developed in the 1940s. During the Second World War there was a broad consensus that major social changes were necessary to meet new hopes and expectations. Together, the Beveridge Report and six Acts of Parliament laid the foundation of the welfare state. They are the:

- Beveridge Report 1942
- Education Act 1944
- Family Allowance Act 1945
- NHS Act 1946
- National Insurance Act 1946
- Children Act 1947
- National Assistance Act 1948.

The Beveridge Report made far-reaching recommendations that formed the foundation of the post-war social welfare services. Underpinning it was an assumption, which lasted until the mid-1970s, that government intervention in economic and social policy was in both the national and the individual's interest.

The report had three central recommendations for social provision:

- family allowances, national insurance and income support
- full employment
- a comprehensive national health service (NHS) – a universal service, free at point of delivery, available to all when needed, at home and in hospital.

UNIVERSALITY VERSUS SELECTIVITY

Ever since 1942 there has been a lively debate as to whether services and benefits should be universal (available to all equally) or selective (directed to those in most need). Beveridge favoured universality. He believed universal benefit would reach those in need since it was automatic and bore no stigma.

Those in favour of a selective system argue that it's wasteful to pay benefits to those not in need, and that spreading resources too thinly fails to benefit those in real need. They suggest that it's better to make adequate payment to those in need and reduce overall cost while allowing taxpayers to spend more of their own money.

DISCUSSION POINT

There continues to be wide public support for child benefit, which is universal. What do you think? Should there be any other universal benefits and services? If so, which ones?

Although there have been many changes in detail and structure, the skeleton of Beveridge's proposal still stands. Opinion polls have consistently indicated the broad popularity of the National Health Service and strong opposition to attempts to 'privatise' it.

Growing extent of services

The Beveridge Report, like many of the measures that stemmed from it, is based on the assumption that it was the proper role of the state to be the major provider. Voluntary agencies were to be supplementary. The private sector was for wealthy people.

The modern state still deals with problems which Beveridge:
- would have been familiar with (illness, accident or unemployment)
- would have expected to be no longer with us (homelessness and large-scale unemployment)
- did not anticipate (the changing nature of the family, large-scale immigration from the 'new' Commonwealth or refugees fleeing wars, the idea of comparative deprivation).

Social policy during the succeeding half-century largely depended on exchanges between four factors:
- the experience of existing systems and their faults
- changing social and economic circumstances
- managing the costs of an increasingly expensive service
- the balance between state and individual responsibility (collectivism versus individualism).

From 1945, local government expanded its services to include major house-building and renovation schemes, leisure and recreation facilities, and an expansion of secondary and further education. Local authorities, using their discretionary powers, expanded health, child and welfare services.

Fragmentation of services

Services were fragmented as social workers worked in different departments with children, older people, adults with sensory impairment or other physical disabilities, those with mental health problems, and hospital patients. The Local Authority Social Services Act 1970 swept away these many separate departments and introduced a new local authority department to manage all personal social services. Initially the Act created generic field social work teams to offer social work interventions for all clients. Subsequently social services departments established specialist teams for adult services, children, under-five services and mental health with close links to residential and day care services.

At the same time, the NHS was reorganised to bring together all health services – primary health services, including mother and child clinics, hospitals and the health functions of the Local Authority Medical Officer of Health.

It was clear that health authorities and social services departments needed to work together. Joint planning committees were created at district and service-planning levels.

Care in the community

Much of the expansion had been through developing community-delivered services. These were increasingly 'preferred' by clients. For example, home helps, luncheon clubs and day centres enabled older people to stay in their homes rather than go into residential homes.

> There was a growing recognition that the best way to meet the needs of people with learning difficulties was with a social care model rather than a medical one. This went hand in hand with changes in attitude towards people with learning difficulties, which included:
>
> - dropping the term 'mental handicap' for 'learning difficulties'
> - moving people from hospitals or residential communities into small hostels and then to shared houses
> - recognising that people with learning difficulties were not 'patients'
> - recognising the right to greater self-determination and advocacy.

Housing

Special needs housing is housing, with social care and other support, which has been specifically provided to meet the needs of groups such as older people, or people with physical disabilities or mental illness.

As social care supported more people in their own homes, working with housing authorities and housing associations became very important. For much of the early post-war period, local authority housing departments provided necessary housing support. From 1985, local authorities were required to provide permanent accommodation for the vulnerable homeless. Housing associations, many started by charities, are increasingly important providers of social housing. The Housing Corporation, which is funded by central government, has promoted a growth in the number of housing associations, including the provision of special needs housing.

Community involvement

The 1960s were characterised by a challenge to existing social, cultural and political norms as the first generation to have benefited from the reforms of the 1940s moved into adulthood. By the 1970s individuals and groups were involved in seeking improvements to services and a voice for clients. Where groups represented clients or their carers, they began to achieve consultative status in planning services. By 1988, such consultation was the norm. At the same time, practitioners in health and local government began to promote the idea of volunteers working with clients. Local authorities increasingly made grants to voluntary groups, and voluntary organisations were funded through central government funding initiatives.

5.1.2 **Radical changes in government policy**

The welfare state proved to be 'popular', and as demand increased and expectations grew so costs steadily rose. Although successive governments, concerned at what they saw as the uncontrolled expansion of costs, did not change the basic structures, they began to put financial constraints on local authorities and the NHS.

At the beginning of the 1970s the long post-war economic boom came to an end and, as unemployment increased, it became clear that the welfare state could no longer be taken for granted. It began to face increasing challenge because of:

- an increasing public and governmental emphasis on individual responsibility and choice
- a series of well-publicised reports into abuses and scandals
- a concern that services were being delivered inefficiently and that the fault might lie in the welfare model itself
- an increasing demand for the right to complain and have access to previously confidential details.

The central debate has therefore been a search by successive governments for the most efficient and cost-effective way of delivering the service.

The introduction of the market

From 1983 successive Conservative governments undertook a radical shift away from the Beveridge arrangements towards a market force approach to health and social care. It resulted in a 'mixed economy' of delivery for clients.

Government policy for health and social care was at two levels:

- **strategic** – the overall philosophies that each government held and sought to implement (for example, the value of the competitive market).
- **tactical** – the practical ways in which those broader philosophies were to be implemented (the structure of the services and the arrangements made for their working).

The Conservatives believed that government took too much control and they therefore sought to reduce the amount of regulation. They saw the role of government as setting the framework – leaving it to health and local authorities to work things out at local level within that framework. They required health and local authorities to identify the needs of their communities and to plan for these. The plans were set out in local documents.

Market forces

The private sector was encouraged to play a greater role in the provision of care and for specified services in local authorities.

CONTRACTING OUT THROUGH COMPETITIVE TENDERING

A local authority took a decision in 1993 to contract out a number of its social services including meals on wheels, day centres and residential homes for older people. The process began with a review of services by an external consultant. The department then drafted specifications for each service, which outlined:

- the care practice required
- the legal requirements
- staffing levels
- quality standards
- monitoring.

The social services committee agreed more detailed service specifications in July 1993 when it was agreed that the contracts would run for three years. The department then:

- asked private and voluntary organisations if they were interested in running any of the services
- placed advertisements for potential contractors with a date for bids to be received
- made decisions on the basis of the tenders received
- allocated a contracts manager to each service provider to monitor the service.

The private sector includes:

- health and other professionals, such as doctors, dentists, osteopaths, counsellors and complementary medical practitioners
- small businesses such as chemists and opticians
- private companies which run nursing or care homes
- national and international companies, such as drug companies and suppliers of special equipment.

In addition, insurance companies were encouraged to play a bigger part in recruiting considerably more people into health schemes linked with private health companies. In the mid-1990s the Government tried to widen the involvement of private and not-for-profit organisations by introducing a voucher scheme where parents of small children could purchase places at an under-school service of their choice.

DISCUSSION POINT

Do you think competition between similar agencies benefits clients? Discuss a range of facilities and different users. Is your conclusion similar in every case?

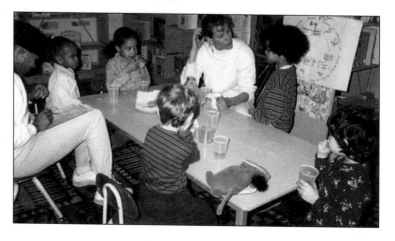

An **internal market** is a competitive system between different parts of the same organisation. It is not open to competition from outside organisations.

ACTIVITY

Find out the main proposals contained in Working for Patients. Look at the Government's web site (http://www.open.gov.uk).

Mixed economy and the purchaser/provider split

Health and social care provision in the UK is now based largely on a mixed economy. The principles for this arrangement were set out in a White Paper Working for Patients (1989) and built into the NHS and Community Care Act 1990. Apart from central purchasing, the NHS services were delivered through an internal mechanism called the internal market. The market was divided with health authorities and GP fundholders purchasing from NHS trusts and primary care services through annual or shorter-term agreements.

66 *My doctor is a fundholder so she was able to allow me to go to the neighbouring hospital for my hip replacement. They had a much shorter waiting list. Our local hospital said I would have to wait nine months.* 99

retired postal worker

Social services departments

The proposals for community care in local authority social services departments were contained within another White Paper: Caring for People. An internal market would not be introduced, but social service departments would introduce the purchaser/provider split by separating those responsible for assessing and purchasing social care from those providing the services. They were also encouraged to purchase services from the voluntary and private sectors. This approach was given the name of 'mixed economy'.

Mixed economy of care describes an approach to providing social services through public, voluntary and private agencies rather than just through social services departments.

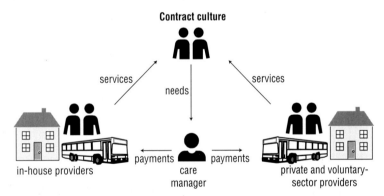

Contract culture

services — needs — services

in-house providers — payments — care manager — payments — private and voluntary-sector providers

At the centre of the purchaser/provider split was the idea of care managers having budgets for their client groups so that they can put together packages of care for an individual from a variety of agencies. Although this way of organising services was intended for social care services, the principle of the split also began to appear within local authority children's services.

Individual choice and responsibility

It was argued that comprehensiveness created a 'nanny state', which stifled individual responsibility and delivered services inefficiently. The Government encouraged the idea that individuals should be able to make choices about their health and social care. In essence managers and professionals purchasing

At the heart of the evolving debate about the role of the welfare state is a conflict between collectivist and individualist values. Taken at their extremes, they mean the following:

- **collectivism** – all provision is made by the state with individuals contributing according to ability and receiving according to their need

- **individualism** – it is no business of the state to interfere in individual choice; people must be free to make their own choices and arrangements.

The NHS is essentially a collectivist model; the state makes arrangements for services, and decisions are made for the patient by the health authorities and GP practices. By going to private medicine, an individualistic model, patients makes their own decision about the services to purchase.

The collectivist believes that, as well as rights, we have obligations to each other and that the rights of the individual must, to a greater or lesser extent, be submerged for the greater good. The individualist regards this as patronising and considers that allowing individual choice encourages enterprise and freedom.

and providing health and care should match these services to individual needs, and clients should expect high standards of care. People should be encouraged to make provision for their own retirement or health needs through private insurance or making a direct payment.

66 *I think contracts for services will give users more choice as we build up a more varied network of providers from the voluntary and private sector.* 99

head of contracting in a social services department

DISCUSSION POINT

Where do you think the balance between collectivist and individualist views should be drawn? Are there some choices which should always be made by the individual? Are there matters on which the collective good must always be more important than individual choice?

Purchasers for individuals

Most purchasing work is aimed at groups specified by age, group, or type of service. But it is possible for purchasing organisations to use a contract to meet a specific individual's need. Individual contracts are used when an individual is living in a residential home. A placement fee was the traditional approach to funding residential care, frequently because residents paid for their care through a mixture of social security, local authority and personal provision. It appears that the provision of home care is being funded through similar means.

DISCUSSION POINT

When people with mental health problems are living in a hostel within the community, what factors may limit their choices of activity and lifestyle?

Clients' rights

Clients were given written statements of their rights and responsibilities and were drawn into the assessment and planning process, being expected to have a say in how their services were provided. Informal carers were also given the right to be assessed and supported. These rights were upheld through initiatives like the Patient's Charter, Charter Marks or Investors in People Award. Clients were also offered opportunities to make their own choices. The voucher scheme for nursery places, already mentioned, was one of these arrangements. Another was the Community Care (Direct Payments) Act 1995 that enabled people under 65 to receive finance to make their own arrangements for their care.

Clients' responsibilities

The Conservative Government believed that individuals should make provision for their future health and care needs through private insurance companies. To encourage this shift, individuals paying into pension schemes and private health insurance were given tax concessions. Additionally, clients were charged for services to a much greater extent.

Accountability

66 *The changes have exposed the inadequacy of financial and managerial systems in many local authorities. Much needs to be done to strengthen financial planning and control, and to improve the use of information for effective management. Evidence has emerged of some authorities abruptly altering the care arrangements of vulnerable people, causing distress and insecurity to them and their carers. Social service departments must work closely with other agencies and the people using their services to manage change with more consideration for service users.* 99

summary of the Annual Report for 1995/6 from the Chief Inspector of the Social Services Inspectorate

The idea behind this increased focus on accountability is that public services should be open to public scrutiny. This enables national and local taxpayers to see that they're getting value for money.

Assessment

The starting point for planning within the market approach in health and social care was the assessment of the needs of the community. In the case of health, need was defined by the NHS Executive as 'the ability to benefit from healthcare', while social services were expected to define need in terms of their population and socioeconomic conditions. This information was then put into an annual health service plan and a community care plan.

Performance targets and league tables

From the mid-1990s the Conservative Government introduced the concept of performance targets against which public services should be measured – for example, national curriculum in education where targets were set for specific age groups. Organisations' success in meeting the targets was published through league tables.

Other changes

By 1997 when the Conservatives left government, it was already possible to see some balancing consequences of the reforms. For example, they have enabled more effective control of allocation and management of budgets, and have devolved responsibility to practitioners working directly with the client, through transferring decision-making about resources from practitioners to managers. They have also increased the participation of independent organisations, and focused services on the needs of clients.

Further changes were made to slim down local authorities to reflect their changed powers and priorities, with many of the services they had traditionally provided moving to outside contractors. These new structures:

- brought social services and another service, such as housing, together

- reorganised services for a clearer focus on a client group or type of service, such as early years provision which started to be grouped together in education departments

- reduced the levels of management and devolved decision-making closer to the client

- reduced central functions such as policy development and training.

5.1.3 Change and modernise

❝ We will be a radical government. But the definition of radical will not be that of doctrine, whether of left or right, but of achievement. ❞

Tony Blair in Labour Party Manifesto (1997)

In 1997 the incoming Labour Government had accepted many of the previous administration's philosophies, most significantly:

- the need to contain expenditure on both the NHS and social care
- the encouragement of a mixed economy in service provision with a shift towards independent providers
- commercial competitiveness and quality
- a focus on services geared towards the needs of clients and their carers.

It therefore looked for a system based on partnership and driven by effective performance. Several government Green and White Papers were published detailing proposals for changing and modernising most public services. The important ones for health, social care and early years are:

The Government Public Service Agenda relevant to health, social care and early years:

Green and White Papers since 1997

Name of Green or White Paper	Date	Outcomes in terms of guidance or legislation
1 Modernising Government (White)	Nov 98	■ Principles incorporated in other public service developments
2 The New NHS (White)	Dec 97	■ 1998 – first primary care groups set up ■ 1999 – NHS Act ■ 1999 – first combined budgets ■ 1999 – first Health Improvement Programme required
3 Meeting the Childcare Challenge (Green)	May 98	■ Sept 98 – first free places for four-year-olds ■ Oct 98 – guidance on childcare priorities ■ Feb 99 – first childcare plan required from local partnerships ■ 1999/2000 – Care Standards Bill
4 Modernising Local Government (White)	July 98	■ 1999 Local Government Act introduces Best Value mechanisms
5 Modernising Social Services (White)	Nov 99	■ Sept 99 Guidance on priorities for both adults and children ■ 1999 Care Leavers Act ■ 1999/2000 – Care Standards Bill

Themes common to all these papers are:

- fair access to national services
- clients and carers at the heart of service
- services delivered against national standards which will be a local responsibility to implement
- safety, protection and inspection standards
- service delivery through partnerships
- cost effectiveness and efficiency.

Each Green and White Paper customises these themes, offers a critique of the current situation, proposes strategic and practical solutions and is supported by government guidance and circulars. As a GNVQ student, you are encouraged to read the material for yourself and keep up to date.

❝ *The methods are pragmatic. But they are a means to an end . . . social justice, quality public services, equality of opportunity and a reassertion that citizens have responsibilities as well as rights.* ❞

Anthony Bevins, New Statesman (17 January 2000)

The Cabinet Office

The Cabinet Office, which operates with direct responsibility to the Prime Minister, became the principal coordinating point for integrating policy. For example, the Better Regulation Task Force oversaw the principles of regulation which needed to be transparent, accountable, targeted, consistent, proportional. The Social Exclusion Unit also is based in the Cabinet Office. Its remit is to help improve government action to reduce social exclusion by producing joined-up solutions to problems.

The NHS

The incoming Government identified the following problems:

- the way that the health authorities, GP fundholders and NHS trusts worked together has caused unnecessary competition and fragmentation of services
- the internal market forced trusts to compete for budgets on a short-term basis
- it encouraged secrecy which meant clients and practitioners did not have access to information.

It proposed to abolish the internal market and replace it with integrated care by:

- keeping the separation between the planning and commissioning of health care and the delivery of care
- building on GP fundholding by creating primary care groups and primary care trusts which will empower doctors and community nurses to plan, commission and deliver services so that all clients are covered
- maintaining decentralised management responsibility by stronger structural and financial arrangements.

Social exclusion is a term for what can happen when people or areas suffer from a combination of linked problems such as unemployment, low incomes, high crime and family breakdown.

Integrated care

Integrated care will replace the internal market through the following:

- the Health Improvement Programme which needs to be agreed by all organisations that are charged with planning and delivering health and social care
- treating patients according to their need, not who their GP is or where they live
- sharing best practice and new performance frameworks to tackle variable standards of quality
- having a broader set of performance measurements and a unified budget
- capping the management cost
- having longer-term service agreements linked with quality
- ending secrecy.

Health Improvement Programme

This is a mechanism for sharing best practice. It is lead by the health authority which pulls together NHS trusts and primary care groups. It involves local authority social services and other relevant organisations in drawing up a progressively updated three-year plan covering:

- important health needs of the local population and how they will be met
- main healthcare requirements and how NHS and other service providers can be developed to meet these
- the range, location and investment required.

Quality

Every part of the NHS and its entire staff take responsibility for improving quality as shown.

Clinical governance sets out to ensure that all staff have responsibility for developing and maintaining standards. NHS trusts will ensure that, for example, quality improvement processes are in place, evidence-based practice is in everyday use, and that good practice is disseminated.

Measures	Mechanisms
National standards and guidelines	National Service Frameworks National Institute of Clinical Excellence (NICE)
Local standards and procedures	Teams of GPs and community nurses working in primary care groups (page 269)
	Quality standards in local service agreements
	Clinical governance in NHS trusts and primary care groups to ensure standards are met and quality improved
An independent organisation to address shortcomings	Commission for Health Improvements to support and oversee quality at local level

Quality will be enhanced and a number of measures aim to improve efficiency such as aligning clinical and financial responsibility, bringing funding together, and having in place action plans where performance falls short.

MODERNISING SOCIAL SERVICES

While some aspects of social services (such as the Care Standards Council) required legislation, other parts (such as Quality Protects) started to be implemented quickly.

The key principles set out in the White Paper were that:

- care should be provided in a way that supports people's independence and respects dignity
- services should meet each individual's specific needs, pulling together social services, health, housing, education and other areas
- care services should be organised, assessed, provided and financed in a fair, open and consistent way in every part of the country
- looked-after children should get a good start in life, including decent education, with the same opportunities to make a success as any child
- every person (child or adult) should be safeguarded against abuse, neglect or poor treatment while receiving care.
- people who receive social services should have assurance that staff are sufficiently trained and skilled for the work they are undertaking
- people should have confidence in their social services.

National performance frameworks

The national performance frameworks are intended to allow a more rounded assessment of NHS performance. They will be used to chart progress for the population of a health authority or primary care group. There are six dimensions:

- health improvement
- fair access
- effective delivery of appropriate health care
- efficiency
- patient/carer experience
- health outcomes of NHS care.

Social services

The White Paper, Modernising Social Services (1998), covered the whole spectrum of the work of social services departments in general as well as adults and children separately. You will need to read the White Paper and follow the progress of the Care Standards Bill 1999 to see how all this will work out.

Critique

In the Government's view, backed up by evidence from Joint Reviews, the pre-1997 situation was deficient in a number of areas:

- protection had failed for children and adults
- coordination – there were barriers to working with health, housing and other authorities
- flexibility – services were based on what is available rather than tailored to the client's needs
- clarity of role – the general public, clients and staff were not clear about what was required
- consistency – although services were local and responding to different needs, there were no mechanisms for ensuring a consistent national quality of care
- efficiency – the costs of particular services varied between similar local authorities highlighting a lack of cost-effectiveness.

Joint Reviews are carried out jointly by the Audit Commission and Social Services Inspectorate on about 20 social services a year. Each review looks at performance across a wide range of factors and publishes its findings.

In its analysis of the situation in adult services, the Government felt that it was unclear who makes decisions about getting a service, and that eligibility criteria were getting tighter and the people who can benefit become more and more dependent.

For children needing care and support from social services, the Government has made links with a wider agenda and particularly with the National Childcare Strategy (page 253). Failures of the system are that:

- too many children are harmed and abused within the care system
- there are gaps in protection of children living at home
- safeguards against the appointment of unsuitable people are not strong enough
- many families caught up in child protection systems/surveillance are at high risk of social exclusion
- young people leaving the care system are not being assisted towards success in adulthood.

The Government aimed to make these improvements:

Across social services	Adults	Children
Protection	Promote independence	Protection
Standards in the workforce	Improve consistency	Quality of care
Partnerships	Provide convenient user-centre services	Improving life chances
Cost-efficiency and effectiveness		

NATIONAL SERVICE FRAMEWORK (NSF) FOR MENTAL HEALTH SERVICES

This is the first of two NSFs. The strategy includes plans for funding over three years, monitoring arrangements and a commitment to review the Mental Health Act.

National Standards

The Labour Government saw national standards as the main means of delivering their objective of providing protection and delivering higher-quality services. It tried to ensure cost-effectiveness and efficiency.

A number of areas are to be covered by standards, including:

- national regulatory standards which will bring consistency to inspection
- codes of standards and practice for workers will be developed by General Social Care Council (page 265)
- national service frameworks, which have been agreed for the NHS, define service models for specific services or groups. The aim is to reduce unacceptable variations in care and standards of treatment.

National Priorities Guidance sets out the key priorities for three years for both social services and health.

National priorities for health and social care 1999/2000–2001/02		
Social services lead	**Shared lead**	**NHS lead**
Children's welfare	Cutting health inequalities	Waiting lists/time
Inter-agency work	Mental health	Primary care
Regulation	Promoting independence	Coronary heart disease and cancer
		Source: Modernising Social Services

Best Value is a rigorous and systematic approach to improving local authority performance. It was described in the White Paper Modern Local Government: In touch with the people (1998) and applies to all local government departments.

Performance assessment framework pulls together key statistical information on performance of social services. This is required for the Best Value arrangements.

Modernising Social Services: extent of the proposals

Objectives	Adults	Children
Protection	■ Regional Commissions for Care Standards which regulate care services (see page 268) ■ General Social Care Council to regulate conduct and practice standards and register social care workers ■ National training strategy drawn up by National Training Organisation – links with National Childcare Strategy ■ Criminal Records Agency to improve access to police checks on people seeking to work with children and vulnerable people	■ Independent regulation strategy bringing in all children services; better complaints procedures
Standards for services and consistency	■ A range of national standards which cover inspection, quality, targets for performance and staff conduct ■ National Priorities Guidance ■ Performance Assessment Frameworks ■ National Service Frameworks (NHS) ■ Fair Access to Care initiative	■ Quality Protects programme ■ Targets set within National Childcare Strategy ■ Health Improvement Programme
Partnerships	■ Better working arrangements with health, housing, employment, education, criminal justice and the voluntary sector	
Cost-effective and efficient	■ National objectives ■ National Priorities Guidance ■ Best Value framework	
Promoting independence and improving life changes	■ Making services client-centred ■ Development of a Long-term Care Charter ■ One-stop shop approach ■ Health Improvement Plan	■ Legislation to ensure local authorities care for 16- to 18-year-olds ■ Assistance for care leavers ■ Better links with further education

Partnerships

Authorities are expected to act corporately in the interests of their citizens, forging partnerships with other services. Main agencies to work alongside social services are:

■ NHS
■ local housing departments
■ employment services
■ criminal justice system
■ education services.

Example of how working together is linked with one of the Government's priorities.

Improving the life chances of young people

Aim	Partner organisations	Means
Improve education for looked-after children	Local authority education department	Targets to be set in the Education Development Plan Authorities required to publish behaviour support plans which cover looked-after young people
Improve health services for children	The NHS	Health services required to work in partnership with social services; looked-after children to be included in Health Improvement Programme When a child or young person enters care they will be offered a health assessment
A statutory obligation to provide for the needs of children leaving care	Housing Careers guidance Higher education Employment services	Assistance to care leavers obtaining suitable and affordable accommodation Links with careers guidance and higher education Exemption from the six months qualifying period for acceptance on New Deal

PARTNERSHIP WITH THE VOLUNTARY SECTOR

Voluntary organisations make an enormous contribution to social care, working alongside and in cooperation with social services. Social services should have good relationships with voluntary organisations, both in service provision partnerships and also in order to help understand the needs and views of clients.

Local authorities should ensure that they know which voluntary organisations are in their area; what the voluntary sector can contribute to meeting the needs of the local population; and where the authority's support for the sector can be used to best effect.

source: Modernising Social Service

The Government wanted the partnerships to continue to involve voluntary organisations and private companies so that policy-making is joined up and strategic, and that clients are the focus.

Client focus

The Government believed it was important that services should have the client and their carers at the centre. It outlined its proposals for promoting independence as follows:

Action	Means
Better preventive services and a stronger focus on rehabilitation	Promoting independence identified as a priority in National Priorities Guidance Requiring jointly agreed plans for improved rehabilitation services (Better Services for Vulnerable People)
Extension of direct payment schemes	Remove the age limit so it applies to over-65 years Consider making it mandatory for the local authority
Better support of clients who are able to work	Build links with the government's welfare-to-work schemes and other employment schemes
Improved review and follow-up to take account of people's changing needs	Care reviews should be carried out within three months and reviewed at least annually. The frequency depends on complexity and the cost of the care package Clients and carers will be expected to take part in planning and reviewing services Guidance should be offered through Fair Access to Care Initiatives (page 312)
More support for carers	Implement the National Carers Strategy (page 277)

Better Services for Vulnerable People (1997) requires health and local authorities to draw up an investment plan to develop services to help people avoid admissions to hospital and to enable them to return home from hospital.

Quality Protects (March 1997) is a three-year programme with a £375 million budget to remedy defects in standards of care offered to looked-after and other children.

ACTIVITY

Find out the most important components of Quality Protects.

Early years services

Before the welfare state was established, responsibility lay with education services for the over-fives, health for babies and nursing mothers and a limited system of welfare where families had broken down. The creation of the welfare state kept this same division of responsibility between the education department and the social services.

Social services generally took on the role of trying to coordinate the various initiatives. In the 1990s local authorities began to focus the services together and several moved their own early years service into education departments to give them more coordination.

The Labour Government picked up this shift of responsibility. It proposed the transfer of early years services nationally to the Department for Education and Employment (DfEE) and locally to the Education Department. This was a major shift in direction which assumes that childcare is more about education than care.

66 *The Government was elected to build a modern Britain and a fair and decent society. Families are at the core of our society, but they are under pressure. Women and men struggle with choices over work and family responsibilities, whether to stay at home with their children full-time or balance home responsibilities with work.* 99

Tony Blair, Prime Minister, in the foreword to
Meeting the Childcare Challenge (1998)

A national childcare strategy

In the consultation document *Meeting the Childcare Challenge (1998)* the Government described its commitment to supporting families and children as building on their work to raise school standards, increase child benefit, help parents back to work, and introduce the Working Families Tax Credit.

Although the document stressed that care within families is the preferred option, it recognises that this type of care is not always available. It planned to take action to fill the gaps through formal care so that parents can take up job opportunities.

The Government's aim in the National Childcare Strategy is to ensure good-quality, affordable childcare for children aged 0 to 14 in every neighbourhood through:

- integration of early years services
- support for parents and informal carers
- consistent regulatory regime
- new qualifications framework and opportunities to train for childcare work
- childcare tax credit which offers help of up to £70 per week
- more help to parents in education and training
- encouraging a diversity of provision
- providing a national helpline linking parents with childcare information
- bringing together local authorities, childcare providers, parents, training and enterprise councils and employers into early years
- development partnerships.

Regulation and inspection

The Children Act 1989 sets out the requirements for registration, inspection and enforcement. A consultation document *Regulation of Early Years Education and Day Care* (1998) has been issued jointly by the DfEE and DoH. This proposes to strengthen protection by:

- transferring responsibility for day care to the DfEE from 1 April 1999; clauses in the Care Standards Bill pass the responsibility for inspection to Ofsted
- a more integrated and consistent system of regulation
- national standards ('Desirable Learning Outcomes') and quality assurance systems
- Early Excellence Centres which can spread good practice and offer support and training to childminders and other providers
- standards for those who work with children, relevant to a recruitment and qualification structure in partnership with the Qualifications and Curriculum Authority and a National Training Organisation.

Support for parents and informal carers

The Government plans to complement raising the quality by supporting parents and informal carers. It is exploring ways of increasing education and support available to parents at key stages in children's development. Encouragement of opportunities for parents to come together will mean supporting mother and toddler groups. Funding will be available for a range of initiatives.

Local partnerships

Local authorities are the key partners because they have responsibilities under the Children Act and are major providers of services. Local authorities have already been convening Early Years Development Partnerships in order to plan and integrate early education and care (Early Years Development Plans). This will be enlarged to create new childcare partnerships.

AN EARLY EXCELLENCE CENTRE

The Centre's purpose is to provide integrated education, health and social services through a one-stop shop approach. It provides nursery education and other childcare services in partnership with the voluntary sector so parents may work. They can offer out-of-school activities too.

5.1.4 Devolution

Since 1997 there have been far-reaching changes to the constitution of the United Kingdom, the results of which are still far from clear. In different ways the constitutional arrangements for Scotland, Wales and Northern Ireland have all changed. The creation in 1999 of the Scottish Parliament and the National Assembly for Wales allowed greater divergence in policy-making to address local needs and priorities. Without close cooperation between all four UK administrations there is the risk that developments in one administration may inadvertently constrain or put pressure on policy or finances of the other administrations.

A *Concordat on Health and Social Care* (December 1999) was produced to provide a framework for cooperation between the Department of Health and the departments or directorates concerned with health and social care in each of the devolved administrations.

Scotland

The constitutional arrangements for Scotland have always been slightly different as a result of Scotland having different laws from England (for example, legislation relating to children). However, in 1999 the first Scottish Parliament for almost 300 years was elected and the powers formerly held by the Secretary of State for Scotland were devolved to the Scottish First Minister and an Executive. The Scottish Parliament not only has responsibility for the budget for health and social services but also has legislative powers over a wide range of areas. This includes:

- health
- social work
- education
- training policy and lifelong learning
- local government
- most aspects of criminal and civil law.

This is likely to mean, as time passes, that there will be an increasing divergence of the Scottish system, with potential conflicts between the United Kingdom Government and Scottish legislators. Although the NHS and Community Care Act applied to the whole of the United Kingdom, Part II refers particularly to Scotland.

In April 1999 primary care trusts came into force as a new kind of trust responsible for the full range of family and community health services. From July 1999 the Scottish Parliament has been responsible for the NHS in Scotland.

Wales

In 1999 the first Welsh Assembly met and the powers formerly held by the Secretary of State for Wales were devolved to the Welsh First Minister and an Executive. Unlike the Scottish Parliament the Welsh Assembly does not have legislative powers, but does have considerable budgetary flexibility. From July

1999 the Welsh Assembly had the power to develop and implement policy in a range of areas which include:

- education and training
- health and health services
- housing
- local government
- social services
- sport and leisure
- the Welsh language.

As the laws of Wales are almost the same as England's, the arrangements for health and social care are very similar. The provisions of the NHS and Community Care Act apply to Wales.

Northern Ireland

Until the beginning of the 1970s Northern Ireland had a separate governmental arrangement from the rest of the United Kingdom with its own parliament (Stormont) and prime minister. This was wound up because of 'the Troubles' and its powers passed to a Secretary of State in the British Cabinet. However, under the Northern Ireland Agreement (commonly known as the 'Good Friday Agreement'), the Northern Ireland Assembly (followed by the Northern Ireland Executive which was a power-sharing arrangement between the main political parties) was established. At the time of publication, the future of this is uncertain. This could have full legislative and executive authority over six departmental areas:

- agriculture
- economic development
- education
- environment (including local government)
- finance and personnel
- health and social services.

In Northern Ireland, health and social services are integrated and are the responsibility of four Health and Social Services Boards which are nominated by, and accountable to, the Secretary of State for Northern Ireland. This arrangement has reduced the need for joint planning and joint financing arrangements as these already exist internally to the organisation.

In Northern Ireland, the DHSS is responsible for an integrated service of health and social welfare delivered by 19 health and social services trusts. Five GP commissioning group pilot schemes commenced in April 1999, though GP fundholding will continue until March 2000.

Neither the NHS and Community Care Act nor the Children Act yet apply to Northern Ireland, although consultations have taken place with the intention of it applying within the province's particular local requirements.

ACTIVITY

Find out the current position in Northern Ireland regarding the Northern Ireland Assembly and Executive and its responsibilities for health and social care and early years provision. Write up your findings in a brief report.

The English regions

It was the expressed policy of the Labour Government that, if pressure developed from the English regions, there would be further devolution to English Regional Assemblies. Nothing has been stated about their form and the powers they would have, but it could be assumed that they would be closer to the Welsh than to the Scottish model. If this takes place then it is possible that organisational approaches across the United Kingdom will diverge, although it is likely that central government would place broad limits on the extent of that divergence, either through the Treasury or through the statutory agencies.

Keeping up with devolution developments

Further information about devolution and the Concordat on Health and Social Care is available from the Department of Health web site (*http://www.doh.gov. uk/devolution.htm*).

For updates about the effects of devolution generally, and on equal opportunities in particular, contact the government information service. See their web site (*http://www.open.gov.uk*). It provides a first entry point to UK public sector information on the Internet and is an easy route to information about progress in the three main devolved countries and other governmental information.

ACTIVITY

If you live in Scotland, Wales or Northern Ireland investigate how the NHS is organised in your country and write a brief account.

5.1.5 **Demographic factors**

When proposing a National Health Service, Beveridge (in common with many others) believed that with proper income support there would be a rapidly rising level of health among the population as a whole. This would then lead to a reduction in demand for health services. In practice this has not been the case. Some of the changes that have taken place are technological but others are demographic – that is, related to the structure of the population.

Some of the demographic factors taken into account are:

- the age profile of the population
- class and income
- family structure and status of women
- the incidence of disease and disability
- geographical location
- employment and unemployment
- migration inwards and outwards.

Age profile

Age profile refers to the numbers of different age groups within the population and the balance between them. The numbers of older and younger people govern the level of services to be provided.

The largest single category of patients and clients are the elderly. In the case of the NHS, over half the beds at any one time are occupied by people over 65, and around 45% of expenditure goes on services for the care and treatment of this age group. A similar proportion of social services expenditure goes on care services for elderly people. Services for children are also extensive and social services and early years services have a high priority.

Class and income

Class and income have an impact on lifestyle, in particular diet and access to, and choices about, recreation. Aspects of poverty, such as poor housing and inadequate heating, may also affect health outcomes.

Family structure and status of women

The last decades of the Twentieth Century saw many changes in the role of women and a consequent change in family structures. As women played a greater role in the workforce there was also a later age of marriage and childbearing, social acceptance of divorce, and an increased incidence of unmarried and single women bringing up their own children. The average size of families decreased to a point below replacement levels – affecting the nation's age profile. The Labour Government's policy of wanting women to be fully in the workforce has brought changes to family support through family credits and childcare allowances.

Incidence of disease and disability

It is essential to plot diseases such as TB, HIV/AIDS, meningitis and leukaemia in order to plan future health needs. Planning on the basis of past health trends means that new developments, such as an unexpected epidemic, can severely strain resources. It is important for purchasers to know the number of people with a disability or who are likely to become disabled. Apart from degenerative disabilities, most support is likely to be by social care, so social services departments look very carefully at these statistics. Information comes from surveys under the Chronically Sick and Disabled Persons Act, the Census, and individual care assessment.

Geographical location

Inner-city areas have a higher incidence of mental illness, accidents and environmental illness such as asthma. Rural areas have scattered populations with resulting poor transport, lower wages than the average, lower percentages of public housing and a smaller percentage of people born outside the UK. For those providing services there are likely to be higher costs and fewer people to offer informal care.

ACTIVITY

Obtain either the community care plan for your social services department or the annual plan from your health authority. Identify how the statistics about disability and disease are presented in these plans and summarise how these statistics are used to reach decisions about future services.

> 66 *Finding ways to get services to clients in rural areas is a major challenge . . . scattered populations, poor public transport and a high proportion of people on low incomes means services are inappropriately based in one location and are inaccessible for the clients they are designed for.* 99
>
> *operational manager for children's services in a Welsh authority*

DISCUSSION POINT

The balance of priority between urban and rural areas has varied over time depending on political considerations. What do you think are the factors that governments should take into account when seeking to meet the needs of rural communities?

COMMUNITY CARE IN RURAL AREAS

During 1998 the Social Services Inspectorate (SSI) conducted an inspection of community care services provided for older people and young adults in eight rural counties. They found evidence of:

- lack of choice and service refusal by users
- services being less accessible
- inappropriate services because they were closer to the user
- services were not changing to reflect actual need.

Employment

Over time the employment profile of Britain has changed greatly. The main changes include:

- the decline of mining and heavy industry with their associated health problems
- longer holidays and a five-day working week for more people
- the raising of the school leaving age from 14 to 16, with a large number of 16- to 18-year-olds in education or employment training
- reduced job security and greater job stress.

Migration

All communities have movements within their populations. Some migration is outwards – often by the economically active or more highly qualified. In other parts of the country, the migration has been inwards such as:

- large-scale immigration from the 'new' Commonwealth in the 1950s and 1960s
- more recently, people fleeing from war and oppression in Eastern Europe and elsewhere.

UNACCOMPANIED MINORS

A series of civil wars in South East Europe in the 1990s brought a new phenomenon – young people and children arriving in Britain as refugees without their parents. For some local authorities this has brought considerable pressures on their care systems with no adults available to take responsibility for decisions about these young people. These pressures have been compounded by differences of language, culture and religion as well as meeting the needs of young people who may have suffered traumatising experiences.

DISCUSSION POINT

The growth in population and the increased demand by single people and couples for accommodation has resulted in a search for land on which to build. Although the Government is encouraging house building on 'brownfield sites' within cities and towns, there will still need to be building within rural communities. What do you think could be the consequences for planning health, social care and early years services in both the urban and the rural communities?

How demographic characteristics affect priorities

Central government bears these characteristics of the population and health in mind when it allocates resources. At a local level, health authority and social services interpret population characteristics when commissioning and purchasing the care for their communities.

HEALTH IMPROVEMENT PROGRAMME (HImP): DEMOGRAPHIC FACTORS

Cambridgeshire HImP analyses some of the factors it has taken into account as follows:

■ a rising population – 6% between 1997/2003 (national rise is 2%); half of the increase is in the 45–64 age range while those over 75 will increase by 8%

■ the extent of deprivation and inequalities varies across the county, with Peterborough City having some areas in the most deprived 10% nationally

■ rural poverty is concealed and made more difficult because of poor transport and communication

■ heart disease and diabetes are identified health risks for ethnic minorities.

Key questions

1 List the six Acts of Parliament that founded the welfare state.

2 What welfare service was provided in the 1930s?

3 What is a universal service?

4 Give three ways in which the NHS and Community Care Act 1990 changed health and social care.

5 What is meant by the 'internal market'?

6 In which year was the Local Authority Social Services Act passed?

7 What is meant by 'individualism'?

8 Give five consequences of the reforms of the 1979–97 Conservative Governments.

9 In what document did the 1997 Labour Government set out its National Childcare Strategy?

10 What is the mixed economy of care?

11 List three major changes in the health of the population since 1946.

12 Give six themes that the 1997 Labour Government felt important in health and social care.

13 What do you understand by 'integrated care'?

14 What can the Scottish Parliament do that the Welsh Assembly cannot?

15 Explain the key components of the Quality Protects programme.

&& We are determined to have a system of health and social care which is convenient to us, can respond quickly to emergencies and provides top quality services . . . Despite the efforts of a lot of very dedicated staff, many services are not provided sufficiently conveniently, promptly or to a good enough standard. 99

Frank Dobson, foreword to Modernising Social Services

&& Childcare has been neglected for too long. There are dedicated childcare providers doing excellent work right across the country, from friends and family providing informal care through to childminders, playgroups and nurseries. But the quality of care can be variable, there are not enough childcare places, and ordinary working parents often cannot afford to take them up. 99

Tony Blair, foreword to Meeting the Childcare Challenge

&& The care my friend is getting is pretty good. They are doing the best they can. You get the impression, though, that they never have quite as much time with each patient as they would like. 99

Guardian (15 January 2000), quoting a relative

&& The public doesn't care how we organise ourselves internally, but people do care about the quality of services. 99

Michael Hake, head of organisation and development, Association of Directors of Social Services

National and local provision of services

This section looks at the structures and responsibilities of agencies at national, regional and local level. It also tells you about some of the individuals who work within these structures. As explained in section 5.1, the organisation of health, social care and early years provision are in the process of a major change. Included here is a description of the arrangements in place, at the time of writing, and those proposed.

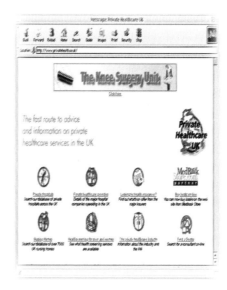

5.2.1 **How national policy is implemented locally**

Different types of organisation provide health, social care and early years services:

- statutory authorities – the NHS, local authorities, criminal services
- voluntary organisations – charities, local voluntary organisations
- private organisations – ranging from individual professionals to multinational companies.

The way in which public services carry out their duties and powers is decided by each health authority, NHS trust or local authority.

Voluntary and private agencies (often called the 'independent sector') can choose what services to deliver. The independent sector's involvement in the health and wellbeing of individuals and communities predates state health and social care services. The concept that the state would take responsibility for services implied that voluntary and private organisations would have a reduced role in providing services. In practice this did not happen. The voluntary sector diversified its activities to find new activities to complement and supplement the state services while the private sector worked alongside governments to offer healthcare.

Voluntary organisations

Voluntary organisations are a collective response to meeting needs. They don't make profits, but put surplus monies back into the activities of the organisation. The majority of voluntary organisations providing local health and social care services are registered charities with legal security to fundraise, employ staff and buy property, with some tax benefits. Their charitable status allows them to receive money from statutory authorities and make contracts for services or facilities.

The private sector

The private sector includes professionals in private practice, sole owner companies, and large national and multinational organisations. Owners and shareholders take profits from the activities of the company. Private insurance companies increasingly contribute to funding healthcare costs. Section 5.4 covers their role in the funding of the health service.

If either the private or voluntary sectors seek financial and other support from health and local authorities, they would also be covered by legislation. Traditionally, the independent sector has offered supplementary and complementary services or has pioneered services and approaches. Over the last 20 years, they've been drawn into closer relationships with statutory authorities because of contracts and service agreements. (This is explored in section 5.5.)

5.2.2 The organisation of health and social care planning and provision

Statutory, voluntary and private organisations operate at national, regional and local level. Each type of statutory organisation commissioning and delivering services (the NHS and local authorities) has functional and accountable relationships with the relevant national departments, while local voluntary and private agencies may be part of a national network.

At national level the DoH has responsibility for ensuring that there is joined-up government so far as health, social care and early years services are concerned. Civil servants from the DoH work with colleagues from the DfEE and provide professional advice to the Department of Environment, Transport and the Regions (DETR) where local authorities are concerned.

At the heart of implementation are local partnerships. The way they fit into social policy is described in section 5.1 and how this works is outlined in section 5.5.

National level: government departments

Government is carried out through a Cabinet system, with Secretaries of State and other ministers coming together to formulate and take forward legislation. Offices of State are usually amalgamations of two or more areas of government activity. Each department has civil servants responsible for implementing government policy, drafting new parliamentary business and monitoring outcomes.

Government departments also set up a range of policy groups, advisory committees and special interest groups.

Department of Health

The DoH brings together health and social services and is responsible for action needed at national level such as:

- integration of health and social care policy
- working with professionals to develop the National Service Frameworks
- undertaking annual surveys of what is happening to compare experiences
- ensuring consistency across the Commissions for Care Standards in each region.

Social Services Inspectorate

For social care the SSI:

- provides professional advice to ministers and central government departments related to personal social services
- assists local government, voluntary organisations and private agencies in planning and delivering services
- runs national inspections and evaluates the quality of services
- monitors the implementation of government policies.

Education Action Zones are clusters of primary, secondary and special schools – working in partnership with local education authorities, parents, businesses, Learning and Skills Councils and others. They're expected to explore imaginative ways of working to improve levels of achievement in literacy and numeracy.

ACTIVITY

Find out if your area is in an Education Action Zone. If so, get information about what is being planned to take forward the objectives of this special initiative.

Department for Education and Employment

The DfEE's aim is: 'to give everyone the chance, through education, training and work, to realise their potential, and thus build an inclusive and fair society and a competitive economy'. One of its objectives is to ensure that all young people reach 16 with the skills, attitudes and personal qualities required for life-long learning and work – this includes support for families through early education and good-quality childcare.

Department of Environment, Transport and the Regions

The DETR is responsible for local government policy in general. It agrees the annual spending round with the Treasury and negotiates with local authorities about their government grant.

Cabinet Office (Social Exclusion Unit)

The Cabinet Office coordinates government policy. The Social Exclusion Unit covers issues which are important for health, social care and early years, such as:

- welfare to work programme
- national childcare strategy
- review of tax and benefits
- truancy and school exclusion
- rough sleeping
- worst estates and poor neighbourhoods
- teenage pregnancies
- 16- to 18-year-olds.

National statutory organisations

Government also acts through non-ministerial government departments or non-departmental public bodies. These are set up by legislation to be independent of ministers. They report to ministers and to parliament but function at arm's length from ministers and are outside the political arena.

NHS Executive

The NHS and Community Care Act 1990 introduced a new structure for the health service by setting up the NHS Executive to manage the service from the centre. Following the 1997 White Paper the structure is still evolving as the Government seeks to simplify the structures and apply the thinking of a changed administration.

The National Health Service Executive is expected to implement the proposals in the 1997 White Paper, in particular:

- investigating major care areas and drawing in the National Services Framework
- coordinating the work of the National Institute for Clinical Excellence and Commission for Health Improvement.

The National Institute for Clinical Excellence

This body provides clinical guidance on relevant evidence and cost-effectiveness, clinical audits and good practice, and a focus for other DoH-funded research. Its membership is drawn from health professionals, NHS academics, health economists and patients' interests. It reports to the NHS Executive.

The Commission for Health Improvement

This body is drawn from professions, NHS academics and patients' interests. It has the powers of inspection of NHS trusts and it:

- monitors, assures and seeks improvements of clinical quality at the local level
- supports local arrangements
- inspects (including unexpected checks) local service delivery
- suggests improvements and resolves problems
- makes recommendations to the NHS Executive; it can suspend NHS trust members.

The Audit Commission

The Audit Commission is the auditing body for the NHS and local authorities in England and Wales. It also publishes comparative information on local authorities. It has four main functions:

- appointing auditors to all health and local authorities
- setting standards for those auditors
- carrying out national studies to promote economy, efficiency and effectiveness (for social services, this is undertaken jointly with the SSI)
- defining comparative indicators of local authority performance – closely linked with the Best Value initiative.

General Social Care Council (GSCC)

Established by the Care Standards Act 2000, it is responsible for social workers' training and qualifications, conduct and practice standards for all social care workers, and registration of those in the most sensitive areas.

Its objectives are to:

- strengthen public protection by relevant and appropriate codes of conduct which apply to all people working in social care services
- expect employers to apply best practice when recruiting or when disciplining unsatisfactory staff
- provide a register for social care workers (to be introduced incrementally).

There is power to deregister, including where workers have not continued their professional development. Some work may be restricted to people who are registered with the GSCC.

The Office of Standards in Education (Ofsted)

This was set up in 1992 to improve the standards of achievement and quality of education through regular independent inspection, public reporting and informed advice. Its head is Her Majesty's Inspector of Education who has teams of inspectors who undertake regular inspections of schools, further education colleges and local education authorities. It reports on:

- the quality of education in schools in England
- standards achieved by pupils
- management of financial resources
- spiritual, moral and cultural development of children.

Ofsted will be responsible for the regulation and inspection of all early years provision, including childminders.

Qualifications Curriculum Authority (QCA)

The QCA's role is to:

- review the school curriculum
- manage the assessment process for schools
- regulate public qualifications
- develop a coherent framework for training and qualifications.

Your Advanced Health and Social Care GNVQ has been agreed by the QCA. It is also responsible for the national vocational qualifications for people working in health, social care and early years.

National Training Organisations (NTOs)

There are 71 National Training Organisations, each representing an individual industry or area of economic activity and covering the whole UK. They bring together employers, government and educators to:

- define and develop learning and skills for their area
- assess the skills needed
- assess the impact of the work situation on training.

They act as a voice for that sector and offer best practice. They can give information to workers and potential workers on the relevant skills and qualifications for specific occupations. There are three NTOs with a particular remit for health, social care and early years – Healthwork UK, Training Organisation for Personal Social Services (TOPSS) and Early Years NTO.

Voluntary and private

Voluntary organisations are involved in all aspects of a community life:

- environmental
- recreational
- educational
- health and social care.

TOPSS – the National Training Organisation for Personal Social Services – was asked to develop a five-year training strategy for social care workers by September 1999. This strategy is closely linked with the ability of the GSCC to set up a register. The strategy aims for the half-million social care workforce to be either qualified or working towards a qualification in 2005.

ACTIVITY

Choose one of the three NTOs mentioned here and collect information about its activities. Choose a specific group of workers in health, social care or early years settings. How do the qualifications promoted or being developed fit with the group of workers?

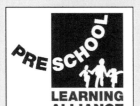 NCVO

voice of the voluntary sector

Some organisations work only at national level, such as the National Council for Voluntary Organisations (NCVO), which acts as a voice for the voluntary sector. The majority working in health, social care and early years settings have links with similarly named local organisations.

ACTIVITY

The NSPCC is a unique voluntary organisation in that it has a statutory role laid down by act of parliament. Find out what this is and write a short report. List any other activities it undertakes.

Private organisations also provide a range of health, social care and early years services. Although much of this activity is likely to be at local level, there are examples of national and international organisations being involved. For example, the NHS can refer patients to private hospitals for treatment. And these are usually linked with health insurance organisations, such as BUPA and PPA. There is a national organisation, which represents the interests of private and independent hospitals – Private Healthcare UK.

The Pre-school Learning Alliance is a national educational charity and umbrella body, linking 17,000 community-based pre-schools. Those pre-schools provide early education and care for nearly three-quarters of a million children under five in England. The charity aims to support the active involvement of parents in their children's early education and to provide opportunities for those same parents to participate in further education and training.

The Alliance offers a wide range of services including comprehensive membership and insurance packages, publications and training courses and a wealth of information and advice on all aspects of the pre-school field.

For more information about the Pre-school Learning Alliance, please contact their national centre at 69 Kings Cross Road, London WC1X 9LL

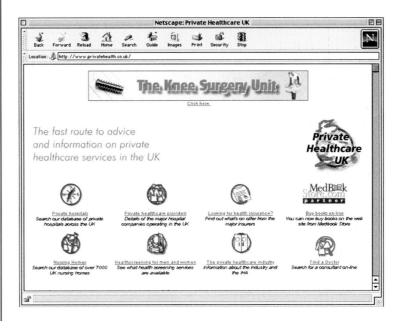

Other private organisations are retail organisations that employ practitioners, such as optometrists and pharmacists. Increasingly the Government is promoting pharmacists as an alternative source of advice on medication for minor conditions, such as a cold.

DISCUSSION POINT

The extent to which the private sector is involved in providing healthcare is the subject of debate. Discussion usually focuses on the issue of private beds within NHS hospitals or the growth of treatment of NHS patients in private hospitals. Discuss why you think this issue may be contentious.

5.2.3 Devolution: organisation of health, social care and early years provision

The devolution of the United Kingdom with the creation of a new parliament and two new assemblies is described in section 5.1. However, the way in which services are organised differs depending on which part of the United Kingdom is being described. The position generally described in this section is that of England although, with a few exceptions, it also applies to Wales.

Regional level

At regional level the DoH is responsible for ensuring that health authorities work with each other, and takes the lead in ensuring creation and continuation of local partnerships between the NHS and local authorities.

NHS regions

Under post-1997 arrangements the NHS Executive regionally is expected to take the lead in bringing about the changes. The responsibilities include holding health authorities and NHS trusts to account for clinical and financial good practice and the achievement of the performance targets. They also commission specialist regional hospital services such as medium-secure psychiatric units, and run national screening programmes such as for breast and cervical cancer.

Regional Commissions for Care Standards

Regional commissions were proposed in Modernising Social Services and are within the Care Standards Act 2000. They will be independent statutory bodies, accountable to the Secretary of State for Health and to Parliament. They will be based on the NHS regions with the chairperson nominated by the Secretary of State and its members coming from local authorities, health authorities, and client and provider representatives.

Each commission's relationship with local social services departments is simple. It will be responsible for inspecting:

- residential homes, nursing homes, and day centres
- children's homes
- domiciliary care providers
- independent foster care agencies
- residential family centres
- boarding schools.

The Government may bring other services, such as field social work, into its remit at a later date. It will not be responsible for the inspection of early years care services (childminding and day nurseries) because they are under the remit of the DfEE and Ofsted.

Local level

Although central government dictates policy and controls budgets, the main responsibility for planning, commissioning and providing services remains

Three levels of regulatory standards

- first level – standards fixed in legislation and non-negotiable (e.g. each person in charge of a nursing home must be a registered nurse or a medical practitioner)

- second level – standards spelled out at national level and applied locally (e.g. procedures for selecting and vetting staff)

- third level – standards which allow interpretation in the local situation (e.g. timescales for upgrading below-standard accommodation).

local. For example, the local statutory agencies have to plan for services to meet the needs of everyone in their communities. In pulling together this plan, health and local authorities:

- identify and assess the needs of the population
- plan how to meet these needs
- encourage and stimulate a range of providers
- monitor and evaluate those services.

Health authorities

With simplification of the structure laid down by the NHS and Community Care Act 1990, and the creation of the primary care groups as the commissioners, and NHS trusts as the providers, health authorities are currently responsible for:

- commissioning services until the primary care group is ready to take over this role
- drawing up a three-year health improvement programme (HImP) by working with local authorities, primary care groups and NHS trusts
- supporting primary care groups and assisting them to become primary care trusts
- allocating funds to primary care groups or primary care trusts on an equitable basis and holding them to account
- taking the lead on workforce planning and training
- strengthening links with social services departments – this is stronger where there is a health action zone.

The members of the health authority are appointed by the Secretary of State.

Health action zones bring together organisations within and beyond the NHS to develop and implement a locally agreed strategy for improving the health of local people. Ten were selected in April 1998.

Community health councils (CHCs)

These scrutinise the health authority and other health services. CHCs were set up in 1974 to represent the views of local health clients.

Primary care groups (PCGs)

PCGs have been formed from April 1999 to replace GP fundholders by involving all GP practices into commissioning services for their communities. Although accountable to health authorities, it is hoped that in time they will become free-standing primary care trusts. Their area should be a natural community and, where possible, be conterminous with the social services department. PCGs:

- contribute to the HImP
- promote the health of the population
- commission health services within the framework of the HImP
- monitor performance through service agreements
- develop primary care services through joint working
- integrate primary and community health care services, particularly for groups where responsibility has been split in the past.

ACTIVITY

Contact your local primary care group and describe its 'area of benefit' (i.e. who it provides its service for). List the services it provides.

ENABLING AUTHORITIES

Social service departments have been described as 'enabling' authorities because they should be going out and encouraging new organisations to offer care. For example, in an area where meals are needed for Asian elders, a social service department negotiated with an Indian restaurant to provide appropriate meals.

An early years development partnership brings together representatives from the local authority (education, social services and district councils), schools, employers, voluntary and private sector, the health service, childminders and parents. It is required to make plans in order to meet the needs of children and their parents and monitor the implementation of these plans. The plan covers the care, play and education of young children and has to be agreed by the local education authority.

ACTIVITY

Contact your local education authority for information about the early years education partnership. List the organisations represented on it. Look at its plan for services and select those that will be available for a parent seeking to return to work.

NHS trusts

These provide hospital and community health services and employ most NHS staff. They are party to the HImP and have service agreements with health authorities and primary care groups.

NHS trusts:
- participate in strategy and planning
- work on standards of quality and efficiency explicit in service agreements
- design service agreements and financial priorities aligned with clinical priorities
- develop clinical governance arrangements
- share and reinvest efficiency gains to improve quality of services.

Local authorities

These are local democratic organisations that are responsible for a wide range of community services, including social care and early years services whose members are elected councillors. They usually stand on a party political ticket. The majority political party makes the decisions about the policy and direction of the council but if there is no clear majority party, these decisions are made by coalitions of councillors.

Social services departments

Since 1970 local authorities have been required to have a social services committee and appoint a Director of Social Services (Director of Social Work in Scotland). There are 150 English local authorities responsible for social services. Social services may be brought together with other services, such as housing and the regrouping of early years into education departments.

Social services departments are responsible for:
- planning to meet the needs of their community
- putting together packages of services to meet individuals' needs
- purchasing services from other agencies
- providing direct services.

Education departments

Local authorities are also responsible for providing for the education of their communities, including services to meet the special needs of children. It is this local authority department which is responsible for bringing together all interests into early years development partnerships under the Schools Standards and Framework Act 1998. These have been in place since April 1999.

Voluntary organisations

Most voluntary organisations which are active in health, social care and early years work at the local level. Many employ staff in the same way as the NHS and social services departments, including those with professional qualifications, such as social workers, nurses and physiotherapists.

Volunteers work on their own or as part of a group within voluntary, statutory or private organisations. They can act as a bridge between services and clients. Their involvement can encourage users to make use of services.

Others may specialise in working in the voluntary sector. For example:

- community workers
- preschool playgroup workers
- advice workers
- volunteers.

66 *I came to work in a voluntary organisation because I wanted to work in partnership with people, the clients. The salary level has been lower and I've had less chance of promotion but I have felt less restricted than social workers in social services.* 99

social worker in a charity for single homeless people

Other voluntary organisations provide emotional and social support to individuals and their families. For example:

- self-help groups
- tenants' associations
- youth organisations
- religious organisations centred around a religious meeting place.

Volunteers make an important contribution to health and social care services. They're usually associated with the voluntary sector but the NHS and local authorities also have volunteers involved in their services where this is agreed with paid staff. In these services their activities are coordinated by a volunteer organiser. Some volunteers may be involved as informal carers through local support groups (see section 5.3).

Private independent organisations

At the local level, the contribution to the provision of care is likely to be from local health professionals (such as GPs or hospital consultants who see their patients outside the NHS), dentists, opticians and pharmacists. Other local private organisations are individuals or small companies that provide residential places or support to clients in their own homes.

Childminding and foster care

Childminders and foster carers offer care in their own homes. Childminders are registered by early years services and are inspected annually to ensure that they continue to comply with the regulations. Inspection will shortly be the responsibility of Ofsted as childminders are being brought into the remit of this agency. Childminders may look after up to three preschool children in their own homes and are usually paid directly by the parents. An important part of their work is to establish and maintain a working relationship with the parents. In each area there will be a network of support and training available from the early years service which ensures they offer good developmental care to their children. Opportunities are being made for childminders to achieve vocational qualifications.

Foster care provides 24-hour support in the foster carer's home to a range of service users. Generally the care is provided for children and young people

Types of intervention

Six broad approaches can be identified:

- diagnosis, assessment and care management
- protection – assessing risks, taking measures to take the individual from harm within legal framework
- treatment and changing behaviour
- educational and developmental
- care and support
- organisational.

ACTIVITY

Look at the six types of intervention listed in the box above and draw up a table cross-referencing which type or types of intervention are provided by a range of health and social care practitioners. You should include doctors, occupational therapists, nurses, health care assistants, social workers, care officers, foster carers, nursery officers, childminders and managers.

but there are schemes which support people with learning disabilities and mental health problems in a home-like setting. Foster carers are assessed, approved and trained by social services. There are also voluntary organisations that run foster care schemes. Groups of foster carer's have joined together to act as an agency.

Foster carers will usually specialise in the type of care or the age or type of user. They can work very closely with the parent or informal carers. Foster carers can offer:

- long-term and permanent care
- respite care
- short-term and emergency care.

There are a number of ways in which people providing services can be categorised, such as by employer, type of intervention which they provide, and their qualifications.

As well as those employed directly by health authorities, social services and private and voluntary agencies, people like the police, education workers and probation officers contribute to things like child protection.

Practitioners can be grouped according to two types of qualifications:

- professional (degree-level and above) – for example doctors, social workers, nurses
- vocational – for example residential workers, healthcare assistants.

Key questions

1 What is the role of the social services inspection unit?

2 What are the five main tasks of the National Health Service Executive?

3 What powers does the Commission for Health Improvement have?

4 Give two responsibilities of the NHS Regional Executive.

5 List the main responsibilities of the health authorities.

6 What is a 'primary health group'?

7 What body employs most NHS staff?

8 What are the main responsibilities of social services departments?

9 Describe the line of accountability in the NHS.

10 What is the 'independent sector'?

11 Which types of worker are employed within a voluntary organisation?

12 Which two workers look after service users in their own homes?

13 What role will Ofsted have in the early years service?

14 What is the purpose of the Early Years Development Plan?

Informal carers

> 66 *Most people had never heard of carers [before the 1990s] . . . We now know that there are six million people who meet the census definition of a carer, and . . . that they save the nation £34 billion – more than the combined budgets of the NHS and local authority social services departments. Most carers want to provide the care themselves and it is help with domestic chores that they most need.* 99
>
> *Baroness Jill Pitkeathley, Past Chief Executive of Carers' National Association*

> 66 *When it comes to looking after my daughter I am the expert. The practitioners are not the experts in her care but they are there to advise me in the particular aspects of her care in which they are expert. I want to be advised by them, not told what to do.* 99
>
> *parent of a child with cerebral palsy*

> 66 *Support for good parenting ought to start early, by example from parents who are the first teachers of parenting for their children, and through effective education in school and elsewhere . . . Parents, informal carers and children can also benefit greatly from the opportunity to come together to share experience.* 99
>
> *from* Meeting the Childcare Challenge

> 66 *Carers need to feel valued and to feel that they are not isolated. There are many hidden carers in our communities who do not think of themselves as carers and may not be aware that help and support are available.* 99
>
> *Strategy for Carers in Scotland, Scottish Executive (November 1999)*

The bulk of health, social care and early years care is not provided by statutory or independent organisations but through unpaid carers: parents, children, other relatives, loved ones, partners and friends. These people are usually referred to as 'informal carers'.

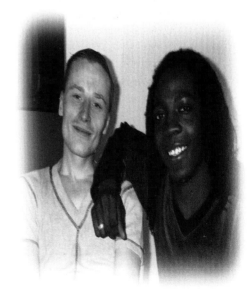

5.3.1 **Who are the informal carers?**

The immediate family is the most likely source of informal care but it may also be provided by friends, neighbours and local support groups.

66 *The UK has an estimated 5.7 million informal carers of people other than children and 17% of households include a carer. 1.7 million carers devote more than 20 hours per week to caring. Most caring is based on a close relationship.* 99

source: Department of Health press release (28 January 2000)

The task of these carers is likely to be:

- long term
- with little expectation that the situation may ease
- in many cases, demanding of time, emotions and physical resources.

Who cares?

- Carers tend to be middle-aged women.
- Most carers look after someone who is elderly.
- Many carers look after more than one person.
- A quarter of carers receive no help from anyone inside or outside the family.
- 50% of those caring for a spouse do so unaided.

source: Carers' National Association

Informal carers and those they care for are likely to include many combinations.

Family

The immediate family includes spouses, parents, children, siblings and other relatives. This care of family members with long-term illness or disability can affect the ability of the carer, frequently a woman, to be employed or have outside interests. Where it is an older parent, this can be undertaken at the same time as bringing up older children and have an effect on family relationships. Where the person receiving the care was the breadwinner or the main pensioner, the family may be living on income support and thus in poverty. A large group of carers support a husband or wife.

Another group of family carers is young carers looking after parents who are ill, disabled or vulnerable. This type of caring is sometimes known as 'reverse caring'. The young carers are particularly disadvantaged because they may face problems at school with attendance and achievements. They can feel isolated from other children because they don't have time to be with their friends.

Carer	Cared for
Parent	Child
Child	Parent
Adult child	Parent
Sibling	Sibling
Spouse	Spouse
Grandparent	Grandchild
Friend	Friend
Neighbour	Neighbour

DISCUSSION POINT

Women take greatest responsibility for care of their children. They're also the bulk of informal carers. The Government's proposals for social care and childcare mean an increase in the number of people working in these services. Women are being encouraged to train for and return to work in these services. What might be the consequences, for informal care, of promoting paid care work?

ANGELA AND HER MOTHER

Angela is 25 and has learning difficulties. Although she stills lives at home, she has successfully been through a training scheme with an employment training project. She works in a local bakery and would like to move into her own home.

Angela's mother has arthritis and her mobility is becoming restricted. The GP refers her to social services because he feels she needs more support to care for Angela. An adult services care manager visits and assesses the needs of both. The practitioner suggests that the best care solution is for Angela to move into a nearby group home and for her mother to have some adaptations to the home, together with practical help with shopping from a local volunteers' group.

ACTIVITY

In the case study, Angela and her mother could both be described as either client or carer. If you were asked to contribute to the care decision, how would you define both women? Give your reasons.

Friends

Friends can support patients and clients by visiting, taking to hospital or social services offices for appointments, shopping or small tasks around the house. The National Carers' Association found that one in five carers are not related to the person they support.

Neighbours

Neighbours may take on assistance and support for clients, either voluntarily or at the request of a social care agency. This concept of neighbourly activity can become more formalised through individuals volunteering to visit patients in hospital or older residents in residential care or their own homes, and groups which offer good neighbour services supporting people in their own homes.

MUTUAL HELP

HIV/AIDS has presented a special challenge as it has certain features that distinguish it from other illnesses:

■ it is a terminal illness

■ its course can be lengthy and unpredictable – with a range of different symptoms

■ 'sufferers' are mainly relatively young

■ it has a high level of social stigma.

One response to the challenge of supporting people with HIV/AIDS has been the 'buddy' scheme. Volunteers are specially trained to work with AIDS sufferers throughout their illness. This is a particularly important intervention for people who may find themselves socially isolated because of the nature of their illness.

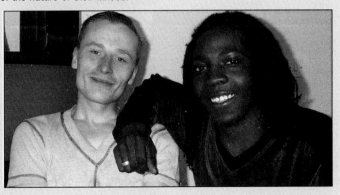

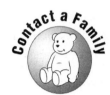

**Support for Families
who Care for Children
with Disabilities and
Special Needs**

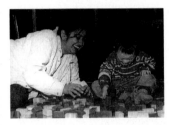

**Information for Parents and
Professional Workers**

Local support groups for carers

Every area has local organisations that exist to support carers. Groups have
been started by:

- voluntary groups (as an extension of their services or community activities)
- practitioners (as an extension of their activities)
- the health or social services department as a means of formally listening to
  carers' views
- carers themselves.

The types of service offered by these networks include:

- providing mutual support to members who share an illness, disability or
  situation
- providing information, advice and representation for individual members
- contributing to the planning and monitoring of services
- commenting on the quality of services and campaigning for better and
  different services.

Some may be established for specific types of carers, such as young carers
with needs of their own.

Two carer networks

Contact a Family is a national organisation that brings together families
with children with special needs to provide mutual support and joint
representation to health and social services.

Local Home Start volunteers offer support, friendship and practical help to
young families under stress in their own homes, helping to prevent family
crisis and breakdown.

5.3.2 National policy for supporting carers

ACTIVITY

Ask a practitioner involved in care
planning about their
organisation's arrangements for
taking carers' needs into account.
Write a report on how carers are
involved in care planning. Suggest
ways in which these
arrangements could be improved.

The NHS and Community Care Act 1990 brought families and other informal
carers into the assessment of a client's needs and the arrangements for
providing care. Local authorities began to ask family members about their
clients' needs and abilities and formalised the caring role as part of the
packages of care to be provided. The work of carers began to be properly
recognised.

CONSULTATION WITH CARERS

Birmingham City Council pioneered consultation with carers in 1987 through its Community Care Special Action Project. The project sought the views of over 300 carers about what it was like to be a carer in Birmingham and what kinds of support they found useful. While practitioners were invited to the meetings, they could only listen, not speak. In this project and other consultations with carers, carers gave this advice to practitioners about how to address their needs:

■ recognise carers' contribution and needs

■ tailor services to individual circumstances, needs and views, through consultation

■ ensure that services reflect an awareness of differing racial, cultural and religious backgrounds

■ give opportunities for short and longer breaks

■ give practical support

■ provide opportunities for talking about feelings.

STRATEGY FOR CARERS IN SCOTLAND

In November 1999 the Scottish Executive published proposals for supporting carers. It acknowledged the contribution made by informal carers and highlighted the difficulty for carers living in rural and remote communities.

The Scottish strategy set out the ways in which the priorities would be met. For example, in relation to better information about and for carers, the strategy includes:

■ putting a question in the 2001 census seeking information about carers

■ identifying hidden carers

■ including carers' needs in the professional training for health and social care staff.

The focus of the NHS and Community Care Act was on better services for patients and clients; there was no responsibility to consider the needs of the carer. National organisations, such as the National Carers' Association, pressed government for better recognition of carers. Research evidence showed the extent to which families and friends cared for clients and the strains that this placed on those carers. As a result the Carers (Recognition and Services) Act 1995 was passed.

Carers (Recognition and Services) Act 1995

This Act gave the right to carers who are being asked to provide a substantial amount of care on a regular basis to request an assessment from the local authority of their ability to provide this care. The local authority must carry out the assessment and take it into account when deciding on the care package. This is relevant whether the care is being provided for an adult or a child with a disability. However, it did not give carers the automatic right to have any service as a result of this assessment. This remains at the discretion of the local authority. The Act covers England, Wales and Scotland but does not extend to Northern Ireland.

National Carers' Strategy 1998

The Labour Government considered that further support should be available, which recognises that carers have as wide a range of needs as the people they care for. The National Carers' Strategy 1998 brings the relevant government departments together; at local level, housing, education and employment agencies take responsibility for meeting carers' needs.

RESPITE CARE

Shared Care UK, an umbrella group for family-based short-term services, offers short breaks which give both relief to carers and a positive experience to the disabled person using the service. It supports adults and children through making lasting links between clients, their carers and the families providing respite. Jessica, ten years old, who has cerebral palsy, spends a weekend every five to six weeks with her support family. There are two children in the support family and they play and share family outings.

Support for carers is an area of social policy that is still developing. The Carers and Disabled Children Bill 2000 will extend carers' rights in England, Wales and Scotland

Key questions

1   Give two examples of informal care.

2   What is the most likely source of informal care?

3   Who do young carers look after?

4   What role can neighbours play as informal carers?

5   What services are offered by local support groups?

6   What Act gives carers the right to request an assessment?

7   When was the National Strategy for Carers announced?

8   What are the key aims of the National Carers' Strategy?

A national insurance scheme means that people in work now pay for people requiring care in the hope that when they need help it will be there.

adviser to the select committee looking at the funding of residential care (1996)

We need to be honest with the public about what we can achieve with the resources we have got and have a completely open debate about how much we as a society are prepared to spend on health care, whether through taxation, other forms of funding or from our own pockets.

Ian Bogle, chairman of the British Medical Association (BMA)

SECTION **5.4**

The funding of services

This section considers the resources needed to provide health and social care services. It looks at where those resources come from and how they are managed. Finally, it explores an issue where the different financial arrangements have brought major challenges for governments – long-term residential care for older people.

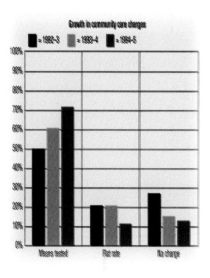

5.4.1 The funding of services

The funding of health and social services is complex, with money coming from a number of sources:

- central government
- local government
- charities
- individuals
- private companies through insurance.

The balance between sources differs according to the organisation or agency concerned, the service being provided, and the ability of clients to pay.

Payment for services

❝ We are faced with a stark choice – we either reduce services or impose charges. [We know] charges alienate service users and threaten the existence of social services by replacing state provision with the economics of the market place. They create poverty traps and are costly to administer. ❞

director of social services

A major aspect of discussion is always how the services are financed. The cost of health and social care is a large percentage of the gross domestic product (GDP). However, spending in Britain, both as a percentage of GDP and per capita, is low compared with other advanced industrialised countries.

Annual spending on health per head of population					
	USA	**Germany**	**France**	**UK**	**Poland**
Public spending	£1,195	£1,146	£943	£740	£219
Private spending	£1,384	£341	£333	£135	£23
Total	£2,579	£1,487	£1,276	£875	£242

source: OECD 1997

Payment in the NHS

The original idea that health and social services would be free to all has been impossible to sustain and there are now variations in the way in which clients are expected to pay a contribution or the full cost of the service. Everyone is able to call on the health services when they're ill and many still have full access to social services. What has changed is that after an initial contact, the patient or client may find that they have to pay for some or all of the service.

- Most primary healthcare, delivered through a GP or a health clinic, is free at the point of delivery. There are exceptions to this, such as a medical conducted for insurance purposes.
- There is a basic charge for each item on a prescription but also a range of exemptions based on age, income or medical condition.
- Opticians charge for eye tests with exemptions similar to those for prescriptions. Glasses and contact lenses are now available at a widening range of retailers with patients, or customers, being encouraged to shop around.

DENTAL TREATMENT ON THE NHS

Dentists in general practice provide most dental treatment. Since the foundation of the NHS they've had contracts to treat NHS patients. They've also had private patients. The contract was based on fees for each item of service. In 1991 a new contract gave a capitation fee. As dentists considered that this reduced the amount they received, many reduced or stopped their NHS work, concentrating on private practice. Consequently, private insurance companies expanded their involvement in this area. The new NHS dentists' contract and arrangements with private insurance companies have promoted preventive work rather than the more costly payment for restorative work.

- There are fees for dental treatment. Changes in the way that dental services are supported mean the service is now only free to those exempt from prescription charges.

66 *Having paid into the system for so long, I now can't find an NHS dentist anywhere. It's not a choice of dentist but a choice between private dental care or no dental care.* 99

man whose dentist retired

Most hospital treatment is free, although patients may opt to be a consultant's private patient or to pay for a private room. There are some charges, however, such as a basic fee charged to the driver in traffic accidents.

DISCUSSION POINT

Some economists argue that people requiring treatment as a result of smoking or drinking should contribute towards the cost. Given the need for prioritising (or rationing) within the health service and the high cost of treatment, what do you think?

Mobility and other aids are also free, provided the patient is prepared to choose from the range available. Payment must be made for additional accessories or specialist equipment. Health authorities have a degree of discretion in some matters. For example, fertility treatment may be free in some areas but only available through private healthcare schemes in others.

Payment for social care

A wide range is provided free, such as information and advice, assessment and care planning. For services provided with a degree of compulsion, such as mental health interventions or child protection work, it would be counter-productive to charge. For example, for some children's services, such as voluntary care, the general practice is not to make charges because the cost of collection is greater than the income generated, although some authorities charge as a disincentive to parents requesting care for their children.

Increasingly, local authorities are introducing charges for all or part of community care packages. With the exception of residential care, local authorities have discretion to set the criteria both for who pays and how much.

66 *The introduction of means-testing for community care is so shocking and dismaying to elderly clients that many are walking away from care.* 99

senior officer with Age Concern England

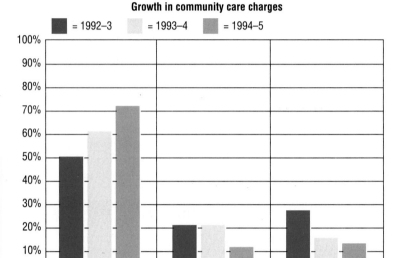

Growth in community care charges

= 1992–3　　= 1993–4　　= 1994–5

Private services

Private medicine has always existed alongside the NHS – BUPA, one of the
largest medical insurance companies, was formed in 1947. In social care there
has been a strong private residential care sector for many years. Since 1990
governments have encouraged private health and social care to take a larger
slice of the market. Private health care is paid for by a combination of the
individual's own income and private insurance.

5.4.2 Statutory funding arrangements

How are the NHS and local government funded? How do they decide how to
spend funds? How is it distributed to organisations providing the service?

The principles of funding for health and social services are laid down by
legislation and directed by government policy. The Government sets limits to
public expenditure through the Comprehensive Spending Review and the
budget. It allocates money from taxation to the NHS and regulates the level of
local authority expenditure in the annual settlement negotiated by the
Department of the Environment.

Central government

Central government funds health and social care services by:

■ taxation – this pays for the NHS through direct payment, supports local
authority social services through revenue support and other special grants,
and supports individuals through the social security system

- borrowing permission – from the City and financial institutions for buildings and other capital expenditure
- private investment and charitable donations – this is encouraged by government to support new buildings and special services
- transfer of funds from one sector to another – e.g. from the social security budget to local authorities, to enable them to implement community care arrangements
- direction to local authorities about allocation of funding, such as the percentage of funding for community care to the independent sector
- regulations setting out how much individuals must pay for health and social care.

NHS funding

The NHS is funded primarily through general taxation, with contributions from National Insurance and charges making up the rest. Traditionally, the amount of money to be allocated each year is decided by the Treasury, in consultation with the Department of Health, and agreed by the Cabinet. This process is both administrative – the NHS needs to know how much it can spend and how – and political. Once the budget is agreed, it's distributed through the regions to district health authorities using a formula based on agreed population criteria and reflecting their budget projections for the next year. At the end of the century, allocation moved to a three-year expenditure allowance which gives greater flexibility. Expenditure is controlled through the different levels of the NHS (see section 5.2). Through this system, Ministers have been able to favour particular service areas or redistribution of resources.

Local government funding

Local government services are funded through:
- central government revenue grants to local government and special grants to encourage activities such as joint funding
- special central government grants for specific services or groups, such as funding for services and facilities for people from minority ethnic communities
- locally raised taxes, such as the council tax and business tax
- charges for services and facilities
- partnership with the private sector
- loans from the City and financial institutions, particularly for capital expenditure.

Increasingly government has used special grants to local authorities to change the direction of local services or to improve or increase services.

Local authorities also raise money through local taxation – the council tax – which is set annually and paid by each household based on the value of their home. Councils' powers to charge are restricted by government-set limits to the level of council tax, and by public opinion expressed through the ballot box at local elections.

In addition to the council tax is a business rate, paid by commerce and business, the level of which is set by the government and distributed on a population basis. Revenue is also raised through charging for services. Government policy is to encourage local authorities to seek new ways of generating income and this now represents a growing part of local authority income.

How are decisions about expenditure made?

Health and local authorities are responsible for deciding how to spend their money. Because the NHS is primarily funded through taxation, it's overseen by the NHS Executive and the DoH. How the lines of accountability work between the NHS Executive, health authorities, primary care groups and NHS trusts is covered in section 5.2. At the local level, health authorities and primary care groups decide how they will allocate their money, and the NHS trusts have authority to decide how they spend the money allocated to them. Whether the health authority is prepared to pay for a service is a key factor in whether the service is available in the locality. Local authority members – elected councillors – make complex decisions about bringing together their central government grant, the level of council tax and how much they charge for services.

Organisations and individuals are accountable for their decisions and actions

The members of the health trust or local authority must ensure that matters prescribed by the Government are implemented and that decisions about services and facilities fall within their legal powers. Where possible, decisions reflect approaches set out in guidance and codes of practice.

The Audit Commission is another national mechanism for checking on the respective standards of financial management and quality of care being provided by health organisations and local authorities. The current system also expects individuals – whether clinicians or managers – to be accountable for the decisions they make.

Health authorities, NHS trusts and local councils are often faced with difficult decisions because the members' wish to offer a service or facility is restricted by other directions from the government. For example, all expenditure on services is subject to government expenditure limits and requirements to demonstrate value for money.

ACTIVITY

All health organisations and local authorities are required to publish information about their annual spending. Choose one – your local authority or health authority – and obtain its information for the last financial year. What are the main budget headings? What does it tell you about the organisation's priorities? Identify differences between services for different groups, such as older people and people with mental health problems, or adults and children's services. Can you tell from the information how much of the budget is used to purchase services from within the organisation (internal market) or from independent organisations (private and voluntary sector)?

CHILD B

When the father of Child B, who suffered from leukaemia, was told that his local health authority would not pay for a second transplant or expensive alternative treatment, he went to court. The case focused around the health authority's decision, which was based on both clinical judgements about the benefits of further treatment and its cost as compared with Child B's right to her choice of treatment. The court found in favour of the health authority.

How is the money allocated to the services?

The internal market and the purchaser/provider split have changed the way that the NHS and local authorities use the money available to them. The split between those who commission and purchase services from those who run them was designed to improve accountability and the delivery of the services in a manner which satisfies the client, purchaser and taxpayer. The 1997 government agenda for modernising and change removed the internal market but did not change the purchaser/provider split.

The primary way in which purchasers ensure that the provider will supply what is required is through:
- clear descriptions of the service required – the 'specifications'
- proper procedures for vetting potential providers
- performance measurements, quality standards and feedback from clients
- proper arrangements for working with the provider, including financial audit
- independent inspection.

Within the NHS there is a split between health authorities and primary care groups that purchase health care from providers. By using surveys and analysing data, health authorities can estimate the future needs of communities within their areas. NHS trusts or other health practitioners provide most services through contracts. The key purpose of NHS contracts is to manage the cost, quantity and quality of services. As such they could more accurately be described as service agreements. Within the NHS a contract is not seen as a legal document but as 'an opportunity to discuss and agree how improvements to patient care can be secured and over what time'. This means that any disputes are dealt with internally and are not subject to court intervention in the event of disagreements.

Other ways in which the health service funds organisations are by:
- contracts with supplies and drug companies
- contracts with independent practitioners such as dentists, opticians and private health and nursing care
- joint funding for projects for community-based services
- grants to voluntary organisations.

66 *Tendering for meals on wheels is not the same as collecting rubbish from the front door; staff hold keys to some of these front doors. It means that we have to make sure that the provider organisation does not go bust or is unsatisfactory. Elderly people have to be able to trust the private contractor with their front door keys.* **99**

social services contract manager

As far as social services are concerned, the NHS and Community Care Act introduced a mixed economy of provision. A policy direction in favour of

A London borough with a large Bangladeshi community has been working actively to encourage organisations within that community to become service providers. They've done so by bringing together community leaders, offering training which covers how to contract to offer services, and linking with its own training programmes so that staff and volunteers can acquire the necessary skills.

ACTIVITY

Select a provider organisation. Write a paragraph describing its services and list the sources of its funding. Estimate the proportions of funding coming from central government, local sources, social security and clients.

involving the independent sector means that purchasers are expected to take steps to find providers outside their own organisation. To do this, local authorities:

- find relevant providers through knowing their area or advertising for providers
- have written procedures for selecting potential providers
- set up or encourage new organisations
- use written contracts or agreements.

Although the purpose of the purchaser/provider split tends to be seen as opening services to external providers, purchasers also look within their own organisation. Each service is expected to be reviewed under Best Value every five years.

In summary, local government has powers to fund other organisations offering social care through:

- contracts with independent providers of services
- grants to voluntary and charitable organisations to provide services and facilities
- payment to individuals to enable them to pay for services, such as direct payment schemes or money to prevent children from coming into care.

DIRECT PAYMENTS TO CLIENTS

The Community Care (Direct Payments) Act 1996 gives local authorities the power to make cash payments for community care direct to individuals assessed as needing care services so that the clients can purchase for themselves the services required. The following are not eligible:

- people over the age of 65
- people with mental health problems
- people needing permanent residential care.

Local authorities have introduced direct payments schemes on an ad hoc basis. The Labour Government intends to widen the scope of the scheme and encourage more people to be given direct payments.

5.4.3 **Other sources of funding**

Although the majority of funds come through statutory sources, there are other sources:

- charities
- national lottery
- private insurance
- direct payments.

Charity

Some national charitable trusts have access to large sums of money which can be used to promote research, disseminate good practice or give grants to organisations to start new initiatives. Examples are:

- Joseph Rowntree Foundation – funds research into housing and social conditions
- Kings Fund – has promoted training for professionals in the health service and promoted good practice
- Family Welfare Association – distributes funds as grants to families in poverty and distress.

However, many charities are involved in providing care services and must look more widely than charitable trusts and fundraising to pay for their services. They have increasingly entered into contracts with the NHS or local authorities for those services. Funding may be supplemented by:

- existing charitably raised funds
- new money collected through donations and covenants
- charging clients
- special grants from central government
- interest from investment.

National Lottery

The National Lottery, which started in 1995, distributes money through a number of boards dealing with National Heritage, arts, sports, charities and the millennium. Although the monies raised for 'good causes' by the National Lottery are intended to provide additional monies and not be used within basic health and social services, the desire of successive governments to reduce public expenditure has meant that the National Lottery monies have started to be allocated towards public services.

> ### ACTIVITY
>
> Find out about the National Lottery Charities Board's criteria for giving grants. Match these criteria with a local voluntary organisation to assess what benefits and disadvantages there would be to receiving funding from the Charities Board.

Private insurance schemes

As government policy has shifted away from comprehensive provision by the state, it has encouraged private insurance to extend its involvement. This is an area for political debate as political parties consider whether the state should provide a universal system or a safety net for those who are unable to provide for themselves.

> ### DISCUSSION POINT
>
> Many people have made insurance contributions since 1948 in the belief that this would entitle them to care when they were ill or old and unable to look after themselves. Some people in employment question why they should be expected to pay, through taxation, for services that will also be used by people who don't contribute. Do you think the state should pay for people who are able to make their own provision through private insurance? What might be the consequences of this for those who can't take out insurance?

Forms of insurance available to support health and social care are:

- retirement pensions through an employer's scheme or private insurance
- insurance to replace income when permanent or long-term ill-health or disability strikes
- health insurance which pays for a variety of healthcare costs such as dental or hospital care
- insurance to meet the costs of community care, particularly residential care, for retired people.

66 *At the moment 11% of the UK population has private health insurance. These people are concentrated in the richest 25% of the population. Those whose policy is paid for by their employer tend to be among the richest of the rich.* 99

Observer *(15 January 2000)*

Not everyone is able to get insurance cover. This may be because of insufficient income, but could be because of ineligibility. Some groups are penalised because they already have long-term or terminal illness or disability. Other disclaimers in policy may mean certain types of treatment or illness won't be covered.

Direct payment by the individual client

66 *There must be greater transparency and fairness in the contribution that people are asked to make towards their social care. The Government believes that the scale of variation in the discretionary charging system, including in how income is assessed, is unacceptable.* 99

Modernising Social Services (1998)

Clients have always been expected to make some contribution to their health and social care services but the extent has increased since the NHS and Community Care Act. Section 5.4.1 gives examples of charges within the NHS and social services. Some charges are defined by government, such as those for prescriptions, eye tests, or the formula for calculating charges for residential care. Other charges are decided by the organisation providing the service, for example, local authorities now make charges for home helps, meals on wheels or day centres. Each local authority decides the amount charged and the criteria for eligibility.

To tackle the variation in charging policies between authorities, the 1997 Labour Government set a national means test for residential and nursing homes. However, the remaining charges are discretionary, with each local authority setting its own rules. The cost varies from 4 per cent to 20 per cent of a local authority's expenditure on services. The Audit Commission has surveyed local authority charging policies to bring consistency.

5.4.4 **Funding and the effects of politics**

Private Finance Initiative
describes the mechanism
through which private money is
brought into public services to
fund capital projects, such as
building new hospitals or
facilities. The Conservative
governments introduced it, when
there was a moratorium on
large building schemes.
Although relaxing restrictions on
capital work, the Labour
Government has continued to
want private finance to
contribute through the same
mechanism.

Because the amount of money available – and the ability of health and social care authorities to raise other finance – is directed by government, funding is sensitive to political direction. Each political party has its own policy for the principles that will underpin the allocation of funds.

Changes since 1997

When the Labour Government published a number of consultation papers setting out their agenda for health, social care and early years services, they included financial arrangements. Some of these changes have been covered earlier in this section and are summarised in Table 1 below.

One important change is a move to a three-year planning cycle – the Comprehensive Spending Review – which allows the DoH and DfEE to plan the funding available to health, social care and early years further ahead than the traditional annual cycle.

NHS funding is intended to promote high quality through:

- fair distribution of resources through health authorities to primary care groups
- a unified budget for primary care groups
- allowing clinicians to influence the use of resources by aligning clinical and financial responsibility
- long-term agreements.

The longer-term arrangements will:

- develop an integrated pattern of care
- address health and quality objectives as well as cost and value
- increase focus on 'programmes of care' for the population, and pathways for patients to cross boundaries
- provide measures to stop activity and funding getting out of step
- share the benefits of greater efficiency
- continue incentives for improvement.

Table 1: Political direction and the impact on funding of health and social care

Political phase	Political philosophy	Effect on funding
The welfare state	Provision by the state of services from the cradle to the grave	Funded through a national insurance scheme and national and local taxes
	Free at the point of access and for the majority of services	Few direct charges for services – the number of these grew over the years as the cost of health and care increased
	Voluntary and private care supplemental to that of the statutory services	Individuals could buy private health and social care; voluntary sector often grant-aided by local authorities to provide services

Internal market and mixed economy	Expenditure on public services should be reduced Services were better provided by private and voluntary sector, sometimes in competition with each other Where services provided in-house, they should be subject to the same rules as for external providers Commissioning/purchasing side split from the providing side Patients and clients should have greater say in their services and a right to a quality service Individuals should make greater provision for their own health and social care	Expenditure capped so that health and local authorities concentrated on those which were mandatory rather than those which were discretionary Limited capital expenditure and introduction of the PFI Greater involvement of other providers through contracts and service agreements Increase in the number of managers required to administer the internal market and contracts Increase in the amount of money patients and service users had to pay towards the cost of their services
Integrated approach	Public services needed to strive for excellence and better value and show they: ■ protect their users and the public ■ meet the patients or services users needs and promote independence or better life chances ■ improve services to meet national standards and performance targets ■ improve the performance of the work force ■ increase the use of IT The purpose is to improve public confidence in the services	Three-year funding arrangements Replacement of the internal market with partnerships and joint working Alignment of clinical and financial planning and accountability Increased funding available through special grants linked to the government's agenda National standards and performance indicators developed, linked with funding arrangements so that services can be monitored and compared with others Review charging policies to make more consistent

Table 2: Social Service Modernisation Fund

	Total for 3 years (£ million)
Promoting independence – partnership grant	647
Promoting independence – prevention grant	100
Children's services (Quality Protects)	375
Mental health	185.2
Training support grant	19.7
Total	1,326.9

Joint funding

There has always been a problem with providing services where health and social services both have responsibility for providing care. The fact that funding has come through two separate routes – with the health service being overseen by central government and social services by locally elected councillors – has not made it easy to resolve. Arrangements for joint funding tried to overcome this. It was usually targeted at services where the patient moved home after hospital discharge, or long-stay patients were relocated into the community, or where clients were no longer seen as needing special health care provision.

The funding was provided by the NHS and tapered down over ten years so that the local authority could take over responsibility. Joint funding was very popular but the point when local authorities were to take over coincided with the government taking measures to curb local authority expenditure.

The NHS and Community Care Act diluted further the benefits of joint funding because the NHS narrowed its definition of services to those which were medical, nursing and acute. Local authorities were left to fund all other services. The DoH issued guidance, which ensured that health and local authorities collaborated on plans for their community but clarified the NHS responsibility to meeting the health needs only. This did not resolve the issue for a number of groups. It had a significant effect on older people requiring long-term residential care, as you will see at the end of this section.

Modernising Social Services sets out the consequences of joint funding, which have sometimes meant:

- services for groups not within the mainstream have been neglected – e.g. the needs of minority ethnic communities
- social services have concentrated on services for those with high dependency needs, not where the level of need is low
- poor development of preventive services or services that would keep clients and their carers in employment.

In recognising the problem, the Government has identified clear responsibility for different services, with shared responsibility for cutting health inequalities, for mental health and for promoting independence. It has also encouraged clear funding arrangements.

Improving commissioning

There is evidence of authorities not using commissioning to secure appropriate services for specific non-mainstream groups – e.g. minority ethnic communities ('They look after their own, don't they?'). The Government has specifically identified concerns as:

- a lack of information on best approaches to commissioning
- budgetary arrangements and their impact on service making tailoring difficult
- less effective relationships with providers – if private, relationships can be adversarial; if public, there can be poor quality control
- the crude system for setting contract prices – there is a poor correlation between quality and the amount paid.

The Government is working on guidance to improve commissioning.

THEY LOOK AFTER THEIR OWN, DON'T THEY?

This SSI report on services for minority ethnic older people showed that:

- the choice of services was limited and basic services were offered inappropriately
- limited information, advice and support was available to enable minority ethnic groups to work with health and social services effectively
- where services were commissioned for minority ethnic older people, they tended to support low dependency elders rather than those with severe needs.

Modernising Social Services

5.4.5 **Funding long-term residential care**

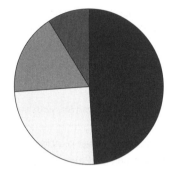

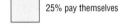 49% paid wholly or partly by local authorities

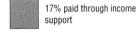 25% pay themselves

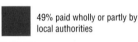 17% paid through income support

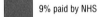 9% paid by NHS

66 My mother wanted to go into the same home as Dad and the only way we could afford this was to sell her flat. The money won't last long and she had wanted to leave it to us so we could support the children through college. This is not what we expected. I always thought that the state would pay for care. We're still trying to decide what to do, and Mum doesn't understand why all her savings are being used up this way. 99

daughter of person in need of residential care

One reason for the escalating costs of health and social care has been the need to provide long-term care, particularly for elderly people. Successive governments have been concerned to cap these costs and have been reluctant to make the service completely free.

Following the NHS and Community Care Act, the Government clarified the different responsibilities for providing long-term care. This meant that the NHS paid for health care within hospital and nursing homes but all other services were the responsibility of local authorities. Where people need residential care and are unable to pay for themselves, then the local authority must be approached. If the local authority supports the placement, then a contribution will be required and a national means test is applied.

RESIDENT'S CONTRIBUTION TO THEIR CARE COSTS

The resident's contribution is calculated using rules laid down by the Government, as follows:

- all income, including state pension, social security benefits and any occupational pension – leaving £14.95 'pocket money'

- the first £10,000 capital or savings is ignored, a percentage taken up to £16,000, and the resident asked to pay the full cost of their care until capital is reduced to £10,000. If the resident owns a home, its value will be taken into account when calculating their capital. This usually means that the resident will be expected to sell the house unless another way is found to meet the charges. Until the property is sold, a 'charge' will be put on the property to be claimed later. If occupied by a partner, relative over 60 or someone who is ill or disabled, the property is not included in the capital.

The funding for long-term care remains unresolved and a highly political issue. It is seen by the public to be an unfair and unacceptable position as elderly people and their families are receiving different treatment.

HELP THE AGED'S HELPLINE 1999

The number of calls about community care was up by 28% and outstripped those about money worries. The charity's SeniorLine received 21,159 calls on this issue, while there were 20,069 on welfare and disability matters and 6,996 on other financial matters.

DISCUSSION POINT

People are living longer, and older people and their families resent putting their savings into paying for residential and community care. The political parties are concerned at the growing cost of community care for older people and are looking at ways to meet it. Discuss what options there might be to meet these costs. Do you feel that older people and their relatives should be expected to pay? In what other ways can this be funded?

A number of attempts have been made to resolve the issue. In 1996 the Commons Health Committee said that: 'People should receive free nursing care in their old age, whether in an NHS hospital or a private nursing home.' While removing the differences between long-term care provided for medical and nursing reasons, it did not resolve the funding of social care provision.

The Labour Government was committed to changing the situation and set up a Royal Commission on Long-Term Care to examine the short-term and long-term options for funding long-term care for elderly people and published its report (*With Respect to Old Age Long-term Care: Rights and Responsibilities*) in 1999.

The commission believed that most of their recommendations could be implemented without legislation. Some of the recommendations, such as extending direct payments, have been included in legislation and the Government is considering others.

ACTIVITY

Find out and summarise the conclusions and recommendations of *With Respect to Old Age Long-term Care.*

Key questions

1   List five sources of funding for health and social care.

2   Name three NHS services for which the patient pays a fee.

3   What do statutory services require funding for?

4   Give three ways in which users pay for residential care.

5   Name six ways in which central government funds services.

6   Name six ways in which local government services are funded.

7   Other than statutory, what sources of funding are available?

8   What forms of insurance support health and social care?

9   What is the social service modernisation fund used for?

10 Give five benefits of joint commissioning.

11 Describe five ways in which charities raise their money.

12 How does local government fund voluntary organisations?

13 How do residents pay for their care?

SECTION **5.5**

The effects of government policies on services

This section looks at ways in which the policies of governments have directly affected the delivery of services and, in particular, at three major pieces of legislation and the changes since their passing. You will consider how legislation and policy become redefined and interpreted by pressure from political parties, pressure groups, the general public and clients.

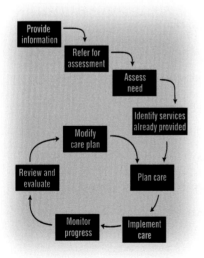

❝ *If good social work practice is really about user advocacy and empowerment, it will inevitably involve risk factors. The legislation is normally referred to when risks seem too great, but where the best long-term outcome must be rehabilitation, the law does not necessarily help. There's never any right or wrong answer – just varying levels of risk: risk to the social services department if anything goes wrong; risk to the professional credibility of the professionals involved; and risk to the clients.* **❞**

social worker, mental health team

❝ *We'd like to think that we were achieving something better than before. The procedures, with our specialised reception and referral teams, should mean that we're less likely to make inappropriate assessments, or to fail to provide essential services. Also, the inclusion of occupational therapists in our team does help to ensure that assessments are comprehensive and speedy.* **❞**

team manager, social services adult services

❝ *We have a duty to ensure that the next generation of children in local authority care get 'five star' protection. We must open up the care system to more independent scrutiny.* **❞**

Neil Hunt, NSPCC Child Protection Director

❝ *We do our own care plans, which cover the next three or four months. They're action plans, which look at all the care and help needed. These are used in conjunction with and inform the health service care plans which are reviewed annually. They're a way of monitoring to see how residents are getting on and any changes which need to be made.* **❞**

project manager, supported housing scheme

5.5.1 How government policies affect services

As governments and political thinking have changed over the life of the welfare state, a number of assumptions have been reviewed and repackaged. Significant changes over this period have been:

- growth in the number of different professional and work groups involved in providing health, social care and early years
- provision of services to prevent ill-health, disability or social distress
- technological advances, such as equipment within the NHS to make diagnoses and treat cancers, widespread introduction of computers
- focus on the needs of patients, clients and carers rather than services
- planning and delivery of services through partnerships between statutory authorities or statutory and independent agencies
- introduction of national standards defining the services and the performance of those working in them.

TREATMENT VERSUS PREVENTION

Earlier legislation focused on treatments or interventions which:

- removed children or mentally ill people from the family or community
- treated rather than prevented dental decay
- concentrated health promotion on mass programmes such as TB or cervical scans rather than general wellbeing
- imprisoned offenders rather than used community-based alternatives.

We are now more concerned with the prevention of illness and disability, recognising that a higher cost for health and social care services is paid if measures to prevent illness and accidents aren't taken.

5.5.2 Major pieces of legislation and their impact

Although many other Acts of Parliament have affected the welfare state and its development, the provision of health, social care and early years services over the last 20 years of the Twentieth Century and onwards have been dominated by three in particular:

- Mental Health Act 1983
- Children Act 1989
- NHS and Community Care Act 1990.

Mental Health Act 1983

66 The current mental health laws have failed. They failed to properly protect the public, patients and staff. They were devised for a time when most patients were treated in hospital . . . It is the community as well as patients who have paid a very high price indeed. The tragic tolls of suicide and homicides graphically illustrate the failure of the old system. 99

Alan Milburn, Secretary of State for Health (November 1999)

295

When people are confused, depressed or psychotic they are unable properly to consider their own or others' best interests. The Mental Health Act lays down procedures designed to draw a balance between the needs of society for protection and the needs of the patient to be protected from abuse of their rights. The Act:

- specifies procedures for the compulsory admission of patients to hospital
- defines their rights while in hospital
- defines the circumstances of their treatment
- lays down procedures for their continued detention and discharge
- sets appeals procedures
- defines who may exercise powers of detention and, in some cases, the training they must have.

A patient may be compulsorily detained if it is judged to be necessary for their health and safety or for the protection of others, with a central assumption that compulsory admission to hospital must be seen as a last resort.

There is a series of safeguards of patients' rights where compulsory treatment is concerned. The more serious the level of medical intervention (e.g. psychosurgery or electro-convulsive therapy, ECT) the stricter the safeguards. Other safeguards of patients' rights are contained in the Mental Health Review Tribunals (which consider applications for discharge) and the Mental Health Commission, which has a general power to review the exercise of the Act's powers.

ACTIVITY

List the various health and social services practitioners involved in mental health work. Find out what specific tasks each has and the various settings in which they might carry out these roles.

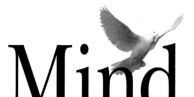

The Mental Health Charity

ROLE OF THE APPROVED SOCIAL WORKER

Under the Mental Health Act 1983 only a social worker who has received specified post-qualifying training is authorised to exercise the extensive powers which are given. This worker is called an 'approved social worker'.

A major development since the Act has been the growth of 'care in the community' as an approach to meeting the needs of people with mental health problems. It is now considered that, for most mentally ill people and people with learning disabilities, hospital is not the best place, and that they are best treated in the community.

ACTIVITY

Find out the type of support voluntary organisations working with people with mental health problems (such as MIND) offer to patients or ex-patients. Write a short report on how they help people to protect their rights to consultation about their treatment or care.

Mental health services are the responsibility of both health and social services. Several mechanisms have been put into place to encourage the organisations to work together:

- representation on each other's planning and joint-funding schemes

CHRISTOPHER ZITO

Schizophrenia is the most commonly recognised severe mental illness, affecting up to one in 100 people during their lifetime. People with schizophrenia can display a range of symptoms including hearing voices and feeling they are subject to persecution. Although violence is not part of the definition of the illness, it can occasionally be present. Christopher Zito was a diagnosed schizophrenic discharged to care in the community. During a severe psychotic episode he stabbed and killed a complete stranger. This case led to public demand for a review of the circumstances in which potentially dangerous patients are readmitted to the community. The publicity may also have contributed to a false perception of the mentally ill as violent and dangerous.

DISCUSSION POINT

According to figures produced by The Zito Trust in 1997, an average of two people a month have been killed by schizophrenics in Great Britain. By contrast 320 people are killed on the roads in the same period. Does society need to be specially protected against people with metal illnesses? Or is the loss of liberty implied by compulsory treatment too high a price to pay for the extra sense of protection and security?

- joint planning with health and community care plans
- community mental health teams which bring together professionals from both health and social services.

66 *People with mental health problems are far more likely to harm themselves than others. The debate needs to focus on people falling through the net in terms of being neglected and not receiving the support they need.* 99

Sue Baker, MIND

66 *Proper risk assessments, medication, monitoring and communication between different health and social services are needed to support mental health workers and to give people the best chance to overcome the terror induced by illness.* 99

Cliff Prior, Chief Executive of the National Schizophrenia Fellowship

Community care has not always worked well, and people with mental health problems sometimes found themselves unsupported and without services. The amount of supportive and sheltered housing was insufficient or didn't come in to place before the closure of hospital wards. The numbers of beds within hospital and crisis centres were also insufficient. The result has been that people with mental health problems form a large proportion of the homeless and the prison population. Consequently they may find themselves without a GP service or social work support and may move in and out of the remaining mental health units in hospitals and prison.

With some illnesses, such as schizophrenia, the reduction of places in hospital has lead to informal carers having to bear the burden of support. Under the Mental Health Act, treatment in a community setting is not compulsory, and so patients can reject their drugs and their mental state can break down. Organisations representing the families of people who are mentally ill have pressed for the services to move back towards a protection model. This view – that the safety of the public is being endangered – has lead to a government rethink.

Current initiatives

The following initiatives have been taken since 1997:

- the National Service Framework for mental health services (see page 250)
- the Mental Health (Public Safety and Appeals) Scotland Act 1999 that deals with loopholes in the discharge of patients detained under the Mental Health (Scotland) Act
- Reform of the Mental Health Act Green Paper, November 1999.

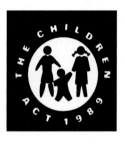

Parental responsibility is defined as 'all the rights, duties, powers, responsibilities and authority which by law a parent of a child has in relation to the child and his or her property'.

REFORM OF THE MENTAL HEALTH ACT

The Green Paper, based on a report from an expert committee, consults on a change of mental health legislation to further protect the public and the patient. It proposes compulsory treatment orders, additional crisis teams, 24-hour access to specialist mental health services for the severely ill, and additional funding available to the NHS and local authorities.

Children Act 1989

From the late 1960s onwards, there was growing criticism of the law relating to children. This came from a number of factors:

- well-publicised child death cases
- poor communication between different services (social services, health, education, housing, police)
- concern that parents' rights were being ignored
- concern that children's views were being disregarded
- a confusing number of routes into the childcare system
- concern (based on research) that children were 'lost in care'
- poor long-term outcomes for many who had been through the care system
- improved understanding of the extent and complexity of child abuse and that most social workers were poorly trained to deal with it.

The Children Act is the response to these concerns and brings together, in a single piece of legislation, the law relating to children. It covers:

- private childcare law (e.g. custody in divorce proceedings)
- public childcare law (e.g. the means by which children are looked after by local authorities)
- the duties of local authorities to children in care
- the powers and duties of local authorities to protect children from abuse
- local authority support for children in need.

The basic principles underlying the Act, together with the guidance that accompanies it, are that:

- 'children are generally best looked after within the family with both parents playing a full part and without resort to legal proceedings'
- the interests of the child are paramount
- parents have parental responsibility which is only given up in the event of the child being adopted.

Although stating that children are best raised in their own families, the Act also recognises that this may not always be possible. It therefore provides means by which a child may be removed from its prime carer. When this occurs there should be a plan either for rehabilitation or for a long-term substitute family.

NATIONAL SOCIETY FOR THE PROTECTION OF CHILDREN (NSPCC)

In 1999 the NSPCC conducted 82 investigations into allegations of physical and sexual abuse of 'looked-after children' in residential and foster care, of which more than half concerned recent cases. As a result of these investigations, more than 50 care workers and others in positions of trust face prosecution.

66 *My experience in care was a sense of not really belonging. You lived in a home and had what was then called aunts and uncles but I was aware of my ethnicity and that having white people looking after me was an anomaly, but having said that, it was my home.* 99

Kriss Akabusi, (Community Care, 1994)

PATRICE

When Patrice, an interior decorator, moved into her flat after being in care for 16 years, she had so little furniture she painted a TV, chairs and a table on the wall.

"*I was pregnant when I was 15, had a baby when I was 16, and was put into a flat when I was 16. All I had was a bed and a cot.*" She recalls that she had no help or support. "*The attitude was 'just get on with it'.*"

Community Care, 1994

Impact on practice

The introduction of the Act coincided with the NHS and Community Care Act and led immediately to an organisational split between adult care and childcare, allowing workers to develop a greater expertise.

The broad impacts of the Act have seen:

- (since 1994) an increase in the number of care orders

- greater independent and judicial supervision of the investigative and assessment process

- more rigorous review processes for looked-after children

- the development of partnership and service level agreements with private and voluntary organisations to deliver specialist assessment work

- closer working partnerships with other services (e.g. health and the police)

- the establishment of specialist teams (e.g. children with disabilities and leaving care)

- (more recently) a split between assessment services and long-term provision

- development of a structured and consistent in-service training

- an increasing emphasis on standardised practice across England and Wales.

An example of the latter is the 'Looking After Children' forms, introduced from 1995, which brought a standard approach to the review and ongoing assessment of children in the care system.

When the Act was first implemented, most of the emphasis on resources related to care and child protection. The powers available in the Act for the assessment and support of 'children in need' was seen as an addendum that enabled social workers to give help in extreme cases. This led to a widespread view that the only path to resources lay through a child's name being placed

AREA CHILD PROTECTION COMMITTEES (ACPC)

Local authorities have a duty to ensure the establishment of an ACPC in their area. It may be established jointly with other local authorities and must contain persons from:

- social services
- education
- health
- police
- probation
- NSPCC (where active in the area)
- armed services (where there is a large service base).

The task is to develop local policies, audit and evaluate the effectiveness of services, develop effective working relationships and ensure common understanding of operational definitions.

A **care plan** is a statement of the service being provided for a client. It is developed through consultation with all concerned and puts together a package of care.

ACTIVITY

Find out and list the information that must be included in the care plan. You will find it helpful to look at the Department of Health's Care Management and Assessment: Practitioners' Guide.

---

on the Child Protection Register, or the child having fairly severe disability. Initiatives from the DoH, most recently a new version of Working Together, have required the assessment of children in need and child protection assessment to be seen as part of a continuum. This has produced a more coherent individual planning framework and a fall in the number of children whose names have been placed on the Child Protection Register.

Current initiatives

Government has sought to raise standards of care and regulate the practice of people working in care through Quality Protects (page 253). It has also, realising that many of the statistics around children in need are unreliable, sought to produce a better quality database through a nationwide census of the work being undertaken. This also ensured that local authorities had detailed and comparable statistics.

The following pieces of legislation, all amending or affecting the Children Act, were passing through parliament in the 1999/2000 session:
- Protection of Children Act 1999
- Care Standards Act 2000
- Children Leaving Care Act 2000
- Carers and Disabled Children Bill.

NHS and Community Care Act 1990

The NHS and Community Care Act had a profound effect on the way local authority social services offered services to adults. Some of the mechanisms put in place also began to be applied to children's services.

66 Community Care means providing the right level of intervention and support to enable people to achieve maximum independence and control over their lives. 99

Caring for People (Department of Health, 1989)

Planning care for an individual

Traditionally, the practitioner's approach to care planning was based on the services being offered by their organisation. The Act introduced a requirement that each individual have a care plan, which aims to put in place the most appropriate and effective support systems for them.

The system linked in with the purchaser/provider split and allowed practitioners to tap into the agreements reached with provider organisations to make the best match for their client. Sometimes the agreement is a one-off (spot contracts) or for provision of a service.

Service agreements are written expressions setting out who does what and how. The agreement can be reached between the purchaser or funder and the provider. It can also be the written agreement between one section of an organisation and another. In local authorities, they're known as 'service level agreements'. Unlike a contract, they're not legally binding.

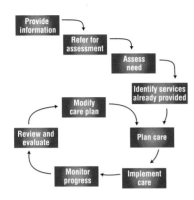

❝ The new system is supposed to mean that professionals work together so that the client gets the service they need. This does seem to fall down when individual professions don't seem to want to cooperate. The division between healthcare and social care can still mean that each service says that it's the other's responsibility. For instance – when is a bath a health bath or a social bath?❞

community worker with Age Concern

A social worker or care manager is responsible for developing the care plan and will work with other practitioners, the client and informal carers to prepare it. Although anyone can request an assessment, not everyone is eligible for one. Health and social services will have criteria for eligibility and procedures for responding to a request for an assessment.

The diagram, based on the DoH's chart, sets out the process through a care planning cycle with nine stages.

To complete the care plan cycle, the care manager will:
- provide information to potential clients and carers
- assess the needs, relate them to the organisation's policies and agree what can be done to help
- identify what services are already being provided, where there is an informal carer, and agree how this assistance can continue
- draw up a care plan to meet immediate and longer-term needs
- ensure that all the service providers are ready to put the plan into action on the agreed date
- monitor progress
- review and evaluate the services
- modify the plan if necessary.

With growing pressure from organisations representing carers to have their needs recognised, the Carers (Recognition and Services) Act 1995 was passed to give carers a right to be assessed with the client (as explained in section 5.3).

Working with a care plan system changed the day-to-day practices of social services departments. It enabled departments to offer a more tailored service for adult clients and be more consistent in their procedures.

Involving clients and carers

❝ Users and carers should be enabled] to exercise genuine choice and participation in the assessment of their care needs. Assessment procedures must be readily accessible by all potential service users and their carers. Authorities will need to take positive steps so that people with communication difficulties arising from sensory impairment, mental incapacity or other disabilities can participate fully in the assessment process and in the determination of service provision.❞

Department of Health Policy Guidance (1990)

The former approach of welfare services of doing things *for* people has had to change to doing things *with* people. The concept of partnership, with client and carer empowerment, is fundamental to implementation of the NHS and Community Care Act.

ACTIVITY

For this activity you will need to work with two others.

It is now six months after the best review of Mrs Moore's care plan. Mrs Moore has generally settled well but has found some of the equipment provided by the occupational therapist difficult to use. However, Polly has been told by her doctor that she is suffering from stress and should reduce the level of her commitment to her mother. With the others, roleplay Mrs Moore, Miss Sharpe and Polly and review the care plan. Write up the new care plan.

5.5.4 # Influence of the general public, clients and others on government policy

Social policy doesn't happen in a vacuum. It comes about because people within political parties and interest groups collect information and form opinions about the principles on which the state should work. Section 5.1 describes the creation and history of the welfare state and charts the shared values and assumptions underpinning the way that people have been supported through health, social care and early years. Although the main instigators of these changes have been Conservative and Labour governments, they've been influenced by a number of different interests.

Political influences

Political parties test their policies through elections – at local, national and European level. Think tanks, which explore, analyse and propagate specific philosophical or political approaches, often support political parties. The election manifestos of political parties indicate their intentions if they achieve power. For example, the NHS is a political battleground between the parties. All parties want to show that 'the NHS is safe in their hands'. Child-centred policies can also be contentious – probably because there is no consensus over the role of women outside the home. Social care is often forgotten but nonetheless is at the centre of discussions around dealing with the ageing population or protection of the community from people with mental health problems.

Professional influences

Another source of influence on governments is groups or individuals that have been established by government as channels of research, consultation or complaint. Although some of these channels have been used for a long time, the past 20 years have seen an increasing emphasis by government on providing formal processes by which academic, professional and client views can be heard. Examples are:
- royal commissions
- when an individual is asked to review a policy area and make recommendations, e.g. Beveridge in 1942, the Griffith's report into community care
- community health councils
- ombudsmen/women have responsibility for investigating individuals' complaints about actions of civil services or central and local government.

An important group of influence on governments can be the organisations providing the services and the professional and trade unions that represent the views of people working in the services. The main grouping for the NHS is the National Health Service Confederation, and for local authorities the Local Government Association. They have been formed to bring together the organisations to promote their interests and meet regularly with government and opposition parties to press their position.

Most professions within the health service have professional groupings. Some, like the British Medical Association, have the role of promoting the interest of doctors, negotiating conditions of service for doctors and regulating the profession through the General Medical Council. Other professional groups, such as the Royal College of Nursing, also act as trade unions. Trade unions, such as UNISON or General Municipal Workers, represent a wide range of

THE NHS CONFEDERATION

The NHS Confederation is a UK-wide membership body for all NHS organisations (trusts, health authorities, health boards, and health and social services boards). Among its aims are to:
- inform the debate on wider health agenda
- promote relationships between the NHS and its partners
- lead the debate on the organisation of the NHS.

DISCUSSION POINT

Professional groups and trade unions have influence on the way services are provided. Some commentators see this as defending their rights rather than those of clients. Others believe they're powerful voices for clients. What do you think?

Voluntary organisations and pressure activity

Following the NHS and Community Care Act, many voluntary organisations have contracts with social services departments for blocks of services. They have offered specialist knowledge and expertise on working with particular client groups. Taking on contracts in a number of districts has created structures similar to those of the statutory authorities. Becoming so closely linked financially with social services departments has affected the ability of these organisations to be independent from the services.

In 1996, The Commission on the Future of the Voluntary Sector was a robust defence of the independence and diversity of the English voluntary sector. It emphasises that voluntary organisations should continue to have a campaigning role even when providing services through contracts with statutory services. It encourages charities to form partnerships with statutory agencies but not to forget that clients should be part of the partnership. It also offers a new definition of charity – benefit to the community – which would widen eligibility.

health, social care and early years workers. Although their role is usually seen as working for higher wages and better working conditions, they offer their members training and qualification opportunities. From time to time, the trade unions promote the services and shared values of collectivism.

Lobbying

Both the private and voluntary sector seek to influence government and potential government policies. In health and social care the focus of this lobbying is as likely to be about better services for a specific client group as for the organisation's own health and financial benefit.

There's a long tradition within the voluntary sector of campaigning for improvements to services. Dr Barnardo was not the only Victorian who used his good work with children to press Parliament to pass laws to protect children.

Voluntary organisations continue to campaign for many causes, both nationally and locally. The role of some is to bring voluntary organisations together to promote and represent the sector. The National Council for Voluntary Organisations (NCVO) does this at a national level. In many districts, councils for voluntary service fulfil a similar function.

If the voluntary organisation is a registered charity, the extent to which they can campaign is carefully monitored by the Charity Commission which ensures that any campaign falls within the charity's main purpose and doesn't occupy too high a percentage of its activities.

ACTIVITY

Arrange to talk to someone involved in a community project. Find out how and why they're involved in the project, what they're trying to achieve and why the project seems an effective way of tackling the issues. With their permission, write up the interview and add an analysis on how the project fits in with the needs of the community and current social policy.

Key questions

1 Give four themes that have characterised the history of the welfare state.

2 Explain the main task of an approved social worker.

3 List six topics covered by the Mental Health Act.

4 How does the Children Act 1989 encourage prevention?

5 What are the three basic values of the Children Act 1989?

6 What is ' parental responsibility'?

7 List the four tasks of the Area Child Protection Committee.

8 Explain the purchaser/provider split.

9 Explain the commissioning role.

10 How do purchasers ensure that providers supply what is required?

11 List the eight elements of the care planning cycle.

12 Give three benefits of joint commissioning.

13 Give four ways in which professionals may influence government policy.

305

SECTION **5.6**

Access to services

With a wide range of services available, there is no single way in which we can gain access to them. This section explains various ways in which clients make contact with services and facilities so that they may receive help and support. It considers the links between services and some of the barriers to access.

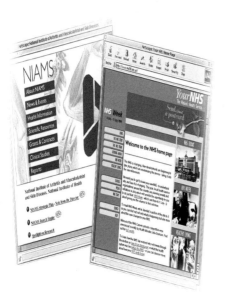

❝ Social services are always saying that access to child and adolescent mental health services is restricted. We think social services is heavily affected by lack of access. Often these specialist services are very isolated from social services and education. ❞

David Browning, Assistant Director, Audit Commission (Community Care, 29 September 1999)

❝ When a person comes on to the bus we play it by ear... Some people come in for leaflets and determinedly walk away, but most have a general or specific enquiry and a conversation starts from this. ❞

project worker with a mobile information project

❝ I didn't get help the last time I asked. I didn't get the chance to talk about my situation. It didn't give me confidence that anyone could help. ❞

potential client

5.6.1   Access routes

There are a number of routes by which clients gain access to the services they seek or need:

- 'open door'
- referral, recall or recommendation
- compulsion.

Open door services

These are where an individual may walk in or telephone for an appointment. Sometimes the service is free or available on payment of a fee. Many primary healthcare services, such as GP surgeries, child welfare clinics or family planning services are offered in this way. Helplines and Internet services are also open door.

Referral, recall or recommendation

Many open door services can be the gateway to other services. The enquirer may be referred on to other services. GP surgeries are the major route to specialist hospital and nursing services. Social service areas or district offices can assess clients for other care services that may, in turn, be supplied by the statutory, voluntary or private sector. Community advice centres can provide information and support.

Some services can only be obtained as a result of referral or recommendation. These are usually at secondary or tertiary level.

Compulsion

People may be 'compelled' to receive services in certain circumstances, such as Child Protection issues or in the case of compulsory mental health admissions. There are also some compulsory powers relating to the control of some contagious diseases. Where compulsion exists it is usually to ensure the protection of either the individual or others to whom they present a risk.

5.6.2   Methods of access

All statutory services are required to publicise their services as part of their quality assurance mechanisms and measures of their performance. Other organisations and professionals also publicise their services.

General publicity

The list of sources of general publicity is long:

- local telephone directories have pages listing health and local authority services
- local newspapers frequently have information about services – such as pharmacy opening hours at bank holiday times
- directories of charity and voluntary services are available in libraries and information centres
- articles in the press or radio and television programmes give contact addresses and telephone numbers.

ACTIVITY

Collect a range of publicity materials. Analyse the material in terms of who it is aimed at, how it is disseminated, how effective it is likely to be and why you think this is. Write a page comparing the likely effectiveness of two examples of the material you have collected.

307

DISCUSSION POINT

Talk about your own experiences of using health or social care services. How did you find out about them? Was it easy?

FINDING A FAMILY SUPPORT SCHEME

Mary is a young single mother, facing up to the challenges of parenthood with some anxiety. She was placed in her flat by a housing association but at some distance from her friends and family. Her health visitor, with whom she shared her fears, told her about a drop-in centre run by the local community association, and produced a cutting from the local newspaper explaining what it does. Mary is now an active member and has gained confidence and made friends at the centre.

Self-referral

Clients may refer themselves, for example when someone makes an appointment to see the doctor or dentist. A mother can visit a playgroup or mother and toddler club to see whether she can join. A child can telephone Childline to discuss their problems.

Recall

Other services operate a recall system, for example screening programmes. Cervical smears are offered to all women over 16 every three years and reminder letters are sent out by the GP or the health service. Dentists and opticians also remind their clients when it is time for a check-up.

Referral

A significant route to a service is referral by one practitioner or organisation to another. The most obvious example is the GP referring patients to specialist hospital services for diagnosis and treatment. Many community care services are made available as a result of a social worker or care manager assessing the client's needs and organising a package of services to support that client.

Referrals may also be a means of accessing more than one service. For example, a community care package may involve a number of different services working together. Equally, a referral to a hospital may involve a number of different services, some medical, others technical (e.g. a visit to a cardiac consultant may also involve blood tests, electrocardiograph tests and an X-ray).

Concerned neighbours or family may sometimes make referrals. There is a requirement on the practitioner to ensure that the intentions behind the referral are genuine rather than malicious.

66 *Anonymous referrals, for example when a neighbour rings up a health visitor about a child, are never very helpful. The health visitor would explain that the caller has to take on the responsibility of talking to social services and will need to give their name. This is because we cannot action unsubstantiated cases.* **99**

child protection adviser

Recommendations

Practitioners or organisations recommend services to clients so that they can refer themselves. For example, parents seeking a childminder may approach the social services department, who will offer a list of registered childminders, but the parents have to make their own contact.

Some recommendations come from other clients. This route is often used where the individual pays for the service, for example the choice of a chiropractor, dentist or an alternative therapy practitioner may occur on the recommendation of a friend already using the service.

5.6.3 Access through new technologies

NHS DIRECT

NHS Direct is a 24-hour nurse-led telephone advice and information service. Nurses give advice on:

- whether illness symptoms can be managed safely at home
- how such illnesses can be managed
- advice if further professional help is needed.

The service was taken up by the public with enthusiasm as an alternative to using their GPs. In January 2000 NHS Direct achieved considerable national publicity during a flu epidemic when it was claimed that so many people had called it that the DoH statistics on the flu outbreak had been seriously skewed.

ACTIVITY

Find out the 16 Department of Health helplines from the Department's web site. Select one which interests you and describe the help offered.

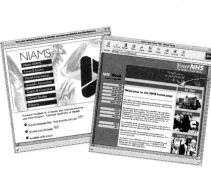

The development of new communications technologies – quick, inexpensive access to the telephone system, sophisticated answering systems, the Internet – has opened new, quick forms of access to health information and diagnosis.

Telephone helplines

Telephone helplines, often using recorded messages and push-button technology, allow access to a range of different services. Some information may be recorded; some may involve discussion with a specially trained professional. Some helplines (such as Childline) offer a minicom service for children who are hearing impaired. Depending on their funding, helplines may be free (0800), charged at a local or normal rate or, in the case of some commercial helplines, charged at premium rates.

A well-known helpline is NHS Direct which was announced in December 1997, with its first pilot taking place in March 1998. Since then it has expanded steadily.

Information technology

There is a developing strategy for the NHS to:

- make patient records electronically available
- use the Internet to give patients their results
- provide accurate information about finance and performance
- provide knowledge about health, illness and treatments.

Although some aspects of this strategy are about the public's right to know, others will require restrictions on access to protect the confidentiality of patients. At present this means that access is restricted to other professionals. Many other organisations now have access to Internet pages with the service varying from information about the service, information about specific conditions and access to personal information.

❝ We're going to have a repeat prescription service on this site, which will hopefully save patients some time... Eventually even registrations will be electronic: obviously you do have to physically examine the person. That will never change. But patients will be able to e-mail us details, and we'll be able to e-mail details of smear tests and so on. ❞

Glasgow GP quoted in the Guardian

❝ I'm sure it's useful, but I don't think it could ever be used for diagnosis or prescription. If you're dealing with a patient with kidney disease or diabetes, you need to see them every couple of months: you need to look at their eyes; you need to remind patients to watch their diet – this is the human mind we're dealing with, and if you don't say it to their face, they forget. The Internet can come up with some interesting diagnoses, but patients still have to discuss them with us. ❞

West London GP quoted in the Guardian

5.6.4 **Rights to services**

The right of access to a service may vary according to the type of service being applied for. For example, education from five to 16 is a universal right, as are certain benefits such as Child Benefit. Others may be restricted according to need (Income Support) or qualification (Higher Education). The same can be true of access to services in health, social care and early years settings.

For users and potential users, some services are available in every geographical area. Who the provider is – NHS or local authority, voluntary or private – may differ locally. However, it is usual for the NHS or local authority to have responsibility for ensuring that the service is there and for monitoring its quality.

Statutory entitlements

Statutory entitlements include:

- being on a GP's list
- attending hospital for a diagnostic check-up and follow-up treatment
- being assessed for a home help
- having a statement of special educational needs.

Statutory entitlement means a legal right to a service.

ACTIVITY

Approach four local organisations and ask about the methods of access to a service. Is there a relationship between the way the service is accessed and the way it's funded?

Mandatory and discretionary services

Clients are entitled to:	Statutory services may provide:
be on a GP's list	counselling services at a GP's surgery
attend a hospital for a diagnostic check-up and follow-up treatment	bathing services for older people
be assessed for community care	concessionary fares for older people
have a statement of special educational needs	drop-in centre for mothers and toddlers

The following table indicates some variations.

Service	Entitlement
General practice	Everyone has a right to be on a GP list and to consult their GP – if a particular GP has removed a patient, the health authority has a duty to find a GP for them
Hospital	Open door right of access to some services, such as Accident and Emergency
	Access to specialist consultant usually indirect from either GP or first point of hospital contact
Dentist	Right of access will depend on local availability as many dentists are private practices and access will depend on ability to pay
Childcare services	Most services can be applied but there isn't necessarily a duty to supply – right of service will generally depend on assessment of need and may vary between authorities
Community care	Right to request an assessment
Voluntary	Will vary – some, such as the Citizens' Advice Bureau (CAB), have an open door policy; some have an assessment of need; others have access restricted to those referred from another service, such as social services
Private	Will generally depend on ability to pay or referral on from another agency which is prepared to pay
Helplines & Internet	Open access, although there may be variations in cost, from free to premium (seen by most as a minor impediment)

5.6.5 Barriers to access

In theory all clients should enjoy equal access but, in practice, there may be barriers.

Barrier	How
Geography	Degree of proximity to service or to means of transport may vary considerably
	Quality of service or length of waiting lists may vary
	There may be local variations between authorities on threshold criteria for service
	Demographic variations may produce local variations in prioritising service development
Finance	Ability to pay for service
	Reluctance to be financially assessed
Class	Research shows there is a correlation between social class and quality of health
	Class differences between the client and provider may affect the rigour with which the service is sought
	Is information supplied in a language that can be understood?
Ethnicity, culture and language	Access to information about service in accessible language
	Ability to ask clearly and understandably for service
	Women from some cultural groups may be reluctant to seek a service from a man
Freedom of information	How available is information about a service?
	Does the service rely on disclosure by or from a third party?
Emotional and psychological	Social acceptability of service being sought (e.g. advice on sexual dysfunction or sexually transmitted diseases)
	Shyness in discussing problem (e.g. someone with severe skin condition)

5.6.6 Actions

While surveys carried out by Joint Reviews of Service Users have shown that 71% rate services as excellent or good, they hide a wide variation between authorities. Two initiatives to deal with this problem are National Service Frameworks and the Fair Access to Care Initiative.

National Service Frameworks (NSFs)

NSFs set NHS standards and define service models for a specific group and establish performance standards against which progress, within a given timescale, can be measured. The aim is to give patients a greater consistency in the availability and quality of services across the NHS. Each NSF is developed with an expert reference group bringing together health professionals, clients and carers, health service managers, partner agencies and others.

311

when you	you can collect evidence for
	information technology
use the Internet to investigate and record the effects of any recent government reforms on your chosen organisation	key skill IT3.1 plan, and use different sources to search for, and select, information required for two different purposes
present the results of the investigations based on the organisations' web sites	key skill IT3.3 present information from different sources for two different purposes and audiences; include at least one example of text, one example of images and one example of numbers
	application of number
investigate demographic characteristics	key skill N3.1 plan, and interpret information from two different types of source, including a large data set
carry out calculations based on large data sets of statistics on age, disability, etc.	key skill N3.2 carry out multistage calculations to do with (a) amounts and sizes (b) scales and proportion (c) handling statistics (d) rearranging and using formulae; work with a large data set on at least one occasion
present the outcomes of the statistical investigation	key skill N3.3 interpret results of calculations, present findings and justify methods; use at least one graph, one chart and one diagram

UNIT **6**

Research perspectives in health and social care

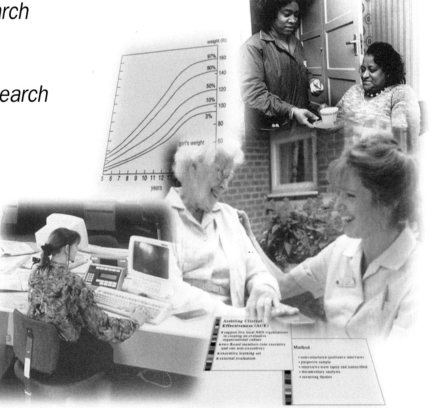

About this unit

Research in health and social care is carried out for a variety of purposes: for reviewing existing knowledge, describing situations and problems, and providing explanations. Research impacts on both the professional life of health and social care professionals and the organisations in which they work.

This unit aims to develop your research knowledge by improving your understanding of the research process. After completing the unit, you should be able to:

- explain the purpose of research in health and social care
- describe how to plan a research project
- design a research study
- describe and apply different research methodologies
- assess the validity of research sources and identify possible sources of error or bias in research that might influence the conclusions
- explain how to present research findings accurately, clearly and coherently in written and oral formats
- identify key ethical issues.

If you do the activities you will design and carry out your own research into an aspect of health and social care that interests you. You can do this on your own or in a group. If you do it in a group, it is important that you keep a record of your personal contribution to the processes of planning, designing, carrying out, analysing and drawing conclusions from your research.

66 *The purpose of research at the Centre is to look at current practice and see how we might develop the service. The age of our client group is wide: 12 to 25. We use research to help us pinpoint the different needs of the different ages. For example, we tried to find out what the word 'confidential' means to a 13-year-old. Do they realise it means the counselling they receive is private and we really won't tell anyone else about it?* 99

counsellor at a young people's counselling and information centre

66 *I don't think you can be an effective practitioner if you're not doing research regularly. I'm not just talking about knowing the latest legal judgements and keeping an eye on the professional journals for new approaches. I'm really saying that you need to be looking at your own practice through the eyes of a researcher as well as a practitioner. Doing research makes you aware of the disciplines of analysis and evaluation. It helps you be a more responsible and reflective person in your work.* 99

social worker

66 *Research is important to my job. Through my recent study on hormone replacement therapy (HRT) I have been able to provide more appropriate counselling. Also, I haven't needed to go away and look things up so it benefits customers because they get the information more quickly.* 99

pharmacist

66 *Research is incredibly important for my job. I couldn't advise people effectively if I didn't keep up to date. I look at research with a view to relating the findings to practice. I think it's equally important to update and extend one's own skills and knowledge. I'm currently doing an MA. One of the things I am looking at is 'disguised compliance' in carers – for example, turning up to the bare minimum of appointments, but not enough to move forward. Cases where this occurs have a high incidence of child abuse so it is an important area to examine.* 99

child protection adviser

66 *Research is very much a part of our work. Every four years we do research in schools, which we use to inform our work. The outcome of the surveys gives us information on trends in young people's health and allows us to track progress.* 99

assistant director, health promotion unit

The purpose of research in health and social care

The Department of Health emphasises the importance of evidence-based practice – good practice drawn from rigorous, ethical research. Practice in social care is derived from research into needs, up-to-date approaches and the nature of effective interventions and support.

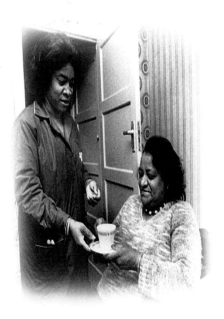

People working in health and social care need to do their own research, and use research from other disciplines (such as medicine, psychology and the law), to keep up to date with practice and policy developments in their professions and services. For example:

- nurses need to know about the latest methods of dressing wounds or how to produce computerised care plans
- social workers involved in child protection need to know how to recognise the signs of distress and possible abuse in children.

Research is also needed when planning services because:

- managers planning services need to know what the needs of the population they serve are
- health service managers and doctors need to know the patterns of illness in their areas
- information is needed on the effectiveness of existing services to ensure their quality.

The purpose of research is mainly to:

- confirm policy and practice
- disprove propositions
- extend knowledge and understanding
- improve care.

Confirming policy and practice

Some research outcomes confirm that the way things are done now is right or acceptable. Even so, beware of claiming too much for the outcomes of research. Researchers can't say that their hypothesis is 'proved' or 'disproved' by the outcomes. All they can say is that it is 'supported' or 'not supported'. If outcomes do show a correlation between the variables in a hypothesis, be careful about identifying cause and effect. The recommendations can suggest further work that could be done to investigate this relationship.

A practice nurse looking at the effects of a planned exercise programme on blood pressure (see page 161) explains:

66 *The outcomes showed more or less what I expected. There does seem to be a connection between taking part in the exercise programme and maintaining reduced blood pressure levels. I am reasonably confident that these reduced levels are a result of the exercise, because the group of patients that didn't join the classes did not show a similar level of reduction. But I can't be certain about the effect of other factors, including the social benefit of coming to the classes and possible reductions in stress.* 99

In this case, the practice nurse is justified in continuing the classes and encouraging other patients with similar conditions to join them. She might also want to carry on the research process by changing the exercise programme and monitoring the effects on blood pressure.

'A **hypothesis** is an idea which has been suggested as a possible explanation for a particular situation or condition but which has not yet been proved to be correct' (*Collins Cobuild English Dictionary*). It is the starting point for research as it spells out exactly what you are setting out to investigate.

Disproving propositions

Sometimes the outcomes of research do not support the hypothesis. In this case, it may be that the hypothesis was wrong. Or there might have been something wrong with the way the study was designed or carried out. If their hypothesis is not supported the first time, researchers often want to try again and check their results. They may use a different method.

Extending knowledge and understanding

Research sometimes breaks new ground and adds to the 'knowledge base' of a profession. Some new knowledge is scientifically valid and significant. For example, the work done in the human genome project is building up a more complete understanding of people's genetic make-up and could provide radically new forms of medical treatment in the future. Much of the knowledge gained through the research carried out by health and social care workers is related to practices and procedures. Most health and social care professions are very practical, and a lot of valuable knowledge gained through research is to do with ways of working more effectively with people using health and social services.

Improving care

A lot of the research carried out by health and social care professionals aims to improve the quality of care provided. People who work in these sectors are in a good position to identify problems or incidents that they do not fully understand. These can often be the starting point for highly practical, relevant research.

IMPROVING CARE FOR PEOPLE WITH ASTHMA

People suffering from asthma can benefit from drugs that dilate the airways. A nebuliser is sometimes used for this, particularly with patients who need high doses. A nebuliser works by converting a solution containing the drug into a fine mist so it is easier to inhale. It can be self-administered.

A clinical nurse specialist in one health trust decided to carry out a survey to see how reliable its nebuliser service was. Around 50 users of the service were identified and sent a questionnaire. Three-quarters of them responded. The questionnaire asked how the patients used their nebulisers and also asked about servicing the equipment.

The study highlighted the need for more and better information about the use and care of nebuliser equipment. It also made several practical recommendations for raising the standard of care, including:

- developing a central register of patients who have the equipment at home
- ensuring the availability of spare equipment 24 hours a day in case of breakdown
- establishing a recall system to ensure equipment is serviced properly
- providing leaflets offering standard and consistent advice.

6.1.2 **The link to health and social care practice**

Research is a practical activity that can have a direct effect on the quality of care. But to be useful, it has to be done properly.

There is a wide variety of purposes for which research in health and social care is carried out. These include:

- evaluating the impact of treatments and interventions for patients and clients and for planning service delivery
- exploring patterns of disease and social problems
- obtaining feedback on services from stakeholders.

The outcomes of research may improve individual and collective knowledge, understanding and practice. They may lead to changes in health and social care policy and practice and the composition of the health and social care workforce.

To improve the quality of care provided, people need to investigate:

- the organisation and delivery of services
- types of treatment and intervention
- the occurrence of different diseases and other health-related problems
- the occurrence of social problems and the need for social support
- health and social care policy, practice and workforces.

There should be a direct link between research and practice. Whether the research is about specific interventions or wider issues of policy, following all the stages of the research process described in this unit allows the outcomes of one person's research to be used by others.

DISCUSSION POINT

How might the practitioners in the case study use the findings from their research to improve practice?

LINKING RESEARCH TO PRACTICE

Here are three examples of research that came out of people's practice.

Youth work

A youth worker felt that she could make a contribution to reducing vandalism on a run-down housing estate. She identified that one of the most significant factors in encouraging vandalism was a lack of recreational opportunities available for teenagers on the estate. She started running an evening youth club, but take-up was not encouraging. She decided to carry out a research project on methods of increasing involvement in such initiatives.

Young people and informed consent

A children's nurse felt strongly that many young people below the age of consent should be allowed more say in important decisions about their treatment. She decided to investigate law and practice in this area.

Pressures on carers

A researcher working for a national charity looked at the pressures on carers, usually family members, who cared for people with dementia. Her findings were used to:

- help health professionals realise the significance of the diagnosis of dementia to individuals and families
- suggest how health professionals could provide more easily accessible information about the condition
- identify the needs of carers for respite care and support.

Key questions

1 What are the main reasons for carrying out research in health and social care?

2 Name three types of research that health and social care practitioners get involved in?

3 What is the relationship between research, policy and practice?

4 How should research in health and social care link to practice?

5 What is a hypothesis?

6 Who uses the findings of health and social care research?

7 What sources of research information are available to health and social care practitioners?

8 Why is reviewing the literature an important part of the research process?

9 Why is it sometimes necessary to repeat research in a different place or at a different time?

SECTION **6.2**

Research methods

Successful research depends upon selecting an appropriate research design and method. Both quantitative and qualitative research methods and their uses are explored in this section. You will have the opportunity to consider the relative merits of primary and secondary sources of data. You will also learn about validity and reliability, how to collect and record data accurately and issues relating to basic sampling.

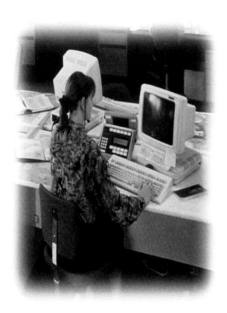

66 We chose action research as the method for our study, which investigated the shift to a health-promoting curriculum in colleges of nursing. Action research emphasises participation and partnership and is compatible with our philosophy of health which promotes participation, equity and empowerment. 99

health promotion researcher

66 The pre-test and post-test research design enabled any changes in practice in the care homes to be measured following the educational interventions with staff. 99

research fellow

66 This qualitative study, carried out on a small group of parents in Scotland whose children have chronic illness, does not justify generalisation. However, it does provide insight into the impact of a child's chronic illness on family functioning in a way that informs practice and moves towards theory development. 99

children's nurse

66 Experimental research is popularly regarded as the 'gold standard' of research. The experiment, which is ideally conducted in a laboratory, has come to be regarded by many as the hallmark of real science. As a method of inquiry, the experiment has been widely used in both the natural and social sciences. 99

university professor

66 When I think back to the beginning of my fieldwork in the outreach project, I am astonished by my naïvety. I assumed that my role would be welcomed and unproblematic. But when I was introduced to the staff they let me know that they were weary of white 'academics' coming in to study their communities. Many of them were reluctant to cooperate with me and although I was allowed to accompany them virtually anywhere, I was often reminded that I was an outsider and that I couldn't possibly be seeing what they saw or interpreting what I saw correctly. They made me realise how difficult it is to truly understand communities with which we have no natural affinity. 99

research student

6.2.1 **Quantitative and qualitative approaches**

Quantitative research approaches involve collecting data in a numerical form, which can be counted and analysed using statistical methods.

Qualitative research approaches involve collecting data in written or spoken form, which is analysed using other methods.

DISCUSSION POINT

Why is it often a good idea to collect both numerical and verbal data? What kinds of things can verbal data tell you that numerical data can't? What about the other way round?

Research approaches can be broadly classified into two main types – quantitative and qualitative.

Some research uses both approaches and collects both kinds of data. For example, a survey of how refugees and asylum-seekers make use of a community centre might collect:

- numerical data from observation – the number of times members of these groups use the community centre, how long they stay for, what they do there
- verbal data from interviews – what members of these groups think about the community centre and the programme of activities on offer, what improvements could be made.

Although many research projects use a combination of approaches, there is a real difference in focus between the two types. An occupational psychologist explains:

66 *Think of yourself outside a crowded, well-lit room, looking in through the window with a notebook in your hand. In quantitative research, you are looking at the world from the outside, as an observer. The aim is to be objective and collect precise, measurable data. Now think of yourself inside that room, talking to people, soaking up the atmosphere. In qualitative research, the aim is to try and get inside the world you are observing.* 99

Research methods

Research is different from ordinary finding out because it is more planned and systematic. It starts with a question or hypothesis and then selects a method that is likely to elicit usable, reliable data. The four main research methods are:

- observation
- interviews
- questionnaires
- experiment.

These methods are considered in more detail in section 6.3.

Variables and control groups

The role of the researcher is to control the environment and change one variable in order to demonstrate the role of that variable. For example, a certain type of bacteria could be sprayed with a particular antibiotic to see whether it kills them. The bacteria are the dependent variable and the antibiotic the independent variable. A separate sample of the same bacteria would be kept in identical circumstances but not sprayed with an antibiotic. The researcher would expect that the antibiotic would kill the bacteria but would not know that they had not been killed by some other factor such as cold unless other bacteria were kept in the same conditions. This second group is called a control group.

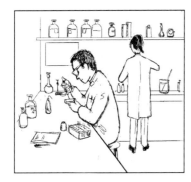

In pharmaceutical research experiments, different drugs are tried out on groups of volunteers. If the only variable is the kind of drug, any differences in the way the volunteers respond can be attributed to the effects of the drug. However, even under laboratory conditions it is difficult to eliminate all other variables. When researchers are studying human behaviour, rather than clinical symptoms, the difficulties of eliminating variables become even greater.

Experiments always start with a research question which suggests a link between two variables, such as the time spent talking to patients on admission to hospital and how satisfied they say they are with their treatment when they leave. There are two ways of carrying out an experiment like this:

- test the 'subject' before and after – if everything else stays the same, any changes which are observed (such as greater satisfaction) have been caused by the change to one variable (talking more to patients when they arrive)
- divide a number of subjects into groups – one group is exposed to an intervention (such as a drug), another group is exposed to a neutral intervention (a placebo), and a third group to no intervention at all.

6.2.3 **Sources of data**

The word **data** refers to all the information, including facts, figures, interview responses, photos, experimental results, collected during the course of a research project. It is sometimes used in the plural – 'data are' – but here you will come across it in the singular, 'data is'. Primary data is collected during the research itself. Someone else collects secondary data, often for a different purpose.

Primary data can be obtained by many methods. There is a great deal of secondary data also available. Much of this may be valuable to a research study even if it has been collected for a different purpose.

Primary sources

Some research projects aim to collect data from primary sources. This means getting data directly from the participants themselves, by interviews, observation, questionnaires or experiments. Other primary sources include demographic data about the people who use health or social services and data about diagnoses collected by health trusts and GPs. Primary sources are valuable because they provide first-hand, up-to-date data.

> **Primary sources** are the original sources of data. They include participants in research projects and first-hand data collected by hospitals, GPs and other organisations. Examples include morbidity and mortality statistics and hospital activity data.

Health authorities and NHS Trusts collect health-related information for their populations, including statistics on morbidity (the incidence of illnesses and disease) and mortality. Much of this information is routinely collected, which means it is done automatically as part of people's work. Some of it is available in individual patient/client records, but much is aggregated (combined) with data from other patients to form larger data sets.

A study was carried out in 1993 to investigate differences in access to heart surgery for men and women. The research was based on data from several hospitals in a health authority region collected over a period of four years. Using various categories of data collected by the hospitals, the researchers selected 24,000 patients with a primary diagnosis of heart disease and compared the management of all cases.

Statistical analysis of the results showed that women were less likely than men to receive surgery for heart disease.

The fall in UK AIDS cases has been mainly in gay men

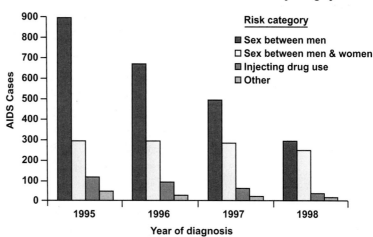

UK cases reported within 15 months of the beginning of the year

Secondary sources

Secondary sources are data that has been collected and analysed for another purpose. They include:

■ quantitative data such as statistics on mortality, morbidity and hospital activity or the number of people with disabilities within a social services area

■ qualitative data such as research reports and case studies.

Some data sets contain large amounts of data, often drawn from representative samples across the whole country or a region, which researchers can analyse for their own purposes or use as comparisons with their own outcomes. For example, the population estimates produced by the Office of Population Censuses and Surveys produce demographic data, which is used to inform funding levels for health and social services.

Most researchers look at secondary sources in the early stages, when they are defining the research question. This is because they need to relate their own idea to research already carried out in the same area. If they find that the same question has already been asked in a similar situation, there may be no need to repeat the research. Or they might decide to:

- carry out a repeat study to check the outcomes of the first study
- build on the outcomes, by looking at one or more of the questions that remained unanswered in the first study or required further investigation.

This is a short selection of some commonly used sources. You should add other secondary sources to your own database of sources.

Sources	Types of information
National Census	age, sex, job, ethnic origin and relationships of people living in all UK households
General Household Survey	many categories of data; data related to health and social services includes chronic sickness, accidents, mobility, sight, hearing, consultations with GP and hospital visits
National Food Survey	resources and expenditure, types of food eaten

Hospital activity data

Information about patients is collected at the start of their stay in hospital. Data is entered from then on at different stages and by a variety of people, including:

- demographic details – things like sex, date of birth, marital status, ethnic origin
- diagnosis – codes from an international classification of diseases (ICD codes) are used
- operative procedures – another set of codes, known as OPCS codes, are used for this.

The number of times a patient sees a consultant, and the outcomes of each 'consultant episode', are also recorded. A simple surgical case such as removal of an appendix may have three consultant episodes (pre-admission, in theatre and post-operative follow-up) compared to five or six for a more complex case such as siting a stoma.

ACTIVITY

Look at a copy of the *Guide to Official Statistics*, published annually by the National Office for Statistics. This describes the various different types of data collected by the government. Use the *Guide* to identify relevant sources of data that you might consult in your own research.

6.2.4 **Sampling**

The ideal way to answer a research question conclusively would be to involve every member of the population (every patient in a hospital, every client on a social work caseload in Britain). This is seldom practical and so researchers have to sample their populations. Careful selection is crucial in order to generate an adequate and representative sample. Market researchers, for example, may question people who pass them in a city street during the day. Such people are unlikely to be typical of the population as a whole as they probably under-represent people in full-time employment and people who shop locally rather than in the city centre. Newspaper surveys are also often based on volunteer samples who have bothered to answer a request for information, or who have written spontaneously about something that excites or annoys them.

> A **sample** is a selection of people from a given population.

Before drawing a sample we must define the population to which it relates and ensure that the sample is drawn from that population and none other. Conclusions can only be drawn in respect of the particular population sampled.

Different populations can be drawn from the same target group. For example, a sample population in a GP practice could be:

- all the patients registered with the practice
- all the patients on a particular doctor's list who have had problems with depression
- all the patients within a particular age range.

Selecting a sample helps to focus the area of study. Who to select depends on the hypothesis being tested and the amount of information already available.

Types of sample

A random sample is one drawn from the complete list of the population of those to whom we want the results to generalise, in such a way that every member has an equal chance of being represented. Because a random sample is drawn by chance it is reasonably likely to be roughly representative of the population – but only roughly.

It is possible to improve the representation by a process known as 'stratification'. This involves separately sampling the strata or layers of the population, using a variable known to be of some importance. If you draw a random sample of a year's hospital admissions, for example, there is every likelihood that your sample will be roughly representative of the population in terms of numbers of men and women – but only roughly. If you know that sex is an important variable in terms of your research question then you can improve the representative nature of your sample in this respect by drawing separate samples of men and women in numbers proportionate to their numbers in the population.

Much research in health and social care is about comparisons between groups of individuals, people in specific circumstances, patients with particular disease conditions. If research participants are drawn from one hospital only, or one geographical area, they are drawn from a limited population – those in that particular hospital or area and the results cannot be generalised to all hospitals or the whole UK. For example, Dr X may be known to be particularly knowledgeable about, or sympathetic to, patients with depression and therefore may particularly attract patients with this type of illness.

Sample size

Some research requires large amounts of data. For example, an analysis of how people acquire HIV infection would need data from several regions (preferably the whole country) and over a period of time to provide meaningful information. Similarly planning services coherently to meet the social care needs of people over 75 years of age requires the collection of data on at least a regional level. Demographic and epidemiological research usually requires large data sets.

Other forms of research do not require large samples. For example, a study into the effects of unemployment on men's self-esteem can produce useful results from just a few participants, as long as the data is obtained in a sensitive way.

ACTIVITY

Who are the participants in your research? What sample size do you need to make the results meaningful? Write the sample size in the third column of your table.

6.2.5 Validity and reliability

'Valid' and 'reliable' are words that we use in everyday conversation. Jot down your understanding of the meaning of each. These words have a specialised meaning in research. Read the definitions below and compare them with your definitions.

> If a method of collecting data is **reliable** it means that anybody else using this method, or the same person using it another time, would come up with the same results.
>
> **Validity** is concerned with establishing whether the data collected offers a true picture of what is being studied. It relates to the extent to which the sample is representative of the total population eligible to be included in the study and the techniques used to collect the data.

Identifying an appropriate method

The research question is a starting point for asking:

- what data should be collected to answer this question
- how the data can be collected.

When researchers select their methods they check:

- that the data collection method is 'fit for purpose' – will it provide the data needed?
- sample size – what size of sample is needed to provide meaningful data? Is it practical to collect data from this sample?
- effect on participants – how will they be affected by the process of carrying out the research and by its outcomes?

Fit for purpose

Some methods are better suited than others to certain types of research with primary sources. For example, the clinical trial of a new drug requires a special form of experiment called a 'double blind randomised controlled trial' so that neither the researcher nor the participants know which of them is trialling the drug and which has a placebo. Research into the experiences of people being discharged from long-stay institutions would require a very different approach.

Experiments are at one end of a 'spectrum' of research methods. They usually produce quantitative data. Other approaches are shown on the diagram below. They may use questionnaires, interviews or observation and tend to produce quantitative data (though they may produce qualitative data as well).

experimental approaches
- testing the validity of a hypothesis

ethnographic approaches
- studying how people interact in particular situations

phenomenological approaches
- describing the experience of being in a particular situation

emancipatory approaches
- helping people ('empowering' them) to examine and improve their own practices

quantitative ── qualitative

DISCUSSION POINT

Which approach would be most suitable for researching into the experiences of people being discharged from long-stay institutions? Why would it be the best approach?

Which approach would be best for a youth worker who wanted to find out why young women on a housing estate do not go to a youth centre?

How to record data

Simply collecting data is only a beginning to an end. The means by which it is recorded will both affect and enhance the understanding and presentation. It may also make a difference to the kind of conclusions which are drawn from it. This is covered in more detail in section 6.3.

Examples of recording

Questionnaires should give clear instructions and be easy to read, with enough space for respondents to write in their comments.

Interview record sheets are for you to fill in. They may contain quantitative and/or qualitative data. If you have identified categories to look out for (such as the number of times people mention a particular issue), the sheet should list the categories and give space for recording how often they occur. If you are taking notes, leave plenty of space to write in between each question. There should be space at the top to write down:

- the name of the person doing the interview
- the code name of the person being interviewed
- the place where the interview was conducted
- the date of the interview, the time it started and the time it ended.

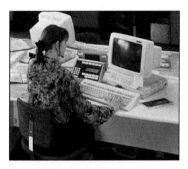

Observation sheets are like interview record sheets. They may have space for recording quantitative data or written notes.

Research data can be collected in two main forms – numbers and words. Quantitative methods such as statistical analysis are used for analysing numerical data; large data sets are usually analysed using computer software packages. Qualitative data analysis involves categorising data to allow themes and patterns to emerge. Now let's see how this applies in an extended case study.

STRESS SUPPORT

Health and social care organisations need to look after their staff as well as care for the people who use their services. A counsellor within a social services department was asked to investigate the high stress levels experienced by staff. He set up and facilitated several support groups for community nurses, district nurses and school nurses.

After the groups had been running for several months, the counsellor was asked to carry out an evaluative study. The aim of the study was 'to evaluate the perceived advantages and disadvantages of attending facilitated staff support groups'.

To answer the research question, data was needed about:

- what expectations people had of the groups
- whether their expectations were met
- the advantages and disadvantages of the groups
- how group members felt about the role of the facilitator.

The counsellor decided to collect this data from primary sources by sending a questionnaire to all 34 members of the groups. A first version of the questionnaire was piloted with a small number of the population, who helped to formulate the questions for the final version. The questionnaire asked respondents to:

- answer a set of closed questions, using a five-point rating scale to record how helpful or unhelpful they felt various aspects of the group were
- write their own open-ended comments on these aspects.

The questionnaire would therefore provide both quantitative and qualitative data.

The counsellor also decided to look at secondary sources to see whether other people in similar situations had tackled stress in the same way, and to draw on others' experiences of facilitating support groups.

ACTIVITY

Look carefully at your research question. What data is needed to answer the question?

Draw four columns on a piece of paper, or use the table function on a wordprocessor. List the data needed in the left-hand column (see the example below).

Stress support: data requirements			
Data needed			
Expectations of groups			
Whether expectations met			
Advantages/disadvantages			
Role of facilitator			
Dealing with stress			
Facilitating support groups			

What data do you need to collect from primary sources to answer your research question? Which sources do you intend to use? What practical difficulties might there be in collecting the primary data?

In the second column of your table, put a P against the data that will come from primary sources. In the third column, note down what the sources are. In the fourth column, note down any practical difficulties you might face in collecting the data.

Stress support: data requirements			
Data needed	*P/S*	*Sources*	*Practical difficulties*
Expectations of groups	P	members of support groups	possible low response rate to questionnaire
Whether expectations met	P	as above	
Advantages/disadvantages	P	as above	
Role of facilitator	P	as above	
Dealing with stress			
Facilitating support groups			

Part of the research itself may involve secondary sources. For example, the counsellor in the case study on page 330 decided to review the outcomes of previous research into dealing with stress and facilitating support groups. The findings of this review were incorporated into the results of his own research with primary sources.

ACTIVITY

Which of the four research methods – experiment, questionnaires, interviews, observation – will you use to collect the data from primary sources? (Remember that you can use a combination of methods.) Add another column to the table you made earlier and note down which collection method(s) you will use.

ACTIVITY

What data do you need to collect from secondary sources to answer your research question? Which sources do you intend to use? What practical difficulties might there be in collecting the secondary data?

Look back at the table you made in the last activity. In the second column, put an S against the data that will come from secondary sources. In the third column, note down what the sources are. In the fourth column, note down any practical difficulties you might face in collecting the data.

Stress support: data requirements			
Data needed	*P/S*	*Sources*	*Practical difficulties*
Expectations of groups	P	members of support groups	possible low response rate
Whether expectations met	P	as above	
Advantages/disadvantages	P	as above	
Role of facilitator	P	as above	
Dealing with stress	S	personnel journals, books on stress, NHSE papers etc.	many sources: need to define search categories closely
Facilitating support groups	S	personnel and psychology journals	not much relevant experience in UK

Key questions

1 What are the two main types of research approach?

2 How does quantitative research data differ from qualitative research data?

3 What are the four main research methods used by health and social care researchers?

4 How do researchers choose which method(s) they should use?

5 What do you understand by 'validity'?

6 What factors are important to consider in designing a research sample?

7 How do primary data sources differ from secondary data sources?

8 What are the benefits of good recording throughout data collection?

9 What should be recorded at the head of an interview sheet?

66 *You need to decide before you start research how best to collect the data. You need a fully worked-out plan of what you want to achieve. It's important to get the right amount of data but limit your research to what is practical. Time is a big factor. So stick to the range you have chosen for all your variables, even if it's tempting to broaden them because of your interest.* 99

optometrist

66 *We do street surveys and use the results in publicity to support our campaigns. One recent one was concerned with people's feelings about smoke-free dining areas.* 99

assistant director, health promotion unit

66 *I am collaborating on a programme with the local teaching hospital, looking at middle-aged women's post-menopausal health and health options. We hope to prove the validity of the role of screening in determining bone mass, to enable a woman to make decisions about looking after her bone health and avoiding a hip fracture.* 99

doctor in charge of health screening

Planning research

In this unit you will learn about six aspects of the research process: defining and planning what research is needed, identifying ethical issues, developing methods, obtaining the data, analysing the data and producing results, and using results to suggest recommendations.

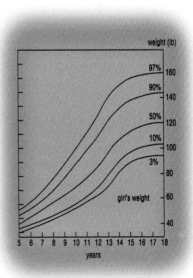

333

6.3.1 **Defining and planning what research is needed**

Health and social care research should be clinically or socially relevant and produce useful information for practitioners and clients. So the first step in doing research is to think carefully about what it is for by stating a hypothesis. This should state clearly what the research aims to do in order to set limits on it, to narrow down the investigation and to provide a clear focus. People who start with a weak hypothesis or poorly constructed research question may find themselves trying to investigate too many things at the same time.

Deciding what to research

When people working in health and social care think about a topic for research, they often start with their own situation. You should do the same when deciding on a topic for your own research. If you have (or have had) a job in the health or social services, that should give you a lead. If not, start by identifying an area of practice that interests you. Find out what the 'hot topics' of discussion are in this area. Which topics interest you?

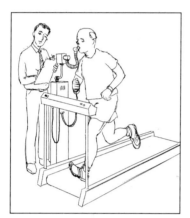

ACTIVITY

Decide if you want to do a research study on your own or with others in a small group. If it's on your own, choose an aspect of health and social care that interests you and make a list of five or six possible topics for research. If you're in a group, agree the broad area of health and social care, then brainstorm some topics.

Choose your topic. Then write your research question or hypothesis. It may take you several goes to get it right. Show it to someone else for an independent view before finalising it.

> ### PRIMARY CARE: THE VALUE OF EXERCISE
>
> One of the jobs of staff in GP practices is to identify new services for their local population and evaluate their success. A practice nurse in a suburban practice set up a three-month programme of exercise classes for people suffering from high blood pressure. She wanted to evaluate their impact. Her hypothesis was that the patients' health had improved as a result of this service.
>
> The hypothesis spelled out:
>
> - what she wanted to investigate – measurable improvements in the health of patients with high blood pressure
>
> - who she wanted to investigate – patients who had high blood pressure and regularly attended the exercise classes
>
> - how she could gain the information – by measuring relevant indicators before the classes started and when the three-month programme had finished.
>
> The practice nurse also decided to compare the patients who had done the classes with a similar group of patients who had not enrolled for the programme. This meant that she could also suggest what is called a 'null hypothesis' – the opposite of the first hypothesis. In this case, the null hypothesis would be that the exercise classes made no difference to the health of people with high blood pressure.

Even though the initial hypothesis is exact, it is important to take account of other factors that may influence the research. For example, if the practice nurse's results showed that the health of patients who did the exercise classes improved over the three-month programme, she would also need to consider what other factors might have contributed to the improvement.

Target audience

Who is the research for? For health and social care workers, one answer is almost certainly themselves. Research results are useful for other people too:

ACTIVITY

List the groups your research is intended for – your target audience. Restrict yourself to a maximum of four groups, one of which should be you and another the assessor for your course. Against each group, write down:

■ what you think they need to know

■ how they would expect the outcomes of the research to be presented.

Look at your completed list. Will your research question produce the information these groups are looking for? Do you need to change the question in any way?

PRIMARY CARE: THE VALUE OF EXERCISE

Following a brief examination of patient records, the practice nurse mentioned on page 334 decides to limit her investigation and adapts her hypothesis.

Hypothesis

A planned exercise schedule for patients between the ages of 50 and 60 suffering from high blood pressure contributes to the improvement of both the overall health of the patient and the lowering of blood pressure when it is carried out as a supplement to other treatments.

The area and scope of study is now clear. The adapted hypothesis:

■ limits the ages of the people being studied to those between 50 and 60

■ allows other factors to be taken into account – for example, the practice nurse could also compare the diets of people in her sample.

The hypothesis also now states the relationship between two variables: improvements in health, such as lowering of blood pressure, and a planned exercise programme.

■ immediate colleagues – especially if the research looks at a local aspect of practice such as appropriate toys to purchase for three-year-old children with mobility problems

■ policy makers, educators and people in similar jobs elsewhere – building a resource pack for a toy library

■ other practitioners – if they know that the research has already been done, it means they don't have to do it again, or that they can build on the results

■ health and social services clients.

Research has to be done properly, following the stages of the research process to ensure that the results are reliable. But knowing who it is for can help in deciding what information is needed and how to publish the results. For example, the outcomes of research into toys could be presented in:

■ a memo or set of guidelines for early years staff

■ a newsletter for parents

■ a training session to staff

■ an article in a professional journal.

Area and scope of study

A research topic may be quite broad. For example, someone involved in childcare may want to look at the way nurses interact with children who are afraid of injections. Several issues could be investigated, such as:

■ the range of tactics nurses use to calm children and how effective these are

■ technical innovations that could make injections less traumatic for children

■ how nurses develop skills in calming distressed children.

The scope of any research should be clearly defined. The person investigating children's fear of injections might need to decide:

■ the setting in which the injections are given

■ whether the injections are routine inoculations or part of the treatment for a medical condition

■ the age of the children.

This decision may be governed by practical considerations, such as the situation in which the person works and their access to data. There may also be other constraints such as the practicalities and ethical issues associated with getting children involved in research (see section 6.5 on page 361).

DISCUSSION POINT

Review the hypothesis you developed in your discussion on page 334. How could you clarify the area of study and scope of your investigation?

DISCUSSION POINT

Why is it sometimes necessary to repeat research in a different place or at a different time? What does repeating or replicating research enable researchers to do?

Previous research

Very little research breaks completely new ground. Most relates in some ways to previous research and is often conducted to:

- build on research that has already been started
- use the previous research findings as a starting point
- check that the outcomes from previous research are applicable in another situation or geographical area – for example, a survey on the link between mental health problems and unemployment might be done in several geographical areas and measured over a period of time.

Looking at the outcomes of previous research can:

- reveal similar investigations and show how the researcher handled these situations
- suggest a method or a technique for dealing with a problematic situation which may help solve similar difficulties
- suggest new or unfamiliar sources of data
- help to put a study in perspective and relate it to earlier investigations of the same problem
- provide new ideas and approaches.

People can find out about previous research by looking at the literature. Or they can ask others. For example, someone interested in a particular type of sports injury might ask staff working in a sports injury clinic or a physiotherapist if they know of any research related to the condition.

Sources of information about research

The sources of information relevant to research in health and social care are very wide-ranging. This is just a selection.

Sources	Types of information
Newspapers and magazines features	short reports of recent research; occasional in-depth
Professional journals, e.g. *Nursing Times, British Journal of Social Work*	more detailed reports of research, summaries of research projects
Specialist journals, e.g. *Journal of Child Psychology and Psychiatry, Community Care*	detailed, often technical reports of research in specific areas, treatments and interventions
Conference reports	papers and records of discussions, often in areas of topical interest and concern

These and other sources are available in libraries, hospital information centres, on-line databases such as Med-Line and on the World Wide Web. There is also a national register of research on health issues, coordinated by the Department of Health.

Searching the literature

Before finalising the research question, researchers look to see what other research has already been done into the aspect of practice they want to research. They do this by carrying out a search of books and articles in journals (sometimes called a 'literature review' or 'literature search').

The standard method of searching the literature has five stages:

1 Identify texts relevant to the subject using databases, indexes and abstracts (many are now available on CD-ROM or the Internet).
2 List the details of relevant texts on cards or a computer database.
3 Get hold of the texts, reading them and making notes.
4 Identify any important references quoted in these texts and adding them to the list.
5 Select the texts which seem most important, then briefly summarising the ideas they contain.

Key words

So as not to waste time, make sure you know the exact subject headings to look for. Do this by examining the hypothesis or research question to find key words. These are words that can be used in the indexes or referencing system to narrow down the field. In the case of the practice nurse investigating the effect of exercise classes, key words could include:

- blood pressure treatment
- planned exercise routines
- 50- to 60-year-olds
- in GP practices.

Sources

It makes sense to start with the most convenient sources – probably the school or college library. There may also be relevant books and journals in the library of a teaching hospital or university. Libraries can borrow books and journals from other collections. There are also services that download the text of articles directly onto a computer. The amount of material available on line is growing all the time and researchers sometimes make contact with others in their field on the Internet.

Reading about other people's research can be fascinating, but it also takes time. The box on page 338 gives hints about how to read quickly.

How general is the research?

Some research is specific to a time and place. For example, if a care home owner undertook a survey to find out whether staff wanted a change in the shift system, the findings would only apply to one specific home at a particular time and may not be of much use to anyone else.

But what if the survey also aimed to find out how staff reacted to the idea of change? That's a much more general question. It would need a different and more complicated research design, but the outcomes might be useful to anyone wanting to bring about change in an organisation.

A tutor in psychology at a college explains the difference:

66 *There is no reason why all research should aim to produce outcomes that can be generalised across a range of situations. A lot of practice-based research may be more useful if it is designed to produce very specific*

Reading quickly

You don't always have to read everything carefully, word by word. Here are two ways of reading quickly:

- scanning
- skimming.

Scanning is when you let your eye run down a page until you see a significant word. You scan a telephone directory to find the name you are looking for. Scanning is useful when you are checking to see whether something is worth reading in more detail.

Skimming is looking quickly through a text to pick out the main ideas. If you get a letter telling you whether or not you've succeeded in getting an interview for a job, you would probably skim it quickly to get the general meaning of what it said before reading it more slowly. Skimming is useful if you think that a text has information that you already know something about. You're just looking for the new bits.

It's useful if you can switch between reading techniques. For example, you can scan an article until you find a word that relates to whatever interests you. You can then skim the section until you find an idea you want to know about. Then it's time to slow down and read carefully.

information. It is usually easier to do as well. Designing a research study that can produce outcomes applicable in different situations can be quite tricky. For most students, I suggest starting with a specific situation and designing their research round that. They can always see whether the outcomes might have a general interest later. 99

The physical activity manager in health education explains how the results of many years of research can be put together to form a health policy:

66 *In 1996, 45 international experts were brought together to review the evidence and arrive at a consensus view on the strategy to adopt. Their report gave the recommendation that everyone should aim to do 30 minutes of moderate-intensity physical activity on at least five days per week, which should ideally be sustained through the 30 minutes. A wide range of activities is suitable for this, including swimming, brisk walking, heavy housework, gardening and climbing stairs.* 99

DISCUSSION POINT

Look at your research question again. Are the outcomes likely to be of general interest or are they specific to a particular time and place? If you wanted the outcomes to be 'generalised across a range of situations', how would you need to alter the question?

Devising research questions

The aim of this phase is to define the problem and answer the question: What exactly will be studied? It may include:

- a review of existing research findings in this area (sometimes called a 'literature review')
- a statement of purpose, giving the reasons for doing the research and indicating its exact area of study (its 'focus')
- identifying ethical issues that affect the research (see section 6.5 Ethical issues)
- selecting the research design – which type of approach is appropriate (quantitative, qualitative or both) and whether the data is to be collected from primary or secondary sources
- selecting the method which will provide valid and reliable data
- selecting the sample – who is going to be involved in the research?

Themes and patterns

If the research has been designed to test a hypothesis, it is usually possible to decide on themes or patterns in advance. Researchers might look for:

- themes in what participants say – for example, a survey to find out the reasons why people fail to stop smoking might establish six themes (including effect on diet, effect on mood or temper, social pressures)
- stages in a process – the same research might categorise participants by

length of time between stopping smoking and starting again
- particular words or phrases – these can be indicators of themes and patterns ('I feel bad-tempered at coffee time if I can't have a cigarette')
- attitudes – for example, how smokers feel about non-smoking flights; attitudes can often be scaled, allowing some numerical analysis.

Researchers sometimes start by looking for a few broad themes and patterns. As they get deeper into the analysis and become familiar with the material, they can make more distinctions.

Codes

Another approach is to code the data. This is a particularly useful method for analysing data from observation. Remember the occupational psychologist's image of looking in through a window at a crowded, well-lit room? How can you make sense of what you see? It's a lot easier if you know exactly what you are looking for.

Codes can be developed to categorise:
- non-verbal behaviour – movements of the body, gestures
- spatial behaviour – the way in which people move towards or away from each other, or in relation to particular locations such as the nursing station
- language – particular phrases or categories of language, e.g. swearing
- verbal behaviour – how quickly people speak, interruptions, loudness.

DISCUSSION POINT

A researcher is investigating the content of the interactions between residents and staff in a group home for people with learning disabilities. Over a period of several weeks the researcher visits the home and videotapes conversations between the staff and the residents. What themes or patterns might be used to analyse the data collected?

6.3.2   **Identifying ethical issues**

No research can be completely value-free. This raises many important ethical questions such as:
- What preconceptions does the researcher bring?
- Who is being researched and how is the research to be explained?
- How might they be affected by the research?
- Who will benefit from the research?

Ethical issues are considered in detail in section 6.5.

6.3.3 **Developing methods**

The aim of this phase of the research process is to collect accurate, relevant data in a form that is easy to analyse. It includes:

- planning how to collect the data – by questionnaire, interview, observation or experiment
- identifying limitations on the study – for example, if the study uses observation there may be limits on certain areas of the building or at certain times
- developing or obtaining the 'instruments' for collecting data – questionnaires, interview questions, tally chart, experimental equipment
- collecting the data.

Methods of obtaining data

Many of the skills you use to find things out in everyday life are similar to the skills used in research. Suppose you are thinking about applying to a particular university and want to find out more about the town or city it is based in. In this situation, you might not be happy with just reading about it in a prospectus or guidebook. You might want to:

- talk to friends who had been there – maybe go out of your way to talk to someone who lives there
- go there yourself for a couple of days
- try finding accommodation in two or three different areas of the city, so you get a feel for the place.

Observation

Watching people in a particular situation and recording what they do can be a useful method of obtaining data for research. There are plenty of opportunities for doing this – for example, you might sit in a café in a railway station and watch how people behave. But you probably wouldn't learn much unless you knew exactly what you were watching for and had a systematic way of collecting the data.

There are four ways that a researcher can observe people systematically:

- by becoming a member of the group and hiding their role as a researcher – this can lead to ethical problems and isn't usually justified (see section 6.5 Ethical issues)
- by becoming a member of a group and telling the others about their role as a researcher – this avoids some ethical problems but it may mean that others don't act normally with the researcher; it may also lead to a conflict of roles
- by watching the participants from outside, but also spending a small amount of time with them
- by becoming a 'fly on the wall' and watching entirely from the outside, with no interaction at all.

UNIT

6

SECTION **6.3**

HEALTH CENTRE APPOINTMENTS

A local health centre on a crowded, inner-city estate has just changed its appointment system to try to avoid the problem of people having to wait a long time before they can see a doctor. Six doctors staff the centre. Five of the doctors have scheduled appointments on a rotational basis, and the other runs an open surgery to which anyone can come along and wait until there is an opportunity for them to be seen. They might have to wait longer than with the appointments system, but they will be seen on the same day.

Another change is to have specialist clinics on regular days so that people do not have to travel long distances to see specialists such as clinical psychologists or gynaecologists.

The health centre manager wants to find out what people think of the changes, and is developing a semi structured interview to use with a sample group of patients.

ACTIVITY

Try preparing a schedule for a semi-structured or unstructured interview. Select a topic. Think about your topic and write down things that you would like to know about it. If you want, do this with one or two other people so you get different ideas. Then sort the questions into three or four themes with a few questions under each theme.

A group leader at a youth centre explains why observation is central to her job:

❝ *Of course I'm always watching the people in my group. It's absolutely vital that I know what's going on between them and can sense the changes of mood. We're dealing with young people who come from difficult, sometimes violent backgrounds. They change moods very quickly. I'm involved with what they do – we agree the programme for each session together and I take part. But I'm also a bit detached. They know that and on the whole they respect my dual role.* ❞

Interviews

Interviews are good for collecting information that is sensitive or can't be predicted in advance. Although they take a lot of time, the information obtained can be of a very high quality. Interviews may also be the only way of getting information from groups such as visually impaired people or children who would not be able to fill in a questionnaire themselves.

An **interview** is a conversation between the researcher and a respondent. Interviews can be done face-to-face or by telephone.

Interviews can be:
- structured – everyone is asked the same questions in the same way
- semi-structured – the same basic questions are asked, but the interviewer can vary the order and 'probe' for more information
- unstructured –the interviewer just has a list of topics to cover and is free to discuss them in any way; it's like a guided conversation.

Questionnaires

A **questionnaire** is a written set of questions which people answer either on their own or with an interviewer to guide them.

Questionnaires are a relatively quick way of collecting a lot of data. But they need designing carefully. There are two types of question: 'open', where people are free to answer in any way they choose; and 'closed', where they select from a limited set of answers. Open questions are more difficult to analyse but often provide more information.

There are four different types of closed question:
- questions with only two answers, like 'yes' or 'no'
- questions with a range of answers, like 'excellent', 'good', 'poor', 'very poor'
- multiple-choice questions which ask people to look at statements and pick the one that best fits their own views
- questions asking people to give a score to several alternatives – these are good for finding out which issues people feel most strongly about.

ACTIVITY

Experiment with different types of question using the situation described in the case study above or another one of your own. First, make sure in your mind that you know what you are aiming to find out. Then start writing the questions. When you have written eight or ten, stop and:

- analyse what types of question they are
- try them out on someone else
- see if you need to change the type of question, e.g. from a question with only two answers to a multiple-choice question
- see if you need to change the wording of the questions to make them clearer.

DISCUSSION POINT

When are the four methods of obtaining data – experiment, questionnaire, interview, observation – used in health and social care research? Discuss some research you know about in various contexts, for example medical, nursing, health education, social work, youth work, community care. Which methods did they use? What made these methods appropriate for the context?

It may sometimes be better to ask indirect questions rather than direct ones. For example, instead of asking 'What do you think about the new open access arrangements at the surgery?' you could ask 'What do you think the general feeling is about the new open access arrangements at the surgery?' People are sometimes more comfortable expressing negative opinions if they can attribute them to others.

Experiments

An experiment is a controlled way of looking at what happens when one or more variables are changed.

A lot of experimental data comes from clinical practice and trials. Some data may come from measurements, like the data on blood pressure and other health indicators collected by the practice nurse in the case study on page 334. Clinical trials of drugs are experiments on a much bigger scale.

Obtaining measurements

Clinical measurements are vital for clinicians – doctors and some other healthcare professionals who work directly with patients – so that they can plan an appropriate treatment. A wide range of equipment is used for collecting data:
- basic equipment, such as thermometers, watches and weigh-scales, used in routine situations
- highly technological equipment, such as scanners and digital imaging techniques to measure blood flows in the brain, used for particular purposes.

The important thing is to choose the equipment most appropriate for the experiment. For example, a research project assessing the effect of changes in diet on body weight might only need an accurate and consistent set of bathroom scales. On the other hand, research which aimed to compare the toxic side-effects of different forms of treatment for breast cancer would need to record far more complex changes in patients' conditions, including their quality of life.

The research question, or hypothesis, determines the most appropriate method to use. In some cases, more than one method is appropriate. For example:
- the practice nurse assessing the effect of exercise on the health of patients with high blood pressure is using experimental methods and observation
- someone finding out about the psychological impact of an unfavourable diagnosis would need to use sensitively managed interviews.

AFTER SURGERY: COLLECTING THE DATA

Data on the experience of patients after being discharged from hospital was collected in a series of face-to-face interviews with six patients in their own homes, two to four days after being discharged.

Data was collected relating to two physical and three personal elements:
- physical elements – pain; movement; posture
- personal elements – communication and information; knowledge and understanding; the process of recovery.

6.3.4 Obtaining the data

If you have completed all the activities outlined so far, you should be almost ready to start collecting the data for your own research project. Before you start, there are four final things to do:

1 Prepare your research instruments.
2 Try them out.
3 Agree a timescale, including review points.
4 Agree a contingency strategy, including an escape route if things go badly.

Timescale and review points

Set a realistic timescale for collecting the data. Bear in mind that:

- people need time to complete and return a questionnaire – if you are sending them by post, allow at least three weeks before they are due to be returned and an extra week to do any chasing necessary
- it takes time to set up interviews – allow three to four weeks between contacting participants and interviewing them
- it also takes time to listen to recordings and write up notes – allow three or four times as long for this as for the interview itself.

Build in times to review progress. This is especially important if you are working in a group.

> ### ACTIVITY
>
> Prepare a timetable for doing the research. If you are working in a group, make sure that everyone can stick to it. Keep a copy of the timetable for yourself and check your own progress regularly.

Contingency strategy

What if the process of collecting data doesn't go to plan? Possible problems include:

- a low response rate to questionnaires
- people are not available for interview in the timescale
- the instruments don't seem to be producing the sort of data required
- too many participants withdraw.

> ### ACTIVITY
>
> Agree with the person supervising your research and your research colleagues (if you are working in a group) what you will do if things go wrong.

There are really only two options. You could start again with a new timetable, a different sample and a revised set of instruments. Or you could carry on, analyse the data that you do manage to obtain and review the problems in your report. A report that is open and honest about the problems and identifies flaws in the design is more useful than one that hides them: it may help other researchers in future to avoid the problems and redesign the research.

6.3.5 Analysing the data and producing results

Quantitative analysis

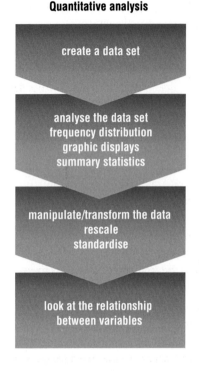

Qualitative analysis

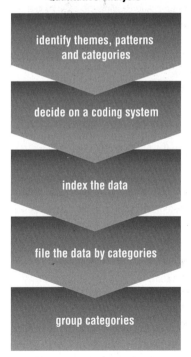

In this phase of the research process, data is analysed and interpreted, the results summarised and recommendations produced. It is likely to include:

- one or more data analysis procedures – statistical procedures for quantitative data and a systematic analysis of themes, patterns, behaviours for qualitative data
- interpretation – does the data support the hypothesis? does the data answer the research question?
- drawing conclusions – what are the conclusions and what do they mean?
- communicating the outcomes, usually in a written report
- forming recommendations – how does this research affect practice? what other questions still need to be asked?

Methods of analysing data

The activities in this section aim to help you try out these different types of analysis. You are shown how to draw valid conclusions and make recommendations for changes in policy and practice from research findings.

Research data takes the form of

- words – interview notes or tapes, notes of observations, comments on questionnaires
- numbers – ticks on a questionnaire, multiple-choice sheet or tally sheet, scores (e.g. 1 to 5), numerical records of observation, such as the number of people asking for a particular piece of information in a period of time.

Quantitative and qualitative analysis

Both primary and secondary data should be analysed. Quantitative methods should be used for numerical data, qualitative methods for other forms of data. The process of analysing the two types of data is summarised in the two flow charts on this page.

Quantitative data is numerical and is analysed using a statistical method. It is usual to analyse using a computer which can do this quickly and accurately. Software packages are available for this purpose. There are two types of statistics:

- descriptive
- inferential, which interpret the data in relation to the hypothesis.

Spreadsheets can also be used to analyse data. Small amounts of numerical data can be analysed by hand, using tally charts and calculators. Data is normally arranged into rows and columns, as in a table of results from an experiment:

- rows correspond to records – such as all the data obtained from one respondent
- columns contain the data for a single variable.

Quantitative analysis often looks at the relationship between variables. For example, the link between smoking and lung cancer is shown quantitatively by the fact that the distribution of scores on one variable (smoker, as opposed to non-smoker) links to the distribution of scores on another variable (lung cancer, no lung cancer). The strength of relationships between variables can be measured using a figure, known as the 'correlation coefficient'.

Once the data has been analysed in this way, it forms a data set. The data set can then be analysed further. Examples of further analysis include:

- frequency distribution – the number of times certain things happen, e.g. the number of respondents who answered Yes to a Yes/No question
- graphical displays – histograms, bar charts, pie charts
- summary statistics – such as the level and spread of distribution (range, inter-quartile range, variance, standard deviation); these can also be shown on graphs and scatter diagrams.

Data can also be manipulated or transformed in various ways. For example, it can be:

- re-scaled, by multiplying by a constant – for example, when imperial weights (lb and oz) are converted into metric equivalents (kg and g)
- standardised – to gain a standardised score from a set of individual scores.

Describing quantitative data

The results of a quantitative survey or experiment are usually in the form of a mass of numbers. To understand what the numbers mean, you have to sort them out. One way of doing this is to work out an average. The three types of average (mean, median and mode) are described in the box below.

The **mean** is the most common type of average. You get it by adding up all the results and dividing the total by the number of results. For example, if three nurses spent 3 minutes, 4.5 minutes and 6 minutes at their work station in one hour, you get the mean by adding up the time (3 + 4.5 + 6 = 13.5) and dividing it by the number of nurses (13.5 ÷ 3 = 4.5 minutes). The mean can give a misleading impression if it is distorted by one or two untypical results – for example, if one of the nurses spent three-quarters of an hour at the work station.

The **median** is the middle value in a set of numbers. You get it by arranging all the results in order and choosing the middle one. It is useful when there are one or two extreme results. If one nurse spent three-quarters of an hour at the work station and the other two spent 3 and 4.5 minutes, the median would be 4.5 (the middle of the three numbers). What would the mean be in this case?

The **mode** is the result that occurs most frequently. If someone asks a nurse how long she usually spends at her work station in an hour, she might say:

66 *If I'm busy with patients, which I usually am, I spend about 5 minutes. If we are short-staffed or under pressure, I might not go there at all, whereas if I'm on nights I can sometimes spend 30 or 40 minutes there catching up. But most of the time, I'd say it's about 5 minutes.* 99

Here, the nurse is giving the mode.

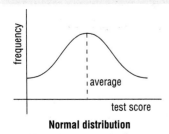

Normal distribution

To describe data, you have to know whether your results fall into a pattern. This is sometimes called the 'distribution' of results. For example, if a health visitor measured the weight of 100 babies of the same age and drew a graph to show the results, it would probably look like the graph below. It is called a graph of 'normal distribution', because data normally falls into this pattern.

Many characteristics of human beings, such as height, birth weight, resting pulse, weight and intelligence, follow a normal distribution curve like this. A midwife in a maternity hospital says:

66 *We measure the weight of all babies when they are born. That means we can calculate the average birth weight of male and female babies in a year. We can also compare this average to the averages in previous years, or the averages in other parts of the country, and see how our average fits in with wider trends in childbirth.* 99

When measuring health indicators, it is often important to know the variability of the results – how much they vary from the mean score. Two measures are useful:

■ the difference between the highest and lowest score – this is called the 'range'

■ how much, on average, the results vary from the mean score – this is known as the 'standard deviation'.

ACTIVITY

A childcare worker has been monitoring the weight of a girl who was born with a digestive disorder. She plots the results on a graph (shown below) which shows the standard weight (the mean) and two deviations from the mean. The standard weight is shown on the graph as 50%. Any weight above or below the first standard deviation, shown as 10% and 90% on the graph, indicates that there might be cause for concern.

Here are the figures she has collected. Plot them on the graph and look at the deviation from the normal range. What conclusion can you draw from the curve?

age	weight (kg)
5	16.3
6	18.1
7	19.5
8	20.9
9	24.9
10	27.2
11	30.8
12	36.3
13	43.5
14	47.2
15	49.9
16	50.8
17	51.7
18	51.7

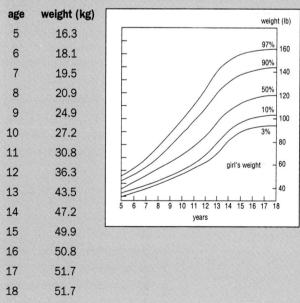

Often, the purpose of a quantitative study is to establish whether there is a relationship between two values, such as a woman's age when she has her first baby and her length of stay in hospital after the birth. The relationship between two values can be expressed as a correlation coefficient.

Interpreting quantitative data

The aim of quantitative research is to establish whether the data supports or fails to support a research hypothesis. This is done by creating a null hypothesis and testing the data against it. In the case study on page 334 (primary care: the value of exercise), the null hypothesis is that a planned exercise programme makes no difference to the blood pressure of men and women between the ages of 50 and 60 who are known to have high blood pressure. If the data supports the null hypothesis, then the research hypothesis is not supported.

The tests that are used fall into two groups:
- comparing results with the normal distribution of the population (as the health visitor did in the activity above)
- carrying out tests to find out the 'statistical significance' of the data.

Statistical significance

Results from epidemiological studies and other studies, which produce large data sets, need to be assessed to see if they contain any statistically significant data. For example, the normal incidence of a particular condition in newborn babies, for mothers between certain ages, might be 1 in 2,000. If the figure is 3 in 2,000 in one area of the country, there is a difference. But it may not be significant either clinically or statistically. To assess whether it is statistically significant, other tests need to be carried out such as the t-test or the chi-square test.

Qualitative data analysis

Researchers collecting qualitative data decide how they are going to analyse the data while the study is still being planned. Verbal data is less straightforward to analyse and make sense of than numerical data. There are two main approaches, which both involve categorising the data in some way:
- looking for themes and patterns
- using codes to record what you see and hear.

Qualitative data usually consists of words: transcripts or notes of interviews with other people, written comments on questionnaires, the researcher's own field notes. It may also include images, such as video recordings and visual records of observation (sketches, diagrams). These can all be very rich – and quite hard to analyse systematically. At the planning stage, researchers normally identify themes, patterns or other categories they are looking for.

Analysing qualitative data means taking something complete – interview notes or a completed questionnaire – and cutting it to bits to identify and categorise recurring themes. It is, sometimes literally, a scissors and paste job. The important things to remember are:

- What are you analysing the data for?
- What categories are you looking out for?
- Where do you put the data you 'cut out' of the complete thing?

Three tips for analysing qualitative data

1 Start analysing as soon as you collect data – don't leave all the analysis to the end. This is because you may see more categories, or groupings of categories, once you start, which could make the process easier from then on.

2 Index the data as you go along – for example, if you are analysing interview notes or written comments on a questionnaire, you could use different coloured highlighter pens to index different categories. File the data by categories. It's much easier to do this if the data is on computer, as you can use the cut and paste functions.

3 Remember that there isn't a single right way of doing the analysis. Follow your own rules, e.g. for categorising data. But don't let that stop you thinking of new, perhaps better ways of categorising it. Keep thinking about what the data is saying to you.

In the planning stage, researchers decide what methods they will use to analyse the data collected. The main analytical techniques for both quantitative and qualitative data are described on page 344.

Data sets

The table below shows the data obtained from four respondents who completed a questionnaire. The first three questions asked them to give a score from 1 to 5. The fourth question required a simple Yes/No answer. The fifth question asked respondents to specify a range from an option of six ranges, coded A to F.

Respondent	Q1 score	Q2 score	Q3 score	Q4	Q5
A	3	4	3	Y	E
B	1	0	2	Y	B
C	2	5	3	n	D
D	4	4	1	Y	C

DISCUSSION POINT

What is the use of being able to analyse data in these ways? See if you can think of examples from health and social care where each of the quantitative methods described above has been used.

COMPARING SHIFTS: DATA ANALYSIS

A clinical nurse manager at a hospital trust carried out a comparative study of staff working twelve-hour and eight-hour shifts to evaluate the effect of the two shift systems on staff and the quality of care. Data was collected through:

■ questionnaires sent to 100 staff on four wards (two working each shift system)

■ semi-structured interviews with 20 staff.

Data from the questionnaires was used to create a data set that compared variables between the twelve-hour and eight-hour wards. An example of a variable was the level of sickness reported in the two types of ward in two different eight-week periods. The figures are expressed in whole-time equivalents.

	12-hour shifts		8-hour shifts	
Ward	A	B	C	D
Period 1	12.89	2.67	6.47	12.22
Period 2	5.36	8.92	11.83	5.5

The semi-structured interviews also generated numerical data in relation to how staff felt about working eight-hour and twelve-hour shifts. Some staff had worked both shifts.

	12-hour shifts	8-hour shifts
Number of staff interviewed	10	10
Tiredness reported working 8-hour shift	8	10
Tiredness reported working 12-hour shift	2	–
Enough time for handover	6	10
Communication between staff could be better	6	8

DISCUSSION POINT

The person who carried out the research described in the case study called it a 'descriptive study'. This explains why she did not analyse the data set using any of the quantitative methods listed in the flow chart. If she had called the study analytical rather than descriptive, what sort of analysis of the figures would you expect to see?

ACTIVITY

What sort of qualitative data will your research produce? Describe the data you expect to get. Then describe:

■ the categories you intend to use for sorting the data (remember these may change once you start the analysis)

■ the method you will use to index the data by categories

■ how you intend to file the data – if you are doing this on a computer, specify the package you will use.

If you are not confident about your ability to analyse written and visual data in the ways described above, now is a good time to practise.

AFTER SURGERY: ANALYSIS AND CONCLUSIONS

The researcher analysed her interviews with patients in relation to the five categories she had determined at the start of the research process. She then grouped the specific experiences of each patient into further categories.

For example, data in the category 'process of recovery' could be analysed into four types:

- patients talked about actions over which they themselves had control
- they also mentioned activities that measured progress to recovery, such as being able to have a bath
- all the patients mentioned disruptions in family life
- they all said they had resumed normal activities too soon.

After completing this detailed level of analysis, the researcher was in a good position to form conclusions and make recommendations for practice. She formed three main conclusions:

- patients need to be provided with better methods of controlling pain
- communication over what to do after being discharged needs to be improved
- personal control over the process is a crucial factor in satisfactory recovery.

Her recommendations were clear:

- doctors should prescribe adequate analgesia and inform patients how to pre-empt pain
- health professionals should have pre-discharge discussions with patients and their families to inform them more clearly about what to expect once they are at home
- further research should investigate how patients can resist pressures to resume tasks in the home and at work until they are sufficiently recovered.

ACTIVITY

Gather together all the data you have collected in your research and make a full list. Group the data into two types:

- numerical data
- data in other forms (words, images).

Which methods of analysis will you use to analyse the data? Attach a note to each type of data. The note should:

- describe which method(s) of analysis you intend to use
- explain why you chose these methods.

Now use the methods you have chosen to analyse the data. Gather the results of your analysis in a folder. Keep all your working papers in a separate folder.

6.3.6 Using results to suggest recommendations

When they have finished analysing data, researchers should be ready to:
- summarise the results
- provide an interpretation of what the results mean
- draw conclusions from the study
- make recommendations based on these conclusions.

This process is the same, whatever the research aimed to do and whatever its conclusions are.

To be valid, conclusions should be:
- consistent with the data
- based on evidence collected during the research
- closely related to the research question
- relevant to the purpose of the research
- within confidence limits.

Valid conclusions

A research supervisor advises how to draw valid conclusions:

All conclusions should derive from the data you have collected, whether they are from primary or secondary sources or a combination of both. You have to be able to justify everything you say on the basis of your analysis and interpretation of the data. That's the first thing. The second is to draw conclusions that relate to your research question and the purpose of the research. Any conclusions that don't do that are irrelevant. Lastly, you have to state the limits of confidence: how reliable and valid are the outcomes of your research?

Conclusions from quantitative analysis

A summary of results from quantitative analysis should start with a general outline of the findings. Where possible, this should be illustrated with:
- tables of results
- statistics derived from the tables, such as averages or standard deviations (see page 346) – these can be in graphical form.

Further quantitative analysis can be used to interpret the data in more detail. If the analysis shows a correlation between the variables in a hypothesis, this may indicate a link. If there are doubts about this – for example, because of other factors – the recommendations can suggest further work that could be done to investigate the relationship between variables.

Conclusions from qualitative analysis

When reporting a qualitative study, the aim is to capture and convey a sense of the particular reality the research was looking at. Conclusions should 'stay close to the data'. In particular, it is important not to draw conclusions that are not supported by the study. It's often not easy to generalise qualitative research to other situations, so avoid the temptation of suggesting that the findings have wider implications than in fact they have.

A qualitative study may not produce definite recommendations. It may be more likely to produce:
- insights which other people may find helpful in their practice
- a theory which could be developed further
- better understanding of how an existing theory applies in a particular context
- a hypothesis which could be tested out in further research.

351

One way to guard against over-interpreting the results is to discuss them with friends and colleagues. Different people may give different explanations based on analysis of the same data.

COMPARING SHIFTS: CONCLUSIONS

After analysing all the data from her questionnaires and interviews, the clinical nurse manager concluded that staff on twelve-hour shifts:

- spend more time on patient care than staff on eight-hour shifts
- make better use of their free time during the shifts
- provide better continuity of care for patients
- get less tired than their colleagues on eight-hour shifts.

On the negative side, she concluded that staff on the longer shifts:

- need more time for hand-over between shifts
- want better communication among themselves.

The researcher then cross-checked her conclusions with findings from other studies. She noted some important differences – for example, previous research had found that twelve-hour shifts reduced rather than increased direct patient care. She explained these differences by the attitude of staff to change: a positive attitude resulted in positive changes and vice versa.

ACTIVITY

Look carefully at the results of your analysis. If you are working in a group, discuss the results with others. What conclusions do they suggest? How do the conclusions relate to your research question? How confident do you feel about them?

Write down your conclusions. Make sure they can all be backed up by the evidence. Add a note explaining any factors that limit the confidence of your results.

Recommendations are the actions that can be taken arising from the outcomes of research.

Confidence limits

How confident can researchers be that their conclusions are valid? It's only possible to be really confident if the results confirm several previous research studies and none of the data points in any other direction. The conclusion that most people benefit from regular, moderate intensity exercise is an example.

Confidence can be reduced by:

- sample size and selection – is the sample big enough to support the conclusions? Is it representative of the population being studied?
- research question or hypothesis – is the question exact and clear? Does the hypothesis make sense?
- methods of collecting and analysing data – are they appropriate? Have they been carried out consistently?
- bias and error – what bias is there in the interpretation? How has the researcher tried to avoid errors in observation?

Recommendations

All recommendations should be:

- derived from the research
- practical.

If the purpose of the research is to inform policy or practice, recommendations can be in the form of actions justified in relation to the outcomes. For example, one of the outcomes of the research into the differences between

What recommendations can be made, based on the outcomes of your research? Do they recommend:

■ changes to policy or practice?

■ further research?

Think carefully about the recommendations you can make. If you are working in a group, discuss them with others. Try writing them down, using the formal language of the recommendations quoted above. You may need several goes before you are sure that the recommendations:

■ arise from the research outcomes

■ are practical.

eight-hour and twelve-hour shifts (see page 349) was that the benefits of the twelve-hour shift are greater if the transition from one type of shift to the other is undertaken by staff themselves. The recommendation could be:

66 *Any decision to change from an 8-hour to a 12-hour shift should be taken on the basis of full consultation with staff and the process of transition should involve staff at all stages.* 99

If the purpose is to test a hypothesis or contribute to knowledge, recommendations often say what further research could be done to:

■ check the results – for example, with a different sample or using other methods

■ extend knowledge and understanding of the subject by building on the outcomes.

One recommendation from the study of patients with ovarian cancer was:

66 *A more detailed investigation is needed into the effects of diagnosis on younger patients, looking at their anxieties about fertility and ageing and focusing on how they deal with problems to do with their sexuality.* 99

DISCUSSION POINT

Which of the two recommendations quoted here can be generalised?

Key questions

1 What are the six aspects of the research process?

2 Why is the hypothesis important for the research?

3 Which methods are appropriate for which situations? (Give two examples showing when each method would be appropriate.)

4 What are the four types of question that can be used in a questionnaire?

5 How would you check that the questions to be asked in a questionnaire or in an interview will give you reliable data?

6 When should statistical methods for analysing data be used?

7 What is the main difference between descriptive and inferential statistics?

8 Define the mean, median and mode.

9 Explain when the mean, median and mode should each be most appropriately used.

10 Describe the stages involved in qualitative data analysis.

11 How can researchers ensure their conclusions are valid?

12 What different types of recommendations do health and social care researchers make?

SECTION **6.4**

Presenting research

Presenting research findings clearly is crucial to their successful communication and implementation in practice. This section explores the presentation of findings in oral and written formats. Presenting research in both of these formats requires that all the relevant information about the process, as well as the outcomes of any research, is included along with recommendations for further research.

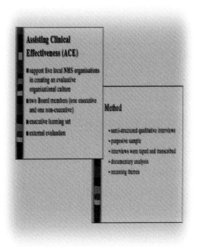

> 66 I was involved in a highly practical research project which looked at particular categories of equipment for people with disabilities, including toilet and bathing aids for children. The rationale was rather like that of a consumer report: to gather the views of respondents and practitioners on the equipment and evaluate it. The resulting data helps practitioners provide an effective service. For those in isolated communities it is an essential reference. 99
>
> *occupational therapy services manager*

> 66 If we know about how child abuse happens, we should be able to formulate procedures on how to avoid it. So I hope the conclusions and recommendations from my research will be of use to other professionals in working more effectively with clients. 99
>
> *child protection adviser*

> 66 Research is vital within psychological services. There is very little research-based evidence available. It is difficult to check outcomes – how do you measure quality of life? Effective psychological services could save the health service money on other care. What we are aiming to show as a result of our research is that access to counselling does work. 99
>
> *head of medical counselling and family support*

> 66 It's essential to read the results of research in places like the Pharmaceutical Journal. 99
>
> *pharmacist*

6.4.1 Producing a written research report

Research reports are special pieces of writing. They are easier to write if you follow guidelines for:

- structure
- writing style
- graphs and tables
- the writing process.

Structure

Most reports follow a structure like the one shown in the table below. Long reports may be divided into sections, with a contents list at the start. Shorter reports may not have separate sections, but they often use headings to show where a new part of the report starts.

Part of report	What's in it
Title	says what kind of study it is, what topic is being studied and the population
Contents	lists the key sections and headings with their page numbers
Summary (abstract)	a brief summary of the aims, methods, results and conclusions
Introduction	explains why the study was done
Literature review	reviews the existing literature on the topic
Objectives	identifies the purpose of the research
Methods	describes methods of collecting and analysing data, giving details of research instruments, sample size, place and dates when data was collected
Results/findings	summarises the analysis of data, using tables, charts and graphs where appropriate
Discussion	presents the interpretation of data and discusses limitations
Conclusion	summarises conclusions and discusses the implications for practice and/or theory
Recommendations	presents suggestions for actions and/or further research
References/bibliography	lists the books and articles consulted for the research
Appendices	includes research instruments and any relevant data such as selection of data

Writing style

Keep the writing simple and direct. Try to express the meaning as clearly and concisely as possible. Don't use colloquial or emotive language, but don't be too formal either. Use technical terms where they are needed, but don't use jargon.

Quantitative studies usually avoid the first person singular or plural ('I' or 'we'). In qualitative research, where the actions and reactions of the researcher are often central to the study, first person sentences are used more often.

When you refer to studies in the text of your report, include the surname of the author(s) and the date of the book or article in brackets, like this:

> 66 *Critics argue that there has been a serious decline in local accountability of NHS organisations (Hunter, 1992).* 99

> 66 *A Carers National Association survey in 1996 identified that very few people think about the possibility of becoming a carer in advance of the event.* 99

List all the references at the end of the report, before the appendices, like this:

- Hunter, D. (1992) Accountability and the NHS. In: Smith, R. (ed.) *The Future of Health Care*. London: BMJ Publishing
- CNA (1996) Who cares? *Perceptions of caring and carers*. London, CNA

DISCUSSION POINT

Have a look at three or four research reports from a range of journals. Concentrate on the writing style. Which of the points mentioned above can you spot in the writing?

Graphs and tables

Use computer software wherever possible to produce graphs and tables. Many wordprocessing and spreadsheet packages include this facility. Keep them simple and straightforward. It's easy to produce 3-D effects or multicoloured pie charts, but they are not always useful and can be confusing. Readers are interested in what the data shows, not in fancy ways of presenting it. Take care not to mislead readers, for example by using different types of scale on two graphs you want them to compare. All graphs, tables and diagrams should be numbered and given a title.

The writing process

Writing is easier if you do it in stages.

Start by doing a plan of what you are going to write about. You already have an overall structure of the report (see page 355). Think about the points you want to cover in each section.

Write a first draft. Don't worry if it's rough and ready. It is much better to get something down on paper, even if it's not exactly what you want to say. Write the whole of your report in draft before you go to the next stage. There is no need to write it in order – some bits that go near the beginning, like the introduction and abstract, are often best written last. Some people start by writing about the methods because they feel confident about describing them. When you have finished the first draft, check it over to see if you have missed out anything important and whether your argument makes sense. Don't worry about spelling or grammar yet.

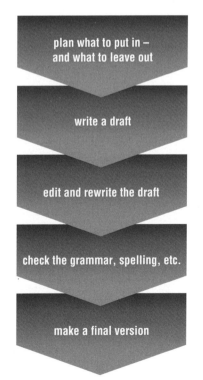

plan what to put in – and what to leave out

write a draft

edit and rewrite the draft

check the grammar, spelling, etc.

make a final version

Now edit the draft. Read the whole draft over with a pen in yo
write notes to yourself about what to do. For example, you migh.
move bits around or make a point more clearly. Then do any rewi
needed. All this is much easier if the draft is on a wordprocessor.

Check the draft for grammar, style, punctuation and spelling. Don't just
putting it through a spell-check, if you are using a wordprocessor, because
mistakes such as the misuse of 'their' and 'there' will not be picked up. Then
check that you have listed all the references, numbered the tables and given
them all a title.

A researcher who has just finished writing her report gives some last-minute
advice:

66 *If you can, leave a day or so between finishing the report and the date you
have scheduled for making a final version. Before you produce the final version,
reread it all. You may find last-minute improvements you can make.* 99

ACTIVITY

Go through the stages listed above to produce a report of your research.
When you have edited the draft, but before making the final version, go
through the checklist below. It lists the things your report should describe.
Tick off each item if you are sure your report contains it. If there isn't a tick,
something is missing and you need to add it.

Make sure your report covers everything on this list.

Report checklist

Research process ☐

Methods you used to obtain the data ☐

Methods you used to analyse the data ☐

Any ethical issues raised by the research ☐

How you handled ethical issues ☐

Impact of the research process on participants ☐

Limitations of the research ☐

Extent to which your conclusions can be generalised ☐

Implications for practice ☐

Recommendations ☐

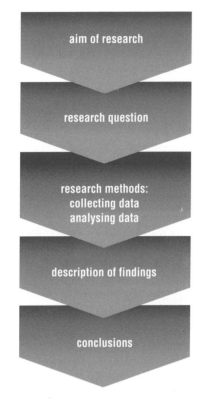

aim of research

research question

research methods:
collecting data
analysing data

description of findings

conclusions

Sometimes researchers are asked to present the results of their research to others at a meeting or conference. The aim of a presentation is to:

- state the conclusions and show how they relate to the data gathered in the research
- summarise the content of the report and its main messages
- communicate in a style and at a level appropriate to the audience.

The order of a presentation is similar to that of a report, as the diagram shows.

Planning

Presentations always go better if prepared in advance. A university research student who studied the psychosocial impact of ovarian cancer diagnosis explains:

66 *I had worked closely with a consultant oncologist during this research. I gave him a copy of my paper and a few days later he rang and asked me if I would present the results at a study day at the hospital. We talked it over and agreed that he would introduce the study and I would present the outcomes. I produced three overhead projector slides that introduced the presentation and summarised the method and findings of my research. I also wrote a page of clear notes – just the headings of what I wanted to say so I would get them in the right order. I was a bit nervous when I saw the number of people attending but the actual presentation went fine. People were interested and asked quite a few questions.* 99

Preparing for a presentation (1)

Make clear, short notes to help you:

- describe the methods used for collecting and analysing data
- explain why these methods were chosen – especially the choice of quantitative and/or qualitative methods
- state the conclusions clearly
- show how the conclusions are justified by the data
- explain the limitations of your research.

Style and level

A presentation is a formal event and should follow a clear structure. The style of communication should also be formal, but not too distant – it's not a lecture. The aim is to present the findings as clearly a possible, not to convince the audience. If the audience knows about the area of study, technical terms can be used. They should be explained briefly the first time they are used. If the audience is not well informed, technical terms should be avoided.

This is a transcript of a short extract from the research student's presentation on the effects of a diagnosis of ovarian cancer:

66 *The effects of the diagnosis on sexual functioning seem to be unrelated to the stage of the disease, the age of the patient or the treatment phase. Of the seven patients I studied, one was sexually inactive before diagnosis, one was more active after the diagnosis, three were less active and two told me there was no change in their sexual activity. The patient who reported increased activity and registered highest on the SAQ [sexual activity questionnaire] was 44 years old, at stage 3 and in treatment. The patient who had the lowest SAQ was aged 26, at stage 1c and in remission.* 99

When the formal presentation is over, people normally want to ask questions. Answers may need to go into more detail than was possible in the presentation – for example, people might want you to describe the sample more fully or justify an aspect of your conclusions.

Content and messages

When a research report or an article based on research is published, readers can look at it several times. They have a chance to focus on the bits that interest or worry them. In a presentation, they – and you – only have one chance, and there isn't usually a lot of time. So:

■ restrict what the presentation contains – its content – to the essentials

■ get the messages across clearly and concisely.

One of the biggest dangers in a presentation is trying to say too much. Speaking always takes a lot longer than reading. As a rule of thumb, it takes a minute to speak aloud 150 words, at moderate speed. So a ten-minute presentation should not be longer than 1,500 words. If time is added in for showing overhead projector (OHP) slides or other images, the number of words goes down to 1,000 or less – between two and three pages of typescript.

OHP slides give the audience something to look at apart from the presenter and help to fix the main points in their minds. They also remind the presenter what to say. Sometimes OHP slides are photocopied and given out either before or just after a presentation. In a ten-minute presentation, the number of slides should be restricted to four or five. Each one should only contain three to five points and a maximum of 20 words. They can be designed on a wordprocessor or presentation package.

Relate conclusions to the data

The conclusions are one of the most interesting parts of a research report for anyone who knows the area of study. They will want to see whether the research has revealed anything new or different from earlier research. They will look closely at how the data was obtained and analysed, to check that:

- the methods used are reliable and valid, and demonstrate good practice
- the data justifies the conclusions.

A well-informed audience is likely to ask questions about these things in a presentation. You can't predict their questions, but you can be well prepared by being confident about the purpose of the research, how it was done and the conclusions.

6.4.3 Critical review

A researcher's work doesn't end when the research report is made available to others or after the presentation. An important part of the research process is critical review by a peer group, including other researchers and practitioners with first-hand knowledge of the area of study. Most specialist journals and some professional journals require research reports to be 'refereed' by others in the research community before accepting them for publication. In any case, once a report is in the public domain, researchers can expect feedback. Even critical feedback should be seen as a constructive contribution to the subject.

Key questions

1 What are the similarities and differences between presenting research orally and in writing?

2 What main sections should a research report contain?

3 What type of writing style is commonly used in qualitative research reports?

4 What is peer review in the context of research reports?

66 *Conflict may arise if the researcher is also a care provider. The Royal College of Nursing addresses this by suggesting that the nurse researcher should be aware of the problem, and plan how potential conflicts can be resolved. In reality it may be difficult to decide at what point the care imperative is being compromised by the research imperative. The researcher aims to generate knowledge to benefit future patients; the carer aims to benefit current patients.* 99

nurse researcher

66 *When applying for a research grant, the funding body likes to know that an application has been submitted for ethical clearance. Funds will not usually be released until the funding body is satisfied that your research has been cleared by the local research ethics committee.* 99

research student

66 *Following the trials between 1946 and 1947 of 20 doctors who conducted extreme human experiments in the concentration camps of the Third Reich, the Nuremburg Ethical Code was formulated. The experiments carried out by these doctors often had fatal consequences and usually involved non-consenting inmates. Participants were exposed to extremes of temperature, given poisons and deliberately injected with bacteria.* 99

historian

66 *The 'Look after your heart' campaign recommends the reduction of saturated fat in the diet. Yet the evidence is far from clear that those with normal levels would reduce their risk of heart disease by reducing their fat consumption. The health professions are guilty of misusing scientific evidence and selectively interpreting data. Although this debate is widely aired in the professional journals, the general public doesn't have access to the debate or necessarily the experience and knowledge to make a decision for themselves as a single message is promoted.* 99

dietician

Ethical issues

It is almost impossible to conduct completely value-free research in health and social care. This section explores the ethical issues that can arise from conducting research and in using the results, including: the possible benefits and negative outcomes of involvement for participants, the need to preserve individual rights and maintain confidentiality, and the importance of avoiding bias.

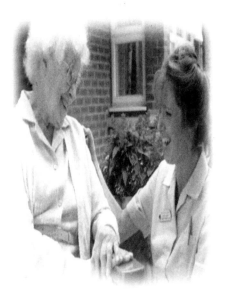

Ethics is a branch of philosophy that considers how people should behave in order to be moral. Ethics is an important practical consideration in health and social care and can't just be left to the philosophers.

All research affects somebody, somehow, even if it is only the person doing the research. When other people are involved, they must:

- know what is going on – the objectives of the research, what they will be doing, how the outcomes will be used
- agree to take part and know that they have the right to withdraw
- be given the chance to comment on the outcomes.

To some extent, ethical considerations apply to all research. They are especially important when the research involves experiments with or observations of other people. An ethical approach should be built in to health and social care research projects at all stages. Ethical considerations should inform the research question and the methods chosen. For example, it would not be ethical for a researcher who knows very little about family relations in Asian communities to carry out comparative research into the influence of family and peer-group pressure on the health or lifestyle choices of teenage Asian girls.

Information obtained from research, which is unethical in any way, is not normally seen as useful or reliable. At the planning stage, researchers should plan how to:

- tell participants about the potential benefits of the research and make sure they have access to these benefits
- anticipate negative effects of the research on participants and take steps to avoid and/or reduce them
- keep information confidential
- tell participants about their rights
- avoid cultural bias.

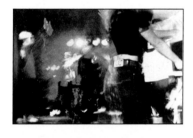

DISCUSSION POINT

In what ways is the student's proposed research study unethical? How might it have damaged the individuals who participated without even knowing? How could similar findings have been obtained in an ethical way?

A research student wants to find out more about how people behave at raves and similar events. She is particularly interested in what drugs people take, why they take them and where they get them from. She would like to establish whether there is a link between patterns of drug use and various social and lifestyle factors, including employment status, educational background and amount of available income.

She plans the research in two phases. In the first phase, she plans to go to a number of raves and get to know five or six people who take drugs. Her aim is to become known to them and accepted as one of the group. She does not intend to reveal her role as a researcher at this point. In the second phase, she plans to visit each of the five or six people individually and ask them a series of questions about drug use and social/lifestyle factors. At this point she will tell them about her research.

Then she goes to discuss the proposed study with her supervisor.

Many professions working with people have ethical standards or codes (see the box below). If researchers in a health-related area of study intend to use patients or clients as research subjects, they may need permission from the ethics committee of the Trust or health authority. In social care organisations there is no formal equivalent to an ethical committee but those undertaking research would need to have the agreement of managers and supervisors. Ethical principles for conducting research with human participants apply to school and college students as well as members of professional bodies.

The British Psychological Society has published a set of ethical principles. They require researchers to:

- get the informed consent of all participants (or their parent or guardian if they are under 16 or have impairments that limit communication)
- not withhold information except where absolutely necessary for the research
- discuss with participants the purpose of the research and their experience of taking part
- make sure that they know of their right to withdraw
- state that information will be treated confidentially
- protect participants from physical or mental harm during the investigation
- respect the privacy and psychological wellbeing of the individuals studied
- be cautious about giving advice.

A student who carried out research in an old people's home into an aspect of care says:

66 *I wasn't sure at first if I should be asking questions of people who are so much older than me. I thought I might come across as intrusive or ignorant. The manager at the home suggested I should ask the residents themselves. So I made a short list of headings that I wanted the interviews to cover and talked to three of the residents about them. One said she wouldn't mind being asked about all those things but two people objected to one of the headings, so I took it out. Then I wrote out the questions I wanted to ask in the interviews and tried them out on the same three people to make sure they weren't upset by anything I asked.* 99

DISCUSSION POINT

Which ethical principles was this student observing?

6.5.2 **Ethics and culture**

Two tips for avoiding culture shock

Choose participants from groups that you know first-hand, in terms of age, sex, social background and ethnic background.

Be aware of any bias or prejudice in yourself and guard against it. Remember that bias is often unconscious, so:

- keep your eyes open for it
- look for signals in others, like being offended or shutting down
- check it out with participants – ask them openly if anything you do or say is causing offence.

People from different cultures have different values. One of the core values of anyone working in health and social care is to respect the values of others. In research, this means:

- identifying any cultural issues in the sample – for example, does the research involve people from different ethnic backgrounds, or does it touch on sensitive issues of belief?
- ensuring that the research question will not be offensive
- checking that the research methods chosen are free from bias.

The ethical principles developed by the British Psychological Society referred to earlier go on to say that: '*in our multicultural and multi-ethnic society . . . the investigators may not have sufficient knowledge of the implications of any investigation for the participants*'. This is also true if a study involves people of different ages, sex or social background from the researcher.

For ethical reasons, it's important to anticipate the effects of the proposed research – on individual participants and on all the people who will benefit – at the earliest stage. It is no use having a brilliant idea about what to study if the only way of getting the results is by breaking ethical principles or codes.

6.5.3 **Ethics and the effects of research**

DISCUSSION POINT

Suppose researchers knew they could make enormous advances in the treatment of AIDS by forcing a small number of patients to become subjects in medical experiments. Many of them would suffer and some might die earlier than otherwise, but the end result could benefit thousands. Would the overall benefit outweigh the individual suffering of a few?

Research has risks and benefits. The main benefit is the knowledge gained from the research, which might help both the participants and everyone else in a similar situation. The risks include any physical or psychological harm to the participants that might result from taking part in the research.

The student researching care in an older people's home said after her first afternoon of interviews:

66 *Many of the old people I interviewed had great difficulty in seeing the point of my questions. They just seemed to accept everything the staff did for them. Two of them seemed to be quite upset that they were being asked about something they took for granted – I think they were frightened that things were going to change. I felt very unsure of myself again and wondered if the research was likely to do more harm than good.* 99

DISCUSSION POINT

What should this student do next? There are several possibilities, so note them down and spend a few moments weighing up the pros and cons of each one.

Benefits

Research aims to benefit the person doing the research and other people as well. To behave ethically, researchers should make sure that participants know how they may benefit from the research. Perhaps they could have access to the outcomes of the research, for example any new and effective clinical procedures that emerge.

> 66 *People who get involved in research as subjects or participants usually do so because they can see it will benefit them as well as others. For example, a radiographer may agree to spend half an hour a day for a period of two weeks completing a record form because she sees that the outcomes of the research might help to improve an aspect of the administrative system. It's a little more tricky with patients. They don't have any sort of obligation to cooperate with researchers. On the whole, if they can see the benefits of the research, they are willing to consider helping. If they are in for treatment we always make sure that the consultant knows what is going on and has agreed.* 99

nurse manager

Risks

People who take part in research might feel negative effects. In health and social care research, the main risks are to:

■ their psychological wellbeing – for example, if research is intrusive or insensitive

■ their health – the clear rule here is that participants should not be exposed to any risks greater than they face in their normal lifestyles or treatment plans

■ their values – the risk of causing offence is greater if researchers come from a different culture, gender or social background from the participants

■ their dignity – for example, if people who have conditions which make them feel uncomfortable, there is a danger that the research process will make them feel worse.

Reducing the risks

How do researchers handle negative effects of the research process? The best way is to avoid them in the first place. A good research design, which follows ethical principles, will reduce the risk of negative effects. Interviews are the most risky from this point of view, because of the close contact between two people and the exploratory nature of the conversation. Two ways of reducing the risk are:

■ being sensitive to how the person being interviewed is feeling – this helps to steer the conversation away from difficult issues

■ regular, frequent debriefing – this helps to identify any issues which may cause a problem if they are explored further.

If the negative effects are too strong, there are two options:

■ participants can withdraw from the research

■ the researcher should reconsider the design.

365

STRESS SUPPORT

This is how the counsellor who carried out an evaluation of the effect of support groups on staff stress levels summarised the positive and negative effects of his research on the participants.

	Process	Outcomes
Positive	1 Made group members think about what they were getting from the groups 2 Encouraged some members to attend meetings more regularly	1 Justified the existence of the groups and helped to maintain funding 2 Provided ideas for improving how the groups work
Negative	1 Emphasised the negative feelings some members had about the group 2 Took a long time to complete the questionnaire	None – yet!

ACTIVITY

What possible effects are there on the participants in your research? Make a table like the one in the case study above to show the possible positive and negative effects of:

- the process of taking part
- the outcomes of the research.

If you are working in a group, discuss the possible effects together first.

A researcher carrying out interviews with women who have recently been diagnosed with ovarian cancer emphasises the need to avoid possible negative effects of the process where possible:

66 *My study is investigating the psychosexual effects of the diagnosis, so the subject matter is especially sensitive. Some people find it very difficult to talk about their feelings, especially feelings about sex. You have to be very sensitive and not push people to talk if they appear to be getting upset. However, some people welcome the opportunity to talk about difficult things even if it does make them upset. The important thing is to let them make the choices all the time, whether to go on talking or turn to another subject.* 99

6.5.4 **Confidentiality**

Confidentiality means respecting the privacy of any information that is disclosed and only using it for the purposes for which it was originally intended.

For a consideration of the law and good practice relating to confidentiality in health and social care, see section 2.5 (page 115).

When participants give their consent to take part in research, it is usual to guarantee confidentiality. This guarantee applies to:

- how the information is kept
- how it is used in the report or other outcomes
- what other use is made of it.

Information should be kept safe and secure, whatever form it is in – handwritten notes, taped recordings of interviews, returned questionnaires or entries on a computer database. The Data Protection Act requires that: 'Appropriate security measures shall be taken against unauthorised access to, or alteration, disclosure or destruction of, personal data and against accidental loss or destruction.'

In a large survey, it is normally easy to hide individual details in the overall results. But in a small sample of subjects, personal details in a report may make individuals readily identifiable. Information about them should not be changed, but it can be presented in such a way as to preserve confidentiality. This can be done by:

■ changing people's names

■ leaving out details that might identify them, such as any distinguishing physical features or behaviours that others might recognise.

Another aspect of confidentiality is the ethical duty only to use information gathered during research for its original purposes. The Data Protection Act states that personal data can only be held for specified purposes and '*shall not be used or disclosed in any manner incompatible with . . . those purposes*'.

Confidentiality conflicts

The ethical duty of confidentiality may sometimes conflict with the ethical duty of care. For example, in some areas all pregnant women are anonymously tested for HIV in order to identify the incidence in the community. Because the tests are anonymous, clinicians are not able to inform their patients and take protective measures for the unborn child.

6.5.5 Participants' rights

In addition to confidentiality, research participants have the right to:

■ agree whether or not to take part in the research, without coercion or pressure – this is called giving 'informed consent'

■ withdraw from the research at any time, for example if it is causing distress or inconvenience.

Obtaining informed consent

In medical research, informed consent is essential. If someone is to be given an experimental drug, or have their treatment withdrawn or changed, they must be aware of the possible consequences. Any research that involves a change in treatment also poses risks and requires informed consent. As the student on page 363 discovered, even talking to people about things relating to their wellbeing may be stressful for them.

DISCUSSION POINT

What examples can you think of where there might be a conflict between someone's role as a researcher and their role as a carer? Look out for cases where this has happened in any reading you do on this subject, or that you hear about on the radio, TV or among practitioners.

There are two difficulties in getting informed consent. First, it is not always possible to describe the research process fully. For example, you might know that you want to interview the subject, but may not know how long the interview will take. Second, if the person doing the research also has a caring role, there may be conflicts between the two roles.

Some people might choose to withdraw from the research process. The student doing interviews in a residential home for older people describes how she offered this option to her participants:

66 *After talking to the manager at the home and my tutor at college, I decided to carry on with the interviews. But I agreed only to talk to people who really didn't mind. I had twelve people on my list and had already interviewed five. So the next afternoon I was there, I talked briefly to the other seven on their own. Two of them dropped out, so I was left with ten interviews altogether. I decided that was enough of a sample, and it meant avoiding all the stress of talking to people who felt uncomfortable about it.* 99

Involving participants

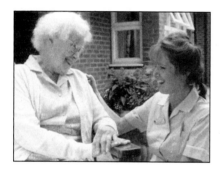

Researchers have an ethical duty to report the findings of their research accurately and fairly. But they should also give participants an opportunity to see the outcomes and comment on them before they are made public. This can be done by:

- discussing the outcomes with participants before writing them up
- giving participants a draft of the report and allowing them to comment – some comments might be included in the final version of the report.

Key questions

1   Why are ethical considerations important in health and social care research?

2   What guidelines should researchers follow to make sure their research is ethical?

3   How can bias related to age, sex, cultural and social background be avoided in research?

4   How can the benefits of taking part in research be maximised for participants?

5   What negative effects can result from taking part in research?

6   How can these potentially negative effects be countered?

7   How can the confidentiality of research participants be preserved?

8   What rights do research participants have?

Assignment

Produce a research report of a research project that you have designed and carried out that is relevant to a health care, social care or early years setting. The report must show your skills in research and your understanding of research methods in this field. It should include:

- a rationale for the research, and the research methods you have chosen
- a review of what is already known in the area of your project
- an exploration of ethical issues that are relevant to your project
- a presentation of findings with conclusions, including appropriate data and statistics, diagrams, charts and a bibliography.

Your work for the written report and an oral presentation of findings may be made to meet the requirements of the key skills in communication and information technology. Opportunities to meet the requirements for the application of number key skills may be met if you undertake a quantitative study.

Key skills

You can use the work you are doing for this part of your GNVQ to collect and develop evidence for the following key skills at level 3.

when you	you can collect evidence for
	communication
take part in brainstorming sessions to help discuss possible topics, interview people to collect information, and have discussions with experts in the field	key skill C3.1a contribute to a group discussion about a complex subject
use relevant literature and current sources	key skill C3.2 read and synthesise information from two extended documents about a complex subject; one of these documents should include a least one image
produce a written report	key skill C3.3 write two different types of document about complex subjects; one piece of writing should be an extended document and include at least one image
	information technology
use the Internet to obtain information	key skill IT3.1 plan, and use different sources to search for, and select, information required for two different purposes
demonstrate your understanding of the Data Protection Act	key skill IT3.3 present information from different sources for two different purposes and audiences; include at least one example of text, one example of images and one example of numbers
	application of number
search for relevant and current sources of data; review and monitor changes in health and social care practice; obtain feedback on services for quality assurance; plan service delivery by establishing the relevant demography	key skill N3.1 plan, and interpret information from two different types of sources, including a large data set

when you	you can collect evidence for
	application of number
make calculations with data to assess changes, quality, etc.; use measures of central tendency	key skill N3.2 carry out multistage calculations to do with (a) amounts and sizes (b) scales and proportion (c) handling statistics (d) rearranging and using formulae; work with a large data set on at least one occasion
present research findings using a range of charts and tables to illustrate data analysis	key skill N3.3 interpret results of calculations, present findings and justify methods; use at least one graph, one chart and one diagram
	improving own learning and performance
prepare a research plan	key skill LP3.1 agree targets and plan how these will be met, using support from appropriate others
implement and monitor the research project; use a standard system for referencing sources; using primary and secondary data sources, qualitative and quantitative methods; learn about basic sampling and how to record data accurately	key skill LP3.2 use the plan, seeking and using feedback and support from relevant sources to help meet the targets, and use different ways of learning to meet new demands
take part in a structured programme of review and monitoring sessions; assess the appropriateness of the measurement tools	key skill LP3.3 review progress in meeting targets, establishing evidence of achievements, and agree action for improving performance
	working with others
work in groups or individually to produce a research design	key skill WO3.1 plan the activity with others, agreeing objectives, responsibilities and working arrangements
	problem-solving
describe a situation or problem, and provide explanations; propose a suitable hypothesis selecting the best method of research to suit your purpose	key skill PS3.1 recognise, explore and describe the problems, and agree the standards for its solution
select suitable research methods that allow appropriate data to be collected	key skill PS3.2 generate and compare at least two options which could be used to solve the problems, and justify the option for taking forward
carry out research using suitable methods to find solutions	key skill PS3.3 plan and implement at least one option for solving the problem, and review progress towards its solution
ensure the validity and reliability of the research	key skill PS3.4 agree and apply methods to check whether the problem has been solved, describe the results and review the approach taken

Index